✻

OXFORD PA...

A Dictionar...
Food an... ...rition

Arnold E. Bender was Professor of Nutrition and ...n and
...sity of London, and ...s... f
...and Nutrition, Queen
...lizabeth College, 1978-82. His publications
include ... Richard Bender ... Calories
... Nutrition (1979).

...aches nutrition and
...ell as of
...ices,

... gether they have written *Food Tables* and *Food*
...belling (OUP, 1986 and 1991) and the forthcoming
...ference Handbook of Nutrition.

Oxford
Paperback
Reference

The most authoritative and up-to-date reference books for both students and the general reader.

Abbreviations
ABC of Music
Accounting
Archaeology*
Architecture*
Art and Artists
Art Terms*
Astronomy
Bible
Biology
British Women Writers
Buddhism*
Business
Card Games
Chemistry
Christian Church
Classical Literature
Classical Mythology*
Colour Medical Dictionary
Colour Science Dictionary
Computing
Dance*
Dates
Earth Sciences
Ecology
Economics
Engineering*
English Etymology
English Folklore*
English Grammar
English Language
English Literature
English Place-Names
Euphemisms
Film*
Finance and Banking
First Names
Food and Nutrition
Fowler's Modern English
  Usage
Geography
Handbook of the World*
Humorous Quotations
Irish Literature*
Jewish Religion
King's and Queens*
King's English
Law

Linguistics
Literary Terms
Mathematics
Medical Dictionary
Medicines*
Modern Design*
Modern Quotations
Modern Slang
Music
Nursing
Opera
Paperback Encyclopedia
Philosophy
Physics
Plant-Lore
Plant Sciences
Political Biography
Political Quotations
Politics
Popes
Proverbs
Psychology*
Quotations
Sailing Terms
Saints
Science
Shakespeare
Ships and the Sea
Sociology
Statistics*
Superstitions
Theatre
Twentieth-Century Art
Twentieth-Century Poetry
Twentieth-Century World
  History
Weather Facts
Who's Who in Opera*
Who's Who in the
  Twentieth Century
Word Games
World Mythology
World Religions*
Writers' Dictionary
Zoology

*forthcoming

A Dictionary of

Food and Nutrition

ARNOLD E. BENDER
Emeritus Professor of Nutrition
University of London

DAVID A. BENDER
Senior Lecturer in Biochemistry
University College London

Oxford   New York

OXFORD UNIVERSITY PRESS

OXFORD
UNIVERSITY PRESS

Great Clarendon Street, Oxford OX2 6DP

Oxford New York
Athens Auckland Bangkok Bogota Bombay
Buenos Aires Calcutta Cape Town Dar es Salaam
Delhi Florence Hong Kong Istanbul Karachi
Kuala Lumpur Madras Madrid Melbourne
Mexico City Nairobi Paris Singapore
Taipei Tokyo Toronto Warsaw

and associated companies in
Berlin Ibadan

Oxford is a trade mark of Oxford University Press

British Library Cataloguing in Publication Data
Data available

Library of Congress Cataloging in Publication Data
Bender, Arnold E. (Arnold Eric)
A dictionary of food and nutrition / Arnold E. Bender & David A.
Bender.
1. Food—Dictionaries.   2. Nutrition—Dictionaries.   3. Cookery—
Dictionaries.   I. Bender, David A.   II. Title.
TX349.B39   1995   641'.03—dc20   95-17405
ISBN 0-19-280006-X

10 9 8 7 6 5 4 3

Printed in Great Britain
by Cox & Wyman Ltd,
Reading, Berkshire

Contents

Preface

This book is intended for all who have an interest in food and nutrition, be it as consumers concerned about the health or otherwise of their diets, as cooks, food manufacturers, and salespeople, concerned about what they produce and sell, or as students of health and human sciences, who must understand, interpret, and communicate information to others.

These days the consumer is faced with dietary advice ranging from government publications to magazines, newspapers, and radio and TV programmes, not to mention food labels that almost require a training in chemistry and physiology to be understood, scare stories in the press, and claims and counter-claims in advertising.

Many of the terms used are technical, and few people can understand all of them. This dictionary is intended to help such understanding. It provides clear, authoritative definitions of some 6,000 terms associated with all aspects of food and nutrition, diet and health that may be encountered on food labels, in advertising, and in the media, as well as culinary terms that may be encountered in menus, cookery books, novels, and films. To help make decisions about which foods are nutritionally valuable, there are notes on those that are good sources of major nutrients.

Most textbooks and reference works list the nutrients present in foods as the amount present in 100 g ($3\frac{1}{2}$ oz), but a portion of some foods, such as bread or potatoes, could be much larger, while for other foods a portion may be only a few grams. Furthermore, the amount of any particular nutrient in a food varies with the agricultural variety of the food, or the breed of the animals, the growing conditions, and how it has been handled and cooked since cropping. The average vitamin and mineral content of some foods, such as bread and milk, varies less than others, such as lettuce and carrots. Therefore, without the analysis (and weight) of the particular samples, the vitamin and mineral contents of food are very approximate.

To help to assess the relative nutritional value of foods, we have taken the averages of the analysed values, and expressed them as rich, good, or simply 'sources' of the nutrients in an average-sized portion or serving, using the reference intakes of nutrients used for food labelling in the European Union (Appendix VI). A rich source of a nutrient provides at least 30%, good sources 20–30%, and sources 10–20% of the reference intake. Foods that are not listed as sources of nutrients, because they supply less than 10% of the reference intake in a serving, may nevertheless make a significant contribution to an overall diet.

Where a word is *starred in the text, this means that you can find further information under that entry.

A

abalone A *shellfish (mollusc), *Haliotus splendens, H. rufescens, H. cracherodii*, also sometimes called ormer, or sea ear. Found especially in waters around Australia, and also California, Japan, the Channel Islands, and France. A 100-g portion is a rich *source of protein and niacin; a source of iron and vitamin B_1; supplies 130 kcal (550 kJ).

abboccato Italian; medium sweet wines.

abdug Iranian; drink made from *vodka and *yoghurt with *soda water.

abocada Spanish; medium sweet wines.

absinthe A herb *liqueur flavoured with wormwood (*Artemisia absinthium*); it is toxic, and banned in many countries. *See also* vermouth.

absolute alcohol Pure ethyl *alcohol.

AC Appellation contrôlée; *see* wine classification, France

acarbose The name of a group of complex *carbohydrates (oligosaccharides) which inhibit the *enzymes of *starch and *disaccharide digestion; used experimentally to reduce the digestion of starch, and so slow the rate of absorption of carbohydrates. It has been marketed for use in association with weight-reducing diet regimes as a 'starch blocker', but there is no evidence that it is of any use whatsoever in weight reduction.

acaricides Pesticides used to kill mites and ticks (the biological family Acaridae) which cause animal diseases and the spoilage of flour and other foods in storage.

accelase A mixture of *enzymes which *hydrolyse *proteins, including an *exopeptidase from the bacterium *Streptococcus lactis*, which is one of the starter organisms in dairy processing. The mixed enzymes are used to shorten the maturation time of cheeses and intensify the flavour of processed cheese.

accelerated freeze drying *See* freeze drying.

Ac'cent Trade name for the flavour enhancer *monosodium glutamate.

Acceptable Daily Intake (ADI) The amount of a food *additive that could be taken daily for an entire life-span without appreciable risk. Determined by measuring the highest dose of the substance that has no effect on experimental animals, then dividing by a safety factor of 100. Substances that are not given an ADI are regarded as having no adverse effect at any level of intake. *See also* no effect level.

accoub Edible thistle (*Goundelia tournefortii*) growing in the Mediterranean region and Middle East. The cooked flower buds have a flavour resembling that of asparagus or globe artichoke; the shoots can be eaten in the same way as *asparagus and the roots as *salsify.

accra Caribbean; heavy batter fritters with salt cod; also known as stamp-and-go, bacalaitos.

accuncciata Corsican; goat, lamb, or mutton stew with potatoes.

acerola *See* cherry, West Indian.

acesulphames (acesulfames) A group of non-nutritive or intense (artificial) *sweeteners. The potassium salt, acesulphame-K, is some 200 times as sweet as *sucrose. It is not metabolized, and is excreted unchanged.

acetic acid One of the simplest organic *acids, also known systematically as ethanoic acid, chemically it is CH_3COOH. It is the acid of *vinegar (which is a solution of acetic acid in water), and is formed, together with *lactic acid, in the fermentation (*pickling) of foods.

Acetobacter A genus of bacteria which oxidize ethyl *alcohol to *acetic acid, used in the manufacture of *vinegar. They also grow as a film on the surface of beer wort, pickle brine, and fruit juices, when they are commonly known as 'mother of vinegar'.

aceto dolce Italian; pickles eaten as an appetizer.

acetoin A precursor of the compound *diacetyl, which is one of the constituents of the flavour of butter. Chemically acetyl methyl carbinol. Acetoin and diacetyl are produced by bacteria during the ripening of *butter.

acétomel Sweet-sour syrup of vinegar and honey used to preserve fruit; also known as agrodolce.

acetomenaphthone Synthetic compound with *vitamin K activity; vitamin K_3, also known as menaquinone-0.

acetone One of the *ketone bodies formed in the body in *fasting. It is a metabolically useless side-product of fat metabolism, but detection of acetone in blood, urine, or breath may be clinically useful in cases of *diabetes, as a means of detecting ketosis. Also used as a solvent, e.g. in varnishes and lacquer. Chemically dimethyl ketone or propan-2-one ($CH_3.C=O.CH_3$)

acetylcholine The acetyl derivative of *choline, produced at some nerve endings (cholinergic nerves) both in the brain, where it acts as a chemical transmitter, and at the junctions between nerves and muscles, where it stimulates muscle contraction.

achene Botanical term for small, dry, one-seeded fruit which does not open to liberate the seed, e.g. a nut.

ACH index Arm, chest, hip index. A method of assessing a person's nutritional status by measuring the arm circumference, chest diameter, and hip width. *See also* anthropometry.

achlorhydria Deficiency of hydrochloric acid in gastric digestive juice. *See also* anaemia; gastric acidity.

achote *See* annatto.

achromotricia Loss of the pigment of hair. One of the signs of *pantothenic acid deficiency in animals, but there is no evidence that pantothenic acid affects loss of hair colour in human beings.

acid Chemically, compounds that dissociate (ionize) in water to give rise to hydrogen ions (H^+); they taste sour. Mineral acids such as hydrochloric, sulphuric, and nitric are more or less completely dissociated and so are strong acids. *Organic acids are generally weak since they are not completely dissociated. *See also* alkali; amino acids; buffers; esters; fatty acids; pH; salt.

acid drops Boiled sweets with sharp flavour from tartaric acid (originally acidulated drops); known as sourballs in USA.

acid foods, basic foods These terms refer to the residue of the *metabolism of foods. The *mineral salts of *sodium, *potassium, *magnesium, and *calcium are base-forming, while *phosphorus, *sulphur, and *chlorine are acid-forming. Which of these predominates in foods determines whether the residue is acidic or basic (alkaline); meat, cheese, eggs, and cereals leave an acidic residue, while milk, vegetables, and some fruits leave a basic residue. Fats and sugars have no mineral content and so leave a neutral residue. Although fruits have an acid taste due to organic acids and their salts, the acids are completely oxidized and the sodium and potassium salts form an alkaline residue.

acid, gastric The acid in the *gastric secretion is hydrochloric acid; *see also* achlorhydria; gastric acidity.

acidity *See* pH.

acidity regulators *See* buffers.

acid number, acid value (of a fat) A measure of its *rancidity due to *hydrolysis, releasing free *fatty acids from the *triacylglycerol of the fat; serves as an index of the efficiency of refining since the fatty acids are removed during refining and increase with deterioration during storage.

acidophilus milk Resembles *yoghurt but is more astringent in taste and cultured only with *Lactobacillus acidophilus*; claimed to enhance the growth of beneficial bacteria in the intestine.

acidophilus therapy A treatment for *constipation based on the consumption of milk containing a high concentration of viable *Lactobacillus acidophilus*, although the milk itself is unfermented. The effect is believed to be due to the implantation of the organisms in the intestine.

acidosis An increase in the acidity of *blood plasma to below the normal range of *pH 7.3–7.45, resulting from a loss of the buffering capacity of the plasma, alteration in the excretion of carbon dioxide, excessive loss of base from the body or metabolic overproduction of acids.

acids, amino *See* amino acids.

acids, fatty *See* fatty acids.

acids, fruit *Organic acids such as citric, malic, tartaric, etc. which give the sharp or sour flavour to fruits; often added to processed foods for taste.

ackee (akee) The fruit of the Caribbean tree *Blighia sapida*. The fruit is toxic when unripe because it contains the toxin hypoglycin.

acne Inflammatory pustular skin eruption occurring around sebaceous glands, especially around the time of puberty. Not known to be caused or exacerbated by diet, although a low-fat diet is sometimes recommended. Severe persistent acne may be treated by topical application of *retinoids (synthetic *vitamin A derivatives).

acorn Fruit of the oak tree (*Quercus* spp.), used both for animal feed and (especially in Spain) to make a flour for baking. Roasted acorns have been used as a coffee substitute (German: *ersatz Kaffee*).

acorn sugar A sweet compound (quercitol) extracted from acorns (*Quercus* spp.).

ACP Acid calcium phosphate, *see* phosphates.

acraldehyde *See* acrolein.

acrodynia A specific type of skin lesion (dermatitis) seen in animals which are deficient in *vitamin B_6. There is no evidence for a similar dermatitis in deficient human beings.

acrolein (acraldehyde) An aldehyde formed when *glycerol is heated to a high temperature. It is responsible for the acrid odour and lachrymatory (tear-causing) vapour produced when fats are overheated. Chemically $CH_2=CH.CHO$.

Acronize Trade name for the *antibiotic chlortetracycline; 'acronized' is used to describe products that have been treated with chlortetracycline, as, e.g. acronized ice.

ACTH *See* adrenocorticotrophic hormone.

actin One of the contractile *proteins of *muscle.

activators Compounds that increase the activity of *enzymes.

active oxygen method A method of measuring the stability of fats and oils to oxidative damage by bubbling air through the heated material and following the formation of peroxides. Also known as the Swift stability test.

actomyosin The combination of the two main contractile *proteins in *muscle, actin and myosin.

Adam's fig *See* plantain.

Addisonian pernicious anaemia *See* anaemia, pernicious.

additive Any compound not commonly regarded or used as a food which is added to foods as an aid in manufacturing or processing, or to improve the keeping properties, flavour, colour, texture, appearance, or stability of the food, or as a convenience to the consumer. The term excludes vitamins, minerals, and other nutrients added to enrich or restore nutritional value. Herbs, spices, hops, salt, yeast, or protein hydrolysates, air and water are usually excluded from this definition. Additives may be extracted from natural sources, synthesized in the laboratory to be chemically the same as the natural materials (and hence known as nature-identical), or may be synthetic compounds that do not occur in nature.

In most countries only additives from a permitted list of compounds which have been extensively tested for safety may legally be added to foods. The additives used must be declared on food labels, using either their chemical names or their numbers in the EU list of permitted additives (*E-numbers). Some additional compounds, numbered in the same sequence but without the preface E-, are permitted in the UK. *See also* Acceptable Daily Intake and Appendix VIII.

adenine A *nucleotide, one of the purine bases of the *nucleic acids (DNA and RNA). The compound formed between adenine and *ribose is the nucleoside adenosine, and can form four phosphorylated derivatives important in metabolism: adenosine monophosphate (AMP, also known as adenylic acid); adenosine diphosphate (ADP); adenosine triphosphate (ATP) and cyclic adenosine monophosphate (cAMP). *See also* ATP; energy metabolism.

adenosine *See* adenine.

adermin An obsolete name for *vitamin B_6.

ADI *See* Acceptable Daily Intake.

adipectomy Surgical removal of subcutaneous fat.

adipocyte A fat-containing cell in *adipose tissue.

adipose tissue Body fat — the cells that synthesize and store *fat, releasing it for *metabolism in *fasting. Also known as white adipose tissue, to distinguish it from the metabolically more active *brown adipose tissue, which is involved in heat production to maintain body temperature. Much of the body fat reserve is subcutaneous; in addition there is adipose tissue around the organs, which serves to protect them from physical damage. In lean people, 20–25% of body weight is adipose tissue, increasing with age; the proportion is greater in people who are *overweight or *obese. Adipose tissue contains 82–88% fat, 2–2.6% protein and 10–14% water. The energy yield of adipose tissue is 8000–9000 kcal (34–38 MJ) per kg or 3600–4000 kcal (15.1–16.8 MJ) per pound.

adipsia Absence of thirst.

Adirondack bread American baked product made from ground *maize, butter, wheat flour, eggs, and sugar.

adlay The seeds of a wild grass (Job's tears, *Coix lachryma-jobi*) botanically related to *maize, growing wild in parts of Africa and Asia and eaten especially in the south-east Pacific region.

adoucir French; to reduce the bitterness of food by prolonged cooking, or to dilute a dish with milk, stock, or water to make it less salty.

ADP Adenosine diphosphate, *see* adenine; ATP.

adrenal glands Also called the suprarenal glands, small *endocrine glands situated just above the kidneys. The inner part (medulla) secretes the *hormones *adrenaline and *noradrenaline, while the outer part (the cortex) secretes *steroid hormones known as corticosteroids, including cortisol and *aldosterone.

adrenaline Also known as epinephrine. A hormone secreted by the medulla of the *adrenal gland, especially in times of stress or in response to fright or shock. Its main actions are to increase blood pressure and to mobilize tissue reserves of *glucose (leading to an increase in the blood glucose concentration) and fat, in preparation for flight or fighting. Derived from the *amino acids *phenylalanine or *tyrosine.

adrenocorticotrophic hormone (ACTH) A *hormone secreted by the anterior part of the pituitary gland which stimulates the *adrenal gland to secrete corticosteroids.

aduki beans *See* bean, adzuki.

adulteration The addition of substances to foods etc. in order to increase the bulk and reduce the cost, with intent to defraud the purchaser. Common adulterants are starch in spices, water in milk and beer, etc. The British Food and Drugs Act (1860) was the first legislation to prevent such practices.

adverse reactions to foods 1 Food aversion, unpleasant reactions caused by emotional responses to certain foods rather than to the foods themselves, which are unlikely to occur in blind testing when the foods are disguised.

2 Food allergy, physiological reactions to specific foods or ingredients due to an immunological response. *Antibodies to the *allergen are formed as a result of previous exposure or sensitization, and cause a variety of symptoms when the food is eaten, including gastro-intestinal disturbances, skin rashes, asthma, and, in severe cases, anaphylactic shock, which may be fatal.

3 Food intolerance, physiological reactions to specific foods or ingredients which are not due to immunological responses, but may result from the irritant action of spices, pharmacological actions of some naturally occurring compounds (e.g. *caffeine), or an inability to metabolize a component of the food as a result of an *enzyme defect. *See also* amino acid disorders; disaccharide intolerance; genetic diseases.

advocaat Dutch; liqueur made from brandy and eggs.

adzuki bean *See* bean, adzuki.

aerobic 1 Aerobic micro-organisms (aerobes) are those that require oxygen for growth; obligate aerobes cannot survive in the absence of oxygen. The opposite are anaerobic organisms, which do not require oxygen for growth; obligate anaerobes cannot survive in the presence of oxygen.

2 Aerobic exercise is physical activity which requires an increase in heart rate and respiration to meet the increased demand of muscle for oxygen, as contrasted with maximum exertion or sprinting, when muscle can metabolize anaerobically, producing *lactic acid, which is metabolized later, creating a need for increased respiration after the exercise has ceased (so-called oxygen debt).

aerosol cream Cream *sterilized and packaged in aerosol canisters with a propellant gas to expel it from the container, giving conveniently available whipped cream. Gelling agents and *stabilizers may also be added.

aerosporin *See* polymyxins.

aesculin (esculin) A glucoside of dihydroxycoumarin found in the leaves and bark of the horse chestnut tree (*Aesculus hippocastanum*) which has an effect on *capillary fragility.

AFD Accelerated freeze drying, *see* freeze drying.

aflatoxins A group of mycotoxins formed by the *mould *Aspergillus flavus*, which can grow on *peanuts and cereal grains when they are stored under damp and warm conditions. Several different aflatoxins are known; in addition to being acutely toxic, many, especially aflatoxin B1, are potent *carcinogens. Fungal spoilage of foods with *A. flavus* is a common problem in many tropical areas, and aflatoxin is believed to be the cause of much primary liver cancer in parts of Africa. Aflatoxins can be secreted in milk, so there is strict control of the level of aflatoxins in cattle feed.

agalactia Failure of the mother to secrete enough milk to feed a suckling infant.

agar Dried extracts from various seaweeds, including *Gelidium* and *Gracilaria* spp. It is a partially soluble *non-starch polysaccharide, composed of *galactose units. It swells with water to form a *gel, and is used in soups, jellies, ice-cream, and meat products. It is also used as the basis of bacteriological culture media, as an adhesive, for sizing silk and as a stabilizer for emulsions. Also called agar-agar, Macassar gum, vegetable gelatine.

ageing 1 As wines age, they develop bouquet and a smooth mellow flavour, associated with slow oxidation and the formation of *esters, as well as losing the harsh yeasty flavour of young wine.
  2 The ageing of meat by hanging in a cool place for several days results in softening of the muscle tissue, which stiffens after death (rigor mortis). This stiffening is due to anaerobic metabolism leading to the formation of lactic acid when the blood flow ceases.
  3 Ageing of wheat flour for bread making is due to oxidation, either by storage for some weeks after milling or by chemical action. Freshly milled flour produces a weaker and less resilient dough, and hence a less 'bold' loaf, than flour which has been aged. Chemicals that are used to age flour include ammonium persulphate, ascorbic acid (*vitamin C), chlorine, *sulphur dioxide, potassium bromate, and *cysteine. In addition, nitrogen peroxide or benzoyl peroxide may be used to bleach flour, and chlorine dioxide both bleaches and ages flour. The use of these chemicals, and the amounts that may be used, is controlled by law in most countries.

agene Nitrogen trichloride, used at one time as a bleaching and improving agent for wheat flour in bread making. It can react with the *amino acid *methionine in proteins to form the toxic compound methionine sulphoximine, and is no longer used.

ageusia Loss or impairment of the sense of *taste.

agglomeration The process of producing a free-flowing, dust-free powder from substances such as dried milk powder and wheat flour, by moistening the powder with droplets of water and then redrying in a stream of air. The resulting agglomerates can readily be wetted.

agglutinins *See* lectins.

Aginomoto Trade name for the flavour enhancer *monosodium glutamate. *See* flavour potentiator.

agnelloto An envelope of *pasta, stuffed with minced meat, cheese, or vegetables, cut into a half-moon shape, and so differing from *ravioli, which is cut into squares.

agneshka churba Bulgarian; whole spring lamb stuffed with rice, offal, and raisins, then roasted. A traditional Easter dish.

agrodolce Italian; sweet and sour. *See* acétomel.

aguardiente Spanish; *see* marc.

aguja Spanish; young wines.

aigre-douce French; sweet and sour. *See* acétomel.

aigrette French; small, light, fried flaky *pastry biscuit.

aiguillette A thin strip or slice of cooked poultry, meat, or fish.

aileron French; wing tip of poultry.

aïllade French; prepared with garlic.

AIN American Institute of Nutrition.

aïoli Garlic-flavoured mayonnaise used in Provençale cooking. *See also* salad dressing.

air classification A way of separating the particles of powdered materials in a current of air, on the basis of their weight and size or density. Particularly applied to the fractionation of the *endosperm of milled wheat flour; smaller particles are richer in protein. Various fractions range from 3% to 25% protein.

aitchbone Cut of *beef from the upper part of the leg. Sometimes incorrectly called the edgebone.

ajada Spanish; sauce made from bread steeped in water and garlic.

ajwain *See* lovage.

akee *See* ackee.

akkra Caribbean (originally West African); fritter made from black-eyed peas or *soya beans. Also known as calas, samsa.

akni Indian; *bouillon, made from water and herbs, used for cooking rice and vegetables.

akutok Inuit (Eskimo); strips of dried caribou meat; the outer part has a crust, but the inside is only partially dry.

akvavit *See* aquavit.

ala *See* bulgur.

alactasia Partial or complete deficiency of the *enzyme *lactase in the small intestine, resulting in an inability to digest the sugar *lactose in milk, and hence intolerance of milk and milk products. *See also* disaccharide intolerance.

alanine A non-essential *amino acid, found in all proteins. β-Alanine is an *isomer of alanine in which the amino group is attached to carbon-3 of the molecule rather than carbon-2 as in alanine; it is important as part of *pantothenic acid, *carnosine, and *anserine.

alant starch *See* inulin.

Alaska, baked *See* baked Alaska.

albacore A long-finned species of tunny fish, *Thynnus alalunga*, usually canned as *tuna fish.

albedo The white pith (mesocarp) of the inner peel of citrus fruits, accounting for some 20–60% of the whole fruit. It consists of sugars, *cellulose, and *pectins, and is used as a commercial source of pectin.

albert French name for English hot *horseradish sauce.

albigeoise, à l' French; garnish for meat consisting of stuffed tomatoes and potato croquettes.

albion French; **1** fish soup made with lobster quenelles and truffles; **2** chicken broth with truffles, asparagus, chicken liver quenelles, and cocks' combs.

albondigas Spanish (Castilian); meat balls or dumplings.

albumin (albumen) A specific class of relatively small *proteins which are soluble in water and readily coagulated by heat. Ovalbumin is the main protein of egg-white, lactalbumin occurs in milk, and plasma or serum albumin is one of the major blood proteins. Serum albumin concentration is sometimes measured as an index of *protein-energy malnutrition.
   Often used as a non-specific term for proteins (e.g. albuminuria is the excretion of proteins in the urine).

albumin index A measure of the quality or freshness of an egg – the height : width ratio of the albumin when the egg is broken onto a flat surface. As the egg deteriorates, so the albumin spreads further, i.e. the albumin index decreases.

albumin milk *See* protein milk.

albuminoids Fibrous proteins that have a structural or protective rather than enzymic role in the body. Also known as scleroproteins. The main proteins of the *connective tissues of the body. There are three main types: (1) collagens in skin, tendons, and bones are resistant to enzymic digestion with trypsin and pepsin, and can be converted to soluble *gelatine by boiling with water; (2) elastins in tendons and arteries, which are not converted to gelatine on boiling; (3) keratins, the proteins of hair, feathers, scales, horns, and hoofs, which are insoluble in dilute acid or alkali, and are resistant to all animal digestive enzymes.

albumin water Beverage made from lightly whisked egg-white and cold water, seasoned with lemon juice and salt.

alcohol Chemically alcohols are compounds with the general formula $C_nH_{(2n+1)}OH$. The alcohol in *alcoholic beverages is ethyl alcohol (ethanol, C_2H_5OH); pure ethyl alcohol is also known as absolute alcohol. The *energy yield of alcohol is 7 kcal (29 kJ)/gram.
   The strength of alcoholic beverages is most often shown as the percentage of alcohol by volume (sometimes shown as % v/v). This is not the same as the percentage of alcohol by weight (% w/v) since alcohol is less dense than water: 5% v/v alcohol = 3.96% by weight (w/v); 10% v/v = 7.93% w/v and 40% v/v = 31.7% w/v. *See also* proof spirit.

alcohol, denatured Drinkable alcohol is subject to tax in most countries and for industrial use it is denatured to render it unfit for consumption, by the addition of 5% methyl alcohol (methanol, CH_3OH, also known as wood alcohol), which is poisonous. This is industrial rectified spirit. For domestic use a purple dye and pyridine (which has an unpleasant odour) are also added; this is methylated spirit.

alcoholic beverages Drinks made by fermenting fruit juices, sugars, and fermentable carbohydrates with *yeast to form *alcohol. These include *beer, *cider, and *perry, 4–6% alcohol by volume; *wines, 9–13% alcohol; *spirits (e.g. *brandy, *gin, *rum, *vodka, *whisky) made by distilling fermented liquor, 38–45% alcohol; *liqueurs made from distilled spirits, sweetened and flavoured, 20–40% alcohol; and fortified wines (aperitif wines, *madeira, *port, *sherry) made by adding spirit to wine, 18–25% alcohol. *See also* alcohol; proof spirit.

alcoholism Physiological addiction to *alcohol, associated with persistent heavy consumption of *alcoholic beverages. In addition to the addiction, there may be damage to the liver (cirrhosis), stomach (gastritis), and pancreas (pancreatitis), as well as behavioural changes and peripheral nerve damage.

alcohol units For convenience in calculating intakes of alcohol, a unit of alcohol is defined as 8 g (10 mL) of absolute alcohol; this is the amount in $^1/_2$ pint (300 mL) beer, a single measure of spirit (25 mL) or a single glass of wine (100 mL).

The Royal College of Physicians of England has set upper limits of prudent consumption of alcohol as 21 units (= 168 g alcohol) per week for men and 14 units (= 112 g alcohol) per week for women.

alcool blanc French; white spirit (silent spirit) or eau de vie. Distilled *spirits from fermented fruit juice.

al dente Firm to the bite, applied to pasta and cooked vegetables (Italian: 'to the tooth').

alderman's walk The name given in London to the longest and finest cut from the haunch of venison or lamb.

aldosterone A *steroid hormone secreted by the *adrenal cortex which controls the excretion of salts and water by the kidneys.

ale *See* beer.

aleatico A *grape variety widely used for *wine making, although not one of the classic varieties; makes fragrant sweet red wines.

alecost An aromatic herbaceous plant, *Tanacetum (Chrysanthemum) balsamita*, related to *tansy, used in salads and formerly used to flavour ale.

aleurone layer The single layer of large cells under the bran coat and outside the endosperm of *cereal grains. About 3% of the weight of the grain, and rich in protein, as well as containing about 20% of the *vitamin B_1, 30% of the *vitamin B_2 and 50% of the *niacin of the grain. Botanically the aleurone layer is part of the endosperm, but in milling it remains attached to the inner layer of the *bran.

alewives River herrings, *Pomolobus pseudoharengus*, commonly used for canning after salting.

alexander A cocktail; usually gin, crème de cacao, and cream, although other spirits may be used.

alexanders A herb, black lovage (*Smyrnium olisatrum*) with a celery-like flavour.

alfalfa Or lucerne, *Medicago sativa*, commonly grown for animal feed and silage; the seeds can be soaked in water to germinate and then eaten as sprouts.

algae Simple (primitive) plants that do not show differentiation into roots, stems, and leaves. They are mostly aquatic — either seaweeds or pond and river-weeds. Some seaweeds, such as *dulse and *Irish moss, have long been eaten, and a number of unicellular algae, including *Chlorella*, *Scenedesmus*, and *Spirulina* spp. have been grown experimentally as novel sources of food (50–60% of the dry weight is protein).

algérienne 1 Garnish for steak consisting of tomatoes and peppers simmered in oil.
   2 Fried eggs served with a purée of tomatoes, peppers, and aubergine.
   3 Salad of courgettes, tomatoes, and cooked sweet potato.
   4 Sautéed chicken and aubergine with sauce of tomatoes, garlic, and onions.
   5 Cream soup made from sweet potatoes and filbert nuts.

alginates Salts of alginic acid found in many seaweeds as calcium salts or the free acid. Chemically, alginic acid is a non-starch *polysaccharide composed of mannuronic acid units.
   Iron, magnesium, and ammonium salts of alginic acid form viscous solutions and hold large amounts of water. They are used as thickeners, stabilizers and gelling, binding, and emulsifying agents in food manufacture, especially in *ice-cream and synthetic cream. Trade name Manucol.

alginic acid *See* alginates.

aligoté A *grape variety widely used for *wine making, although not one of the classic varieties. Burgundy's second-ranking white grape; the wines need drinking within three years.

alimentary canal The digestive tract, comprising (in man) the mouth, oesophagus, stomach, duodenum, and small and large intestines.
See also gastro-intestinal tract.

alimentary pastes *See* pasta.

alkali (or base) A compound that takes up hydrogen ions and so raises the *pH of a solution; *see also* acid; buffers; salt.

alkali formers *See* acid foods.

alkali reserve *See* buffers.

alkaloids Naturally occurring organic bases which have marked pharmacological actions in man and other animals. Many are found in plant foods, including potatoes and tomatoes (the *Solanum* alkaloids), or as the products of fungal action (e.g. ergot), although they also occur in animal foods (e.g. tetrodotoxin in *puffer fish, tetramine in *shellfish), and some are formed in the body (e.g. tryptamine, tyramine, phenylethylamine, and histamine are *amines formed by the decarboxylation of *amino acids). A number of alkaloids are used medically, e.g. morphine, colchicine, quinine, and atropine.

alkalosis *See* acidosis.

alkannet (alkanet, alkannin, alkanna) A colouring obtained from the root of *Anchusa (Alkanna) tinctoria* which is insoluble in water but soluble in alcohol and oils. It is blue in alkali (or in the presence of lead), crimson with tin and violet with iron. Used for colouring fats, cheese, essences, and inferior *port wine. Also known as orcanella.

allantoin The oxidation product of *uric acid which is the end-product of *purine metabolism in most animals apart from man and apes, which excrete uric acid.

All-Bran Trade name for a breakfast cereal prepared from wheat *bran, and hence a rich source of *non-starch polysaccharide. A 60-g portion is a rich *source of vitamins B_1, B_2, B_6, B_{12}, niacin, folate, iron, and copper; a source of protein; contains 1.5 g of fat of which 24% is saturated; provides 18 g of dietary fibre; supplies 160 kcal (670 kJ).

allemande Classic French *sauce, velouté blended with egg yolks and cream. Also known as sauce blonde or parisienne. Named for its light colour, as opposed to sauce *espagnole, which is dark.

allemande, à l' German style; dishes finished or garnished with German specialities such as sauerkraut, smoked sausage, or pickled pork.

allergen A chemical compound, commonly a protein, which causes the production of antibodies, and hence an allergic reaction. *See also* adverse reactions to foods.

allergy *Adverse reaction to foods caused by the production of antibodies.

alliance French; *sauce made from reduced (partially concentrated) white wine with tarragon vinegar and egg yolk.

allicin A sulphur-containing compound partially responsible for the flavour of *garlic.

alligator pear *See* avocado.

Allinson bread A wholewheat *bread named after Allinson, who advocated its consumption in England at the end of the nineteenth century, as did Graham in the USA (hence *Graham bread). Now trade name for a wholemeal loaf.

all-i-olli Spanish (Catalan); oil and garlic sauce prepared by pounding garlic in olive oil.

allotriophagy An unnatural desire for abnormal foods; also known as cissa, cittosis, and pica.

allspice Dried fruits of the evergreen plant *Pimenta officinalis*, also known as pimento (as distinct from *pimiento) or Jamaican pepper. The name allspice derives from the aromatic oil, which has an aroma similar to a mixture of *cloves, *cinnamon, and *nutmeg. Used to flavour meat and in baking.

allumettes Potatoes cut into thin 'matchsticks' and fried, also known as straw potatoes. Also used sometimes for narrow fingers of pastry.

almond A nut, the seeds of *Prunus amygdalus* var. *dulcis*. All varieties contain the *glycoside *amygdalin, which forms hydrogen cyanide when the nuts are crushed. The bitter almond, used for *almond oil, (*P. amygdalus* var. *amara*) may yield dangerous amounts of cyanide.

A 60-g portion (36 nuts) is a rich *source of protein, copper, niacin, and vitamins B_2, E; a good source of iron and zinc; a source of vitamin B_1; contains 35 g of fat of which 10% is *saturated and 70% mono-unsaturated; provides 8.4 g of dietary fibre; supplies 370 kcal (1550 kJ).

almond oil, bitter Essential oil from the seeds of either the almond tree (*Prunus amygdalis*) or more commonly the apricot tree (*Prunus armeniaca*), containing benzaldehyde, hydrogen cyanide, and benzaldehyde cyanohydrin. After removal of the hydrogen cyanide, used as a flavour and in perfumes and cosmetics.

almond paste Ground *almonds mixed with powdered sugar, bound with egg, used to decorate cakes and make *petits fours. Also known as marzipan.

almorta Spanish; flour made from seeds of common vetch or tare, *Vicia sativa*.

aloe Dried juice from the leaves of *Aloe perryi*, used in medicines. Contains a *glycoside, aloe-emodin or rhabarberone, aloe oil, and aloin or barbaloin.

aloo Hindi; *see* potatoes.

Alpha-Laval centrifuge A continuous bowl centrifuge for separating liquids of different densities and for clarifying. Widely used for cream separation.

alpine strawberry *See* strawberry.

alsacienne, à l' Dishes garnished with smoked sausages, ham, and peas.

aluminium The third most abundant element in the earth's crust (after oxygen and silicon) but with no known biological function. Present in small amounts in many foods but only a small proportion is absorbed. Aluminium salts are found in the abnormal nerve tangles in the brain in Alzheimer's disease, and it has been suggested that aluminium poisoning may be a factor in the development of the disease, although there is little evidence.

Aluminium is used in cooking vessels and as foil for wrapping food, as well as in cans and tubes; it is a soft flexible metal, resistant to oxidation and deterioration, although it is dissolved by alkalis. The 'silver' beads used to decorate confectionery are coated with either silver foil or an alloy of aluminium and *copper.

*Baking powders containing sodium aluminium sulphate as the acid agent were used at one time (alum baking powders), and aluminium hydroxide and silicates are commonly used in *antacid medications.

alveographe A device for measuring the stretching quality of *dough as an index of its protein quality for baking. A standard disc of dough is blown into a bubble and the pressure curve and bursting pressure are measured to give the stability, extensibility, and strength of the dough.

amabile Italian; wines intermediate between medium sweet (abboccato) and sweet (dulce).

amaranth A burgundy red colour, stable to light (E-123).

Amaranthus A genus of plants cultivated for their leaves and sometimes for their seeds also. The leaves are promoted in South East Asia as a good source of *carotene.

amaretti Italian; *macaroon.

amaretto Almond-flavoured *liqueur made by infusion of apricot kernels.

amazone French garnish for meat; lentil fritters, hollowed out and stuffed with morel mushrooms and chestnut purée.

ambergris A waxy concretion obtained from the intestine of the sperm whale, containing *cholesterol, ambrein, and benzoic acid. Used in drugs and perfumery.

Amberlite Group of polystyrene resins (*ion-exchange resins) used to absorb specific ions in water softening and purification in general.

ambigu French; cold collation or substantial snack eaten between meals or after midnight.

amenorrhoea Cessation of menstruation, normally occurring between the ages of 40 and 55 (the menopause), but sometimes at an early age, especially as a result of severe under-nutrition (as in *anorexia nervosa) when body weight falls below about 45 kg.

américaine, à l' Various methods of preparing meat, game, fish, vegetables, and eggs, the best-known example being homard à l'américaine, lobster in a sauce based on tomato, onion, and herbs, cooked in wine or brandy.

American icing *See* sugar, icing.

Amer Picon Trade name; pungent *bitters invented in 1830 by Gaston Picon; contains quinine, gentian, and orange.

Ames test An *in vitro* test for the ability of chemicals, including potential food *additives, to cause mutation in bacteria (the mutagenic potential). Commonly used as a preliminary screening method to detect substances likely to be carcinogenic.

amines Formed by the decarboxylation of *amino acids. Three are potentially important in foods: phenylethylamine (formed from *phenylalanine), tyramine (from *tyrosine), and tryptamine (from *tryptophan). They are found in ripened cheese, chocolate, yeast, wines, and fermented foods. They all stimulate the sympathetic nervous system and can cause increased blood pressure. In sensitive people they are one of the possible dietary causes of migraine.

Amines from foods are normally inactivated by the enzyme monoamine oxidase in the liver, but some drugs used as antidepressant medication (monoamine oxidase inhibitors) inhibit the enzyme; patients receiving such drugs must avoid foods that contain relatively large amounts of amines.

amino acid disorders A number of extremely rare *genetic diseases, occurring in 1–80 per million live births which affect the metabolism of individual *amino acids; if untreated many result in mental retardation. Screening for those conditions that can be treated is carried out shortly after birth in most countries. Treatment is generally by feeding specially formulated diets providing minimal amounts of the amino acid involved. *See also* argininaemia; argininosuccinic aciduria; citrullinaemia, cystinuria; cystathioninuria; Hartnup disease; homocystinuria; hyperammonaemia; maple syrup urine disease; phenylketonuria.

amino acid profile The *amino acid composition of a *protein.

amino acids The basic units from which *proteins are made. Chemically compounds with an amino group (–NH₂) and a carboxyl group (–COOH) attached to the same carbon atom.

Thirteen of the amino acids involved in proteins can be synthesized in the body, and so are called non-essential or dispensable amino acids, since they do not have to be provided in the diet. They are alanine, arginine, aspartic acid, asparagine, cysteine, cystine, glutamic acid, glutamine, glycine, hydroxyproline, proline, serine, and tyrosine.

Eight amino acids cannot be synthesized in the body at all and so must be provided in the diet; they are called the essential or indispensable amino acids — isoleucine, leucine, lysine, methionine, phenylalanine, threonine, tryptophan, and valine. In addition, histidine is partially essential, since it cannot be synthesized in adequate amounts to meet requirements without some dietary intake, and arginine may be essential for infants, since their requirement is greater than their ability to synthesize this amino acid. Two of the non-essential amino acids are made in the body from essential amino acids: cysteine (and cystine) from methionine, and tyrosine from phenylalanine.

The limiting amino acid of a protein is that essential *amino acid present in least amount relative to the requirement for that amino acid. The ratio between the amount of the limiting amino acid in a protein and the requirement for that amino acid provides a chemical estimation of the nutritional value (*protein quality) of that protein, termed chemical score. Most cereal proteins are limited by *lysine, and most animal and other vegetable proteins by the sum of *methionine + *cysteine (the *sulphur amino acids). In whole diets it is usually the sulphur amino acids that are limiting.

A number of other amino acids also occur in proteins, including hydroxyproline, hydroxylysine, γ-carboxyglutamate and methylhistidine, but are nutritionally unimportant since they cannot be re-utilized for protein synthesis. Other amino acids occur as intermediates in metabolic pathways, but are not required for protein synthesis, and are nutritionally unimportant, although they may occur in foods. These include *homocysteine, citrulline, and ornithine. Some of the non-protein amino acids that occur in plants are toxic in excess.

The amino acids are sometimes classified by the chemical nature of the side-chain. Two are acidic: glutamic acid (glutamate) and aspartic acid (aspartate) and have a carboxylic acid (–COOH) group in the side-chain. Three, lysine, arginine and histidine, have basic groups in the side-chain. Three, phenylalanine, tyrosine, and tryptophan, have an *aromatic group in the side-chain. Three, leucine, isoleucine, and valine, have a branched chain structure. These three have very similar metabolism, and a rare *genetic disease affecting their metabolism results in *maple syrup urine disease. Two, methionine and cysteine, contain sulphur in the side-chain; although cysteine is not an essential amino acid, it can only be synthesized from methionine, and it is conventional to consider the sum of methionine plus cysteine (the sulphur amino acids) in consideration of *protein quality.

An alternative classification of the amino acids is by their metabolic fate; whether they can be utilized for glucose synthesis or not. Those that can give rise to glucose are termed glucogenic (or sometimes antiketogenic); those that give rise to *ketones or *acetate when they are metabolized are termed ketogenic. Only leucine and lysine are purely ketogenic; isoleucine, phenylalanine, tyrosine, and tryptophan give rise to both ketogenic and glucogenic fragments; the remainder are purely glucogenic.

aminoaciduria Excretion of abnormal amounts of one or more *amino acids in the urine, usually as a result of a *genetic disease. *See also* amino acid disorders.

aminogram A diagrammatic representation of the *amino acid composition of a *peptide or *protein. A plasma aminogram is the composition of the free amino acid pool in blood plasma.

amino group Chemically the CH—NH$_2$ group of *amino acids and amines, among other compounds. The amino acid *lysine has a second amino group in its side-chain.

aminopeptidase An *enzyme secreted in the *pancreatic juice which removes amino acids sequentially from the free amino terminal of a peptide or protein (i.e. the end which has a free amino group exposed), until the final product is a *dipeptide. Since it works at the end of the peptide chain, it is an *exopeptidase.

aminotransferase Any *enzyme that catalyses the reaction of *transamination.

amla Indian gooseberry, *Emblica officinalis Gaertn*, important in Ayurvedic medicine and reported to reduce *hypercholesterolaemia. An extremely rich source of vitamin C (600 mg/100 g).

amoebiasis (amoebic dysentery) Infection of the intestinal tract with pathogenic amoeba (commonly *Entamoeba histolytica*) from contaminated food or water, causing profuse diarrhoea, intestinal bleeding, pain, jaundice, anorexia, and weight loss.

amomum A group of tropical plants including *cardamom and melegueta *pepper, which have pungent and aromatic seeds.

amontillado, amoroso *See* sherry.

amour (parfait amour) Purple-coloured liqueur, flavoured with citrus fruits and violets.

amourettes French; marrow from calves' bones, normally cooked as a garnish.

AMP Adenosine monophosphate; *see* adenine.

amphetamine A chemical at one time used as an appetite suppressant; addictive, and a common drug of abuse ('speed'), its use is strictly controlled by law.

amphoteric *See* isoelectric point.

amtlicher Prüfungsnummer (AP) German; batch number on labels of quality wines. *See* wine classification, Germany.

amydon A traditional starchy material made by steeping wheat flour in water, then drying the starch sediment in the sun, used for thickening broths, etc.

amygdalin 1 A *glycoside in *almonds and apricot and cherry stones which is hydrolysed by the enzyme emulsin to yield glucose, hydrocyanic acid, and benzaldehyde. It is therefore highly poisonous, although it has been promoted, with no evidence, as a nutrient, laetrile or so-called vitamin B_{17}. Unfounded claims have been made for its value in treating cancer.
   2 French name for cakes and sweets made with almonds.

amylases *Enzymes that hydrolyse *starch and *glycogen. α-Amylase (dextrinogenic amylase or diastase) acts to produce small *dextrin fragments from starch, while β-amylase (maltogenic amylase) liberates maltose, some free glucose, and isomaltose from the branch points in *amylopectin.
   Salivary amylase (sometimes called by its obsolete name of ptyalin) and pancreatic amylase are both α-amylases. *See also* Z-enzyme.

amyli Dried *tamarind.

amyloamylose Old name for *amylose, as distinct from erythroamylose, the old name for *amylopectin.

amylodyspepsia An inability to digest starch.

amylograph A device to measure the viscosity of flour paste as it is heated from 25 ˚C to 90 ˚C (the same increase in temperature as occurs in baking), which serves as a measure of the *diastatic activity of the flour.

amyloins Carbohydrates that are complexes of dextrins with varying proportions of maltose.

amylopectin The branched chain form of *starch. About 75–80% of starch is in this form, the remainder is *amylose.

amylopeptic A general description of enzymes that are able to split *starch to give soluble products.

amylopsin Alternative name for pancreatic *amylase.

amylose The straight chain form of *starch. About 20–25% of starch is in this form, the remainder is *amylopectin.

anabolic hormones Those *hormones (and hormone-like drugs) that stimulate growth and the development of muscle tissue.

anabolism The process of building up or synthesizing. *See* metabolism.

anacard Brazilian; vinegar made by fermentation of the pulp surrounding the cashew nut.

anaemia A shortage of red *blood cells, leading to pallor and shortness of breath, especially on exertion. Most commonly due to a dietary deficiency of *iron, or excessive blood losses resulting in iron losses greater than can be met from the diet. Other dietary deficiencies can also result in anaemia, including deficiency of *vitamin B_{12} or *folic acid (megaloblastic anaemia), *vitamin E (haemolytic anaemia), and rarely *vitamin C or *vitamin B_6.

anaemia, haemolytic *Anaemia caused by premature and excessive destruction of red blood cells; not normally due to nutritional deficiency, but can occur as a result of vitamin E deficiency in premature infants.

anaemia, megaloblastic Release into the circulation of immature precursors of red *blood cells, due to deficiency of either *folic acid or *vitamin B_{12}. *See also* anaemia, pernicious.

anaemia, pernicious *Anaemia due to deficiency of *vitamin B_{12}, most commonly as a result of failure to absorb the vitamin from the diet. There is release into the circulation of immature precursors of red *blood cells, the same type of megaloblastic anaemia as is seen in *folic acid deficiency. There is also progressive damage to the spinal cord (sub-acute combined degeneration), which is not reversed on restoring the vitamin. The underlying cause of the condition may be the production of *antibodies against either the *intrinsic factor that is required for absorption of the vitamin, or the cells of the gastric mucosa that secrete intrinsic factor. Atrophy of the gastric mucosa with ageing also impairs vitamin B_{12} absorption, and causes pernicious anaemia. Dietary deficiency of vitamin B_{12}, leading to a similar anaemia with spinal cord degeneration, may occur in strict vegetarians.

anaerobes Micro-organisms that grow in the absence of oxygen. Obligate anaerobes cannot survive in the presence of oxygen, facultative anaerobes normally grow in the presence of oxygen but can also grow in its absence.

analysis, gastric *See* fractional test meal.

analysis, proximate *See* proximate analysis.

ananas *See* pineapple.

anatto *See* annatto.

anchovy (French: *anchois*; German: *Sardelle*.) Small oily *fish, *Engraulis* spp., usually semi-preserved with 10–12% salt and sometimes *benzoic acid. A 50-g portion (canned, drained) is a good *source of protein and niacin; a source of calcium, iron, and zinc; contains 10 g of fat; supplies 140 kcal (590 kJ). Anchovy butter is prepared from pounded fillets of anchovy mixed with butter as a savoury spread; anchovy paste from pounded fillets of anchovy mixed with vinegar and spices.

anchoyade French (Provençale); anchovies puréed with garlic and olive oil.

ancienne, à l' Literally, 'old-style'. Usually a dish with a mixed garnish of beans, cooked lettuce, and hard-boiled egg.

andalouse 1 Dishes with rice and tomatoes.
    2 French sauce based on mayonnaise with tomato purée and diced peppers.
    3 Garnish of tomatoes stuffed with rice, aubergine, and tomatoes.
    4 Clear chicken soup garnished with tomatoes, rice, ham, and beaten egg.

andouille French sausage made from pork and pork intestines (chitterlings); smaller versions are andouillettes.

andruty Polish; *waffle.

aneurine Obsolete name for *vitamin B$_1$.

aneurysm Local dilatation (swelling and weakening) of the wall of a blood vessel, usually the result of *atherosclerosis and *hypertension; especially serious when occurring in the aorta, when rupture may prove fatal.

angelica Crystallized young stalks of the umbelliferous herb *Angelica archangelica*, which grows in southern Europe. They are bright green in colour, and are used to decorate and flavour confectionery goods. The roots are used together with *juniper berries to flavour *gin, and the seeds are used in *vermouth and *Chartreuse. *Essential oils are distilled from the roots, stem, and leaves.

angel's hair (Spanish: *cabello de angel*.) Jam made from the fibrous part of mature pumpkin or squash, preferably kept from the previous year's harvest.

angels on horseback Oysters wrapped in bacon, skewered, and grilled.

anghiti Indian; charcoal brazier used for grilling *kebabs.

angina (angina pectoris) Paroxysmal thoracic pain and choking sensation, especially during exercise or stress, due to partial blockage of the coronary artery (the blood vessel supplying the heart), as a result of *atherosclerosis.

anglaise 1 Plainly cooked in stock or water;
    2 coating of eggs on foods that are then dipped in breadcrumbs and fried;
    3 garnish for boiled salt beef consisting of boiled vegetables.

Angostura The best known of the *bitters, widely used in cocktails; a secret blend of herbs and spices, including the bitter aromatic bark of either of two trees of the orange family (*Galipea officinalis, Cusparia felorifuga*). Invented in 1824 by Dr Siegert in the town of Angostura in Bolivia, originally as a medicine, and now made in Trinidad. A few drops of Angostura in *gin makes a 'pink gin'.

Ångstrom A unit of length equal to 10^{-8} cm (10^{-10} m) and hence = 10 nm; not an official SI unit, but still commonly used in structural chemistry and crystallography. *See* Appendix I.

angular stomatitis A characteristic cracking and fissuring of the skin at the angles of the mouth, a symptom of *vitamin B_2 deficiency, but also seen in other conditions.

animal charcoal *See* bone charcoal.

animal protein factor A name given to a growth factor or factors which were found to be present in animal but not vegetable proteins. *Vitamin B_{12} was identified as one of these.

anion A negatively charged *ion.

anise (anis) *Liqueur made by infusion of *aniseed berries (not star anise) in *spirit; may be sweet or dry. French sweet anise liqueur is anisette. *Pastis is prepared by distillation of anise and liquorice rather than infusion.

aniseed (anise) The dried fruit of *Pimpinella anisum*, a member of the parsley family, which is used to flavour baked goods, meat dishes, and drinks, including *anise, *anisette, and *ouzo. *See also* anise, star.

aniseed milk Dutch (*anijs melk*); hot milk drink flavoured with aniseed, traditionally drunk when one is ice skating.

anise pepper A pungent spice from the Sichuan region of China (the fruit of *Zanthoxylum piperitum*); the flavour develops gradually after biting into the pepper.

anise, star A spice, the seeds of *Illicium verum*, widely used in Chinese cooking. Distinct from *aniseed.

anisette A sweet *liqueur flavoured with aniseed.

annata Year of vintage on Italian wine labels. *See* wine classification, Italy.

annatto (anatto) Also known as bixin, butter colour, or rocou; a yellow colouring (E-160(b)) extracted from the pericarp of the fruit of the tropical shrub *Bixa orellana*. The main component is the *carotenoid bixin, which is fat-soluble. It is used to colour cheese, dairy produce, and baked goods. The seeds are used for flavouring in Caribbean foods.

anona *See* custard apple.

anorectic drugs (anorexigenic drugs) Drugs that depress the appetite, used as an aid to weight reduction. The most commonly used are diethylpropion, fenfluramine (and dexfenfluramine), phenmetrazine hydrochloride, and mazindol. *Amphetamines were used at one time, but are addictive and subject to special control.

anorexia Lack of appetite.

anorexia nervosa A psychological disturbance resulting in a refusal to eat, possibly with restriction to a very limited range of foods, and often accompanied by a rigid programme of vigorous physical exercise, to the point of exhaustion. Anorectic subjects generally do not feel sensations of hunger. The result is a very considerable loss of weight, with tissue atrophy and a fall in *basal metabolic rate. It is especially prevalent among adolescent girls; when body weight falls below about 45 kg there is a cessation of menstruation.

anosmia Lack or impairment of the sense of smell.

anserine A *dipeptide found in *muscle, of unknown function. It consists of β-alanine and *methylhistidine.

Antabuse Trade name for the drug disulfiram, used in the treatment of *alcoholism. It inhibits the further metabolism of acetaldehyde arising from the metabolism of alcohol, and so causes headache, nausea, vomiting, and palpitations if alcohol is consumed.

antacids *Bases or *buffers that neutralize acids, used generally to counteract excessive *gastric acidity and to treat *indigestion. Antacid preparations generally contain such compounds as *sodium bicarbonate, aluminium hydroxide, magnesium carbonate, or magnesium hydroxide.

anthocyanins Violet, red, and blue water-soluble colours extracted from flowers, fruits, and leaves (E-163). They can react with *iron or *tin, and so may cause discoloration in canned foods.

anthoxanthins Alternative name for *flavonoids.

anthropometry Body measurements used as an index of physiological development and nutritional status; a non-invasive way of assessing body composition. Weight for age provides information about the overall nutritional status of children; weight for height is used to detect acute malnutrition (wasting); height for age to detect chronic malnutrition (stunting). Mid-upper arm circumference provides an index of muscle wastage in undernutrition. *Skinfold thickness is related to the amount of subcutaneous fat as an index of over- or under-nutrition. *See also* body mass index; cristal height; stunting; Wetzel grid.

antibiotics Substances produced by living organisms which inhibit the growth of other organisms. The first antibiotic to be discovered was *penicillin, which is produced by the *mould *Penicillium notatum* and inhibits the growth of sensitive bacteria. Many antibiotics are used to treat bacterial infections in human beings and animals; different compounds affect different bacteria. Small amounts of antibiotics may be added to animal feed (a few grams/tonne), resulting in improved growth, possibly by controlling mild infections or changing the population of intestinal bacteria and so altering the digestion and absorption of food. To prevent the development of antibiotic-resistant strains of disease-causing bacteria, only those antibiotics that are not used clinically are permitted in animal feed (e.g. *nisin, which is also used as a food preservative (E-234)).

antibodies A class of proteins formed in the body in response to the presence of *antigens (foreign proteins and other compounds), which bind to the antigen, so inactivating it. Immunity to infection is due to the production of antibodies against specific proteins of bacteria, viruses, or other disease-causing organisms, and immunization is the process of giving these marker proteins, generally in an inactivated form, to stimulate the production of antibodies. *Adverse reactions to foods (food allergies) may be due to the production of antibodies against specific food proteins. Chemically the antibodies form a class of proteins known as the γ-globulins or immunoglobulins; there are five types, classified as IgA, IgD, IgE, IgG, and IgM.

anti-caking agents Compounds added in small amounts to powdered foodstuffs to prevent clumping or caking — e.g. anhydrous disodium hydrogen phosphate is added to salt and icing sugar, aluminium calcium silicate or calcium or magnesium carbonate to table salt, calcium silicate to *baking powder.

anticoagulants Compounds that prevent or slow the process of blood clotting or coagulation, either in samples of blood taken for analysis or in the body. One of the most commonly used such substances is heparin, which is formed in the body (especially the lungs and liver).

People at risk of thrombosis are often treated with Warfarin and similar compounds as an anticoagulant, to reduce the risk of intravenous blood clot formation. These act by antagonizing the action of *vitamin K in the synthesis of blood clotting proteins, and people taking anticoagulants should be careful not to take supplements containing large amounts of vitamin K. It is most unlikely that the vitamin K in foods would be enough to have any such adverse effect.

antidiarrhoeal Drug used to treat *diarrhoea by absorbing water from the intestine, altering intestinal motility, or adsorbing (bacterial) toxins.

antidiuretic Drug used to reduce the formation of urine and so conserve fluid in the body. *See also* water balance.

antiemetic Drug used to prevent or alleviate nausea and vomiting.

antigalactic Drug that reduces or prevents the secretion of milk in women after parturition.

antigen Any compound that is foreign to the body (e.g. bacterial, food, or pollen protein, or some complex carbohydrates) which, when introduced into the circulation, stimulates the formation of an *antibody. *See also* adverse reactions to foods.

anti-grey-hair factor Deficiency of the *vitamin *pantothenic acid causes loss of hair colour in black and brown rats, and at one time the vitamin was known as the anti-grey-hair factor. It is not related to the loss of hair pigment in human beings.

antihaemorrhagic vitamin *See* vitamin K.

antihistamine Drug that antagonizes the actions of *histamine; those that block histamine H_1 receptors are used to treat allergic reactions; those that block H_2 receptors are used to treat peptic *ulcers.

antihypertensive Drug, diet, or other treatment used to treat *hypertension by lowering blood pressure.

antilipidaemic Drug, diet, or other treatment used to treat *hyperlipidaemia by lowering blood lipids.

antimetabolite Compound that inhibits a normal metabolic process, acting as an analogue of a normal metabolite. Some are useful in chemotherapy of cancer, others are naturally occurring toxins in foods, frequently causing vitamin deficiency diseases by inhibiting the normal metabolism of the vitamin. *See also* antivitamin.

antimony Toxic metal of no known metabolic function, and therefore not a dietary essential. Antimony compounds are used in treatment of some parasitic diseases.

anti-mould agents *See* antimycotics.

antimycotics Substances that inhibit the growth of *moulds and *fungi, such as sodium and calcium propionates, methyl hydroxybenzoate, quaternary ammonium chloride, sodium benzoate, sorbic acid.

antioxidant A substance that retards the oxidative *rancidity of fats in stored foods. Many fats, and especially vegetable oils, contain naturally occurring antioxidants, including *vitamin E (E-306–309), which protect them against rancidity for some time. Synthetic antioxidants include propyl, octyl, and dodecyl gallates (E-310, 311, 312), butylated hydroxyanisole (BHA, E-320) and butylated hydroxytoluene (BHT, E-321). *See also* antioxidant nutrients; induction period.

antioxidant nutrients Highly reactive oxygen *radicals are formed both during normal oxidative *metabolism and in response to infection and some chemicals. They cause damage to *fatty acids in cell membranes, and the products of this damage can then cause damage to proteins and *DNA. The most widely accepted theory of the biochemical basis of much *cancer, and also of *atherosclerosis and possibly *kwashiorkor, is that the key factor in precipitating the condition is tissue damage by such radicals. A number of different mechanisms are involved in protection against, or repair after, oxygen radical damage, including a number of nutrients, especially *vitamin E, *carotene, *vitamin C, and *selenium. Collectively these are known as antioxidant nutrients.

antipasto Italian; dishes served before the main meal, hors d'œuvre.

antiscorbutic vitamin *See* vitamin C.

antisialagogues Substances that reduce the flow of *saliva.

anti-spattering agents Compounds such as *lecithin, sucrose esters of *fatty acids, and sodium sulpho-acetate derivatives of *mono- and *diglycerides, which are added to oils and fats used for frying to prevent potentially dangerous spattering. They function by preventing the coalescence of water droplets.

anti-staling agents Substances that retard the *staling of baked products, and soften the crumb, e.g. sucrose stearate, polyoxyethylene monostearate, glyceryl monostearate, stearoyl tartrate.

antivitamins Substances that interfere with the normal metabolism or function of *vitamins, or destroy them. Dicoumarol in spoiled sweet clover antagonizes the function of *vitamin K, thiaminase in raw fish destroys *vitamin B_1, the drug methotrexate antagonizes folic acid action (this is part of its mechanism of action in treating cancer), the drug isoniazid antagonizes the action of *vitamin B_6.

antixerophthalmic vitamin *See* vitamin A.

AOC Appellation d'origine contrôlée; *see* wine classification, France.

aortic aneurysm *See* aneurysm.

AP Amtlicher Prüfungsnummer, German; batch number on labels of quality wines. *See* wine classification, Germany.

apastia Refusal to take food, as an expression of a psychiatric disturbance. *See also* anorexia nervosa.

aperient *See* laxative.

aperitif wines *See* wine, aperitif.

apfelstrudel *See* strudel.

aphagia Inability to swallow. Difficulty in swallowing is dysphagia.

aphagosis Inability to eat.

apo-carotenal *See* carotene.

apoenzyme The protein part of an *enzyme which requires a *coenzyme for activity, and is therefore inactive if the coenzyme is absent. *See also* coenzyme; enzyme activation; prosthetic group.

apokreo Greek: literally 'fast from meat'; the three weeks of abstinence from meat ordained by the Greek Orthodox Church during Lent.

apolipoprotein The protein part of *lipoproteins without the associated lipid. *See also* lipids, plasma.

Apollinaris water An alkaline, highly aerated, *mineral water containing sodium chloride and calcium, sodium, and magnesium carbonates, from a spring in the valley of Ahr (in Germany).

aporrhegma *Ptomaine or other toxic substance formed from an *amino acid during the bacterial decomposition of a protein.

aposia Absence of sensation of thirst.

apositia Aversion to food.

apparent digestibility *See* digestibility.

appellation contrôlée (AC) Or appellation d'origine contrôlée (AOC); *see* wine classification, France.

appendix (vermiform appendix) A residual part of the intestinal tract, a small sac-like process extending from the caecum, some 4–8 cm long. Acute inflammation, caused by an obstruction (appendicitis) can lead to perforation and peritonitis if surgery is not performed in time. *See also* gastro-intestinal tract.

appertization French term for the process of destroying all the micro-organisms of significance in food, i.e. 'commercial sterility'; a few organisms remain alive but quiescent. Named after Nicholas Appert (1752–1841), a Paris confectioner who invented the process of *canning.

apple Fruit of the tree *Malus sylvestris* and its many cultivars and hybrids; there are more than 2000 varieties in the British National Fruit Collection. Crab apples are grown mainly for decoration, and for pollination of fruit-bearing trees, although the sour fruit can be used for making jelly. Cooking apples are generally sourer varieties than dessert apples, and normally have flesh which crumbles on cooking; cider apples are sour varieties especially suited to the making of *cider. One apple (110 g) provides 2.2 g of dietary fibre and supplies 40 kcal (165 kJ).

apple brandy *Spirit made by distillation of *cider, known in France as Calvados. See also apple jack.

apple butter Apple that has been boiled in an open pan to a thick consistency; similar to *apple sauce, but darker in colour due to the prolonged boiling.

apple jack American name for *apple brandy, normally distilled, but traditionally prepared by leaving cider outside in winter, when the water froze out as ice crystals, leaving the alcoholic spirit.

apple, liquid American preparation of apple juice with pulverized apple pulp in suspension.

apple mint A herb, *Mentha rotundifolia. See also* mint.

apple nuggets Crisp granules of apple of low moisture content, used commercially for manufacture of *apple sauce.

apple-pear Not a cross between apple and pear but a distinctive varietal type of pear-shaped fruit with apple texture. Also called Japanese pear, pear-apple, and shalea or chalea.

apple sauce Pulped stewed apple; in the UK it is made from sour apples, as an accompaniment to pork and goose; in the USA also used for stewed apple as a dessert.

apricot Fruit of the tree *Prunus armeniaca*. Apricot kernels are used to prepare *almond oil. One apricot (60 g) is a *source of vitamins A (as carotene) and C; provides 1.2 g of dietary fibre and supplies 18 kcal (75 kJ). A 60-g portion of dried apricots is a rich source of vitamin A (as carotene); a good source of copper; a source of niacin and iron; provides 14.4 g of dietary fibre; supplies 110 kcal (470 kJ).

aquamiel See pulque.

aquavit (akvavit or akavit) Scandinavian; spirit flavoured with herbs (commonly caraway, cumin, dill, or fennel). Also known as snaps, and in Germany as schnapps.

araboascorbic acid See erythorbic acid.

arachidonic acid A *fatty acid with twenty carbon atoms and four double bonds (20:4 ω6). Not strictly an essential fatty acid, since it can be formed from *linoleic acid, but three times more potent than linoleic acid in curing the signs of essential fatty acid deficiency. Found in animal tissues, especially fish, eggs, liver, and brain.

arachin One of the globulin proteins from the *peanut.

arachis oil Oil extracted from the groundnut or *peanut, *Arachis hypogea*, 20% *saturated, 50% mono-unsaturated (*oleic acid), 30% polyunsaturated (*linolenic acid), less than 1% linolenic acid.

arak (arack) (Greek: *ouzo*; Turkish: *raki*.) Arabic; *anise- and *liquorice-flavoured spirit. Also used generally in the Middle and Far East to mean any one of a variety of spirits, often distilled from fermented dates or palm wine.

Arbroath smokie Smoked haddock; unlike *finnan haddock in that it is not split but smoked whole to a dull copper colour.

arbute Fruit of the southern European strawberry tree (*Arbutus unedo*); resemble strawberries in appearance but have a grainy texture and little taste.

archiduc, à l' Dishes seasoned with paprika and blended with cream.

Arctons *See* refrigerants.

ard bhoona *See* bhoona.

areca nut *See* betel.

argininaemia A *genetic disease affecting the metabolism of the *amino acid arginine, and hence the normal formation of urea and elimination of end-products of protein metabolism. Depending on the severity of the condition, affected infants may become comatose and die after a moderately high intake of protein. Treatment is by severe restriction of protein intake. Sodium benzoate may be given to increase the excretion of nitrogenous waste as hippuric acid. *See also* benzoic acid.

arginine A basic *amino acid. Not a dietary essential for adult human beings, but infants may not be able to synthesize enough to meet the high demands of growth so some may be required in infant diets.

argininosuccinic aciduria A *genetic disease affecting the formation of urea, and hence the elimination of end-products of protein metabolism. Depending on the severity of the condition, affected infants may become comatose and die after a moderately high intake of protein. Treatment is by restriction of protein intake and feeding supplements of the amino acid arginine, which permits elimination of nitrogenous waste as argininosuccinic acid. Sodium benzoate may be given to increase the excretion of nitrogenous waste as hippuric acid. *See also* benzoic acid.

argol Crust of crude *cream of tartar (potassium acid tartrate) which forms on the sides of wine vats, also called wine stone. It consists of 50–85% potassium hydrogen tartrate and 6–12% calcium tartrate, and will be coloured by the grapes, so white argol comes from white grapes and red argol from red grapes. Used in *vinegar fermentation, in the manufacture of *tartaric acid and as a mordant in dyeing.

ariboflavinosis Deficiency of riboflavin (*vitamin B_2) characterized by swollen, cracked, bright red lips (cheilosis), an enlarged, tender, magenta-red tongue (glossitis), cracking at the corners of the mouth (angular stomatitis), congestion of the blood vessels of the conjunctiva and a characteristic dermatitis with filiform (wire-like) excrescences.

arkshell *See* cockles.

arlesienne, à l' French garnishes: (1) aubergine, onions, and tomatoes; (2) fried small whole tomatoes and pickled chicory hearts; (3) tomatoes stuffed with rice and large olives stuffed with minced chicken.

armagnac *Brandy made from white wine from one of three defined areas of France: Bas-Armagnac, Haut-Armagnac, or Ténarèze. *See also* cognac.

Armenian bole Ferric oxide (iron oxide), either occurring naturally as haematite or prepared by heating ferrous sulphate and other iron salts. Used in metallurgy, polishing compounds, paint pigment, and as a food colour (E-172).

Arogel Trade name for a potato starch preparation which is stable to heating and is used as a thickener in gravies, sauces, and canned foods.

Aros *See* P-4000.

arrak (arak) *See* ouzo.

arrowroot Tuber of the Caribbean plant *Maranta arundinacea*, mainly used to prepare arrowroot starch, a particularly pure form of starch, which contains only a trace of protein (0.2%) and is free from vitamins. It is used to thicken sauces and in bland, low-salt, and protein-restricted diets, and as an infant food in some Caribbean islands.

arsenic A toxic metal, with no known metabolic function. Organic arsenic derivatives (arsenicals) have been used as pesticides and in treatment of diseases such as syphilis, leprosy, and yaws. Arsenic can accumulate in crops treated with arsenical pesticides, and in fish and shellfish living in arsenic-polluted water.

arteriosclerosis Thickening and calcification of the arterial walls, leading to loss of elasticity, occurring with ageing and especially in *hypertension. *See also* atheroma; atherosclerosis.

artichoke, Chinese Tubers of *Stachys affinis*, similar to Jerusalem artichoke but smaller.

artichoke, globe Young flower heads of *Cynara scolymus*; the edible parts the fleshy bracts and the base; the choke is the inedible filaments. A 110-g portion (two artichoke hearts) is a *source of vitamin C; provides 1.1 g of dietary fibre; supplies 17 kcal (70 kJ).

artichoke, Japanese Tubers of the perennial plant *Stachys sieboldi*, similar to Jerusalem artichoke.

artichoke, Jerusalem Tubers of *Helianthus tuberosus* introduced into Europe from Canada in the seventeenth century; the origin of the name Jerusalem is from the Italian *girasole* (sunflower). A 170-g portion is a good *source of copper; a source of vitamin B_1; provides 1.7 g of dietary fibre; supplies 30 kcal (125 kJ). Much of the carbohydrate is the *non-starch polysaccharide *inulin.

artificial cream A non-dairy substitute for *cream, made from vegetable oils, with *stabilizers, *emulsifiers, and sometimes flavourings and colours added.

artificial sweeteners *See* sweeteners, intense.

asafoetida A resin extracted from the oriental umbelliferous plant *Narthex asafoetida*, with a bitter flavour and strong garlic-like odour, used widely in oriental and Middle-Eastern cooking, and in small amounts in sauces and pickles. (The strength of its aroma is suggested by its French and German names: respectively, *merde du diable* and *Teufelsdreck*.)

ascites Abnormal accumulation of fluid in the peritoneal cavity, occurring as a complication of cirrhosis of the liver, congestive heart failure, cancer, and infectious diseases. Depending on the underlying cause, treatment may sometimes consist of a high-energy, high-protein, low-sodium diet, together with diuretic drugs and fluid restriction.

ascorbic acid *Vitamin C, chemically L-xyloascorbic acid, to distinguish it from the *isomer D-araboascorbic acid (isoascorbic acid or erythorbic acid), which has only slight vitamin C activity. Both ascorbic acid and erythorbic acid have strong chemical-reducing properties, and are used as *antioxidants in foods and to preserve the red colour of fresh and preserved meats, and in the curing of hams.

ascorbic acid oxidase An *enzyme in plant tissues that oxidizes ascorbic acid to dehydro-ascorbic acid. In the intact fresh plant the enzyme is separated from the ascorbic acid, and is only released when the plant wilts or is cut. To preserve the vitamin in cooked vegetables, it is generally recommended that they be plunged into boiling water, to denature and therefore inactivate the enzyme, as soon as possible after cutting.

ascorbin stearate An ester of *ascorbic acid and *stearic acid; a fat-soluble form of the vitamin which is used as an *antioxidant.

ascorbyl palmitate An ester of *ascorbic acid and *palmitic acid which is used as an *anti-staling compound in bakery goods (E-304).

aseptic filling The filling of cans or other containers with food that has already been sterilized, the process thus having to be carried out under aseptic conditions. Continuous sterilization as the food passes along narrow pipes (followed by aseptic filling) allows more rapid heating, with less effect on the quality of the food, than sterilization by heating after *canning.

ash The residue left behind after all organic matter has been burnt off, a measure of the total content of mineral salts in a food.

asparagine A non-essential *amino acid, chemically the β-amide of *aspartic acid.

asparagus The young shoots of the plant *Asparagus officinalis*. A 110-g portion (four spears) is a rich *source of folate; a source of vitamin C and copper; provides 1.1 g of dietary fibre; supplies 8 kcal (33 kJ).

aspartame An artificial *sweetener, aspartyl-phenylalanine methyl ester, some 200 times as sweet as sucrose. Stable for a limited time (a few months) in solution, when it gradually breaks down. Used in soft drinks, dessert mixes, and as a 'table top sweetener'. The major trade names are Canderel, Equal, Nutrasweet, and Sanecta.

  Because aspartame contains *phenylalanine, it is specifically recommended that children with *phenylketonuria avoid consuming it, although the amounts that would be consumed are extremely small.

aspartic acid (aspartate) A non-essential *amino acid.

aspartyl-phenylalanine methyl ester *See* aspartame.

ASPEN American Society for Parenteral and Enteral Nutrition.

Aspergillus A family of moulds, important in the spoiling of stored nuts and grains because *A. flavus* produces *aflatoxins. *A. oryzae* is grown commercially as a source of *takadiastase.

aspic jelly A clear jelly made from fish, chicken, or meat stock, sometimes with added *gelatine, flavoured with lemon, tarragon, vinegar, sherry, peppercorns, and vegetables, used to glaze foods such as meat, fish, and game. The name may be derived from the herb espic or spikenard.

assiette anglaise French; plate of cold assorted meats (literally 'English plate').

astaxanthin One of the *carotenoids, the pink colour of salmon and trout muscle; has no *vitamin A activity.

asti spumante Italian; sparkling wines (generally sweet) made from muscat grapes.

astringency The action of unripe fruits and cider apples, among other foods, to cause a contraction of the epithelial tissues of the tongue (literally astringency means 'a drawing together'). It is believed to result from a destruction of the lubricant properties of *saliva by precipitation by *tannins.

atheroma The fatty deposit composed of various lipids, complex carbohydrates, and fibrous tissue which forms on the inner wall of blood vessels in *atherosclerosis.

atherosclerosis Degenerative disease of the arteries in which there is accumulation on the inner wall of lipids together with complex carbohydrates and fibrous tissue, called *atheroma. This leads to narrowing of the lumen of the arteries. When it occurs in the coronary artery it can lead to failure of the blood supply to the heart muscle (ischaemia). *See also* arteriosclerosis.

atholl brose Scottish beverage made from malt whisky, honey, cream, and oatmeal.

ATP Adenosine triphosphate, the coenzyme that acts as an intermediate between energy-yielding (catabolic) *metabolism (the oxidation of metabolic fuels) and *energy expenditure as physical work and in synthetic (anabolic) reactions. ADP (adenosine diphosphate) is phosphorylated to ATP linked to oxidations; in energy expenditure ATP is hydrolysed to ADP and phosphate ions.

atta Indian; wholewheat flour or dough made from it for preparation of *chapattis.

attelette Or hâtelet, ornamental skewers used to decorate cold meats and fish.

Atwater factors *See* energy factors.

aubergine The fruit of *Solanum melongena*, a native of South East Asia, widely cultivated and eaten as a vegetable, also known as egg-plant and (in West Africa) field egg. Half a medium-sized aubergine (140 g) is a

*source of folate and vitamin C; provides 2.8 g of dietary fibre; supplies 20 kcal (85 kJ).

audit ale Strong *beer originally brewed at Oxford and Cambridge Universities to be drunk on 'audit days'.

auguiser French; to sharpen a *sauce by adding lemon juice or citric acid.

aurantiamarin A *glucoside present in the *albedo of the bitter orange which is partly responsible for its flavour.

aureomycin Oxytetracycline, one of the tetracycline group of *antibiotics.

aurora sauce Danish; *béchamel sauce with tomato purée.

aurore, à l' Dishes served with tomato-flavoured aurora sauce or yellow-coloured garnishes, suggesting the rising sun.

aurum potabile Italian liqueur (literally 'drinkable gold'), made from brandy coloured with saffron, flavoured with oranges, orange zest, and herbs; probably the forerunner of *Goldwasser.

ausbruch *See* wine classification, German.

auslese *See* wine classification, German.

autoclave A vessel in which high temperatures can be achieved by using high pressure; the domestic pressure cooker is an example. At atmospheric pressure water boils at 100 °C; at 5 lb (35 kPa) above atmospheric pressure the boiling point is 109 °C; at 10 lb (70 kPa), 115 °C; at 15 lb (105 kPa), 121 °C, and at 20 lb (140 kPa), 126 °C.

Autoclaves have two major uses. In cooking, the higher temperature reduces the time needed. At these higher temperatures, and under moist conditions, bacteria are destroyed more rapidly, so permitting sterilization of foods, surgical dressing and instruments, etc.

autolysis The process of self-digestion by the enzymes naturally present in tissues. For example, the tenderizing of *game while hanging is due to autolysis of *connective tissue. *Yeast extract is produced by autolysis of yeast.

autotrophes Organisms that can synthesize all the compounds required for growth from simple inorganic salts, as distinct from heterotrophes, which must be supplied with complex organic compounds. Plants are autotrophes, whereas animals are heterotrophes. Bacteria may be of either type; heterotrophic bacteria are responsible for food spoilage and disease.

autrichienne, à l' French; used synonymously with à l'hongroise for dishes seasoned with paprika, fennel, and sour cream.

auvergnate French; soup made from pig's head broth with lentils, leeks, and potatoes.

availability Also known as bioavailability or biological availability. In some foodstuffs, nutrients that can be demonstrated to be present chemically may not be available, or only partially so, when they are eaten. This is because the nutrients are chemically bound in a form that is not susceptible to enzymic digestion, although it is susceptible to the strong acid or alkali *hydrolysis used in chemical analysis. For example, the *niacin in cereal grains, *calcium bound to *phytate, and *lysine combined with sugars in the *Maillard complex, are all biologically unavailable. *See also* available lysine.

available carbon dioxide *See* baking powder; flour, self-raising.

available lysine Not all of the *lysine in proteins is biologically available, since some is linked through its side-chain *amino group, either to sugars in the *Maillard complex, or to other *amino acids. These linkages are not *hydrolysed by digestive enzymes, and so the lysine cannot be absorbed. Available lysine is that proportion of the protein-bound lysine in which the side-chain amino group is free, so that it can be absorbed after digestion of the protein.

available nutrients *See* availability.

avenalin, avenin *Proteins present in *oats.

avern jelly Scottish; jelly made from wild strawberries.

aversion to foods *See* adverse reactions to foods.

avgolemono Greek; egg and lemon soup or sauce.

Avicel Trade name for microcrystalline α-cellulose. It is natural *cellulose which has been partially *hydrolysed with *acid, and reduced to a fine powder. It disperses in water and has the properties of a *gum. It is used in oily foods such as *cheese and *peanut butter, as well as in *syrups and *honey, sauces and dressings.

avidin A protein in egg white which binds the *vitamin *biotin, so rendering it unavailable to the body. Cooking denatures proteins, and denatured avidin in cooked eggs does not bind biotin.

avitaminosis The absence of a vitamin; may be used specifically, as, for example, avitaminosis A, or generally, to mean a vitamin deficiency disease.

avocado Fruit of the tree *Persica americana*, also known as the avocado pear or alligator pear, because of its rough skin and pear shape, although it is not related to the *pear. It is unusual among fruits for its high fat content (17–27%), of which 7–14% is *linoleic acid, and also for the fact that it does not ripen until after it has been removed from the tree.

Half an avocado (130 g) is a rich *source of vitamin C and copper; a good source of vitamin B_6; a source of protein and iron; contains 26 g of fat of which 20% is saturated; provides 2.6 g of dietary fibre; supplies 265 kcal (1110 kJ).

avron *See* cloudberry.

azienda Italian; estate or vineyard on wine labels. *See* wine classification, Italy.

azlon Textile fibres produced from proteins such as *casein and *zein.

azo dyes Synthetic chemicals used as dye-stuffs and food colours, made by reacting a diazonium salt (which has two nitrogen atoms linked to each other) with a phenol or *aromatic amine. Also known as diazo or diazonium compounds.

azorubin(e) A red colour, carmoisine (E-122).

baba A French cake supposedly invented by King Stanislas I of Poland and named after Ali Baba. 'Rum baba' is flavoured with rum; a French modification using a 'secret' syrup was called brillat-savarin or savarin.

babaco The seedless fruit of the tree *Carica pentagona*, related to the *pawpaw, discovered in Ecuador in the 1920s, introduced into New Zealand in 1973, and more recently into the Channel Islands. A 100-g portion is a rich *source of vitamin C.

babassu oil Edible oil from the Brazilian palm nut, similar in fatty acid composition to *coconut oil, and used for food and in soaps and cosmetics.

Babcock test A test for the fat content of milk.

babka 1 Russian; yeast cake with grated carrot or potato and flour.
2 Polish; a cake similar to *baba, but baked without yeast.

baby foods General term to include *infant formula milk and *weaning foods.

bacalaitos *See* accra.

bacalao Spanish and South American name for dried salted cod; Portuguese is bacalhau. *See* klipfish.

backerbsen German; garnish for soup, batter mixture poured through a colander into hot oil and fried to resemble dried peas.

bäckerei German for baked goods; Austrian name for a variety of different types of biscuit made with baking powder.

baclava *See* baklava.

bacon (French: *lard*; German: *Schweinespeck*.) Cured (and usually smoked) meat from the back, sides, and belly of a pig; variety of cuts with differing fat contents.

A 100-g portion of boiled collar joint is a rich *source of protein, niacin, and vitamin B_1, a source of vitamin B_2 and iron; contains 30 g of fat of which 40% is saturated; supplies 320 kcal (1345 kJ). A 100-g grilled gammon rasher is exceptionally rich in vitamin B_1 (0.9 mg); a rich source of protein and niacin; a good source of iron; a source of vitamin B_2; contains 12 g of fat of which 40% is saturated; supplies 230 kcal (970 kJ). A 100-g portion of fried, streaky bacon is a rich source of protein, niacin, and vitamin B_1; a source of vitamin B_2 and iron; contains 45 g of fat of which 40% is saturated; supplies 500 kcal (2100 kJ). Also a source of zinc, copper, and selenium.

Gammon is bacon made from the top of the hind legs; green bacon has been cured but not smoked.

bacon weed *See* fat hen.

bacoreta A variety of *tuna fish with dark flesh.

bacteria Unicellular micro-organisms, ranging between 0.5 and 5 μm in size. They may be classified on the basis of their shape: spherical (coccus), rodlike (bacilli), spiral (spirillum), comma-shaped (vibrio), corkscrew-shaped (spirochaetes), or filamentous. Other classifications are based on whether or not they are stained by Gram's stain, *aerobic or *anaerobic, and *autotrophic or *heterotrophic. Some bacteria form spores which are relatively resistant to heat and sterilizing agents.

Bacteria are responsible for much food spoilage, and for disease (pathogenic bacteria which produce toxins), but they are also made use of, for example in the *pickling process and *fermentation of milk, as well as in the manufacture of *vitamins and *amino acids and a variety of *enzymes and *hormones.

Between 45 and 85% of the dry matter of bacteria is protein, and some can be grown on petroleum residues, methane, or methanol for use in animal feed.

bacterial count *See* plate count.

bacterial filter A filter fine enough to prevent the passage of *bacteria (0.5–5 μm in diameter), which permits removal of bacteria from solutions. *Viruses are considerably smaller, and will pass through a bacterial filter.

bacteriophage *Viruses which attack bacteria, commonly known as phages. They pass through *bacterial filters, and can be a cause of considerable trouble in bacterial cultures (for example milk starter cultures).

Bacterium aceti *See* Acetobacter.

bactofugation A Belgian process for removing bacteria from milk by high speed *centrifugation.

bactometer A device for the rapid estimation of bacterial contamination (within a few hours) based on measuring the early stages of breakdown of nutrients by the bacteria through changes in the electrical impedance of the medium.

badam *See* almonds.

badderlocks Edible seaweed (*Alaria esculenta*) found on northern British coasts and around the Faroe Islands. Known as honeyware in Scotland.

badminton A drink prepared with *claret, sugar, and *soda water.

bagaciera *See* marc.

bagasse The residues from sugar-cane milling, consisting of the crushed stalks from which the juice has been expressed; it consists of 50% *cellulose, 25% *hemicelluloses, and 25% *lignin. It is used as a fuel, for cattle feed, and in the manufacture of paper and fibre board. The name is sometimes also applied to the residues of other plants, such as beet, which is sometimes incorporated into foods as a source of *dietary fibre.

bagel A circular bread roll with a hole in the middle, made from fermented wheat flour dough (including egg), which is boiled before being baked. A Jewish speciality; variants include onion bagels, which are topped with crisply fried onion before baking and poppy-seed bagels, which are topped with *poppy seeds.

bagna cauda Italian (Piedmontese); sauce made from olive oil and butter flavoured with garlic and anchovy, small pieces of raw vegetables are dipped into the hot sauce.

baguette A French *bread, a long thin loaf (about 60 cm long) and weighing 250 g, with a crisp crust.

baingan *See* aubergine.

bain marie A double saucepan (from the French for 'water bath').

baiser French; two small meringues joined together with cream or jam.

bajoa *See* millet.

baked Alaska Dessert of ice cream on a sponge base and covered with meringue, baked in a hot oven for a very short time, so that the meringue is cooked but the ice cream remains frozen. Earlier called omelette norvégienne or Norwegian omelette.

baked apple berry *See* cloudberry.

baker's cheese *See* cheese, cottage.

bakes Caribbean (Trinidadian); fried biscuits made with baking powder dough. *See also* floats.

Bakewell tart An open pastry tart with an almond-flavoured cake filling, originally made in Bakewell in Derbyshire, England.

baking *Cooking in an oven by dry heat.

baking additives Materials added to flour products for a variety of purposes, including bleaching the flour, *ageing, slowing the rate of staling, and improving the texture of the finished product.

baking blind Making a pastry case for a tart or flan, which is baked empty and then filled.

baking powder A mixture that liberates carbon dioxide when moistened and heated. The source of carbon dioxide is sodium bicarbonate, and an acid is required. This may be *cream of tartar (in fast-acting baking powders which liberate carbon dioxide in the dough before heating) or calcium acid phosphate, sodium pyrophosphate, or sodium aluminium sulphate (in slow-acting powders, which liberate most of the carbon dioxide during heating).

Legally, baking powder must contain not less than 8% available, and not more than 1.5% residual, carbon dioxide. Golden raising powder (formerly known as egg substitute) is similar, but is coloured yellow, and must contain not less than 6% available, and not more than 1.5% residual, carbon dioxide.

baking soda Or bicarbonate of soda, chemically sodium bicarbonate ($NaHCO_3$), the source of carbon dioxide in *baking powder.

baklava (baclava) Middle-Eastern; sweet made from *phyllo pastry filled with nuts and honey, baked and served drenched with syrup.

balance 1 With reference to diet, positive balance is a net gain to the body and negative balance a net loss from the body. When intake equals excretion the body is in equilibrium or balance with respect to the nutrient in question. Used in reference to nitrogen (protein), mineral salts, and energy.

2 A balanced diet is one containing all nutrients in appropriate amounts.

3 A weighing device.

balil pilâki Turkish Jewish; fish grilled lightly then baked with sliced onions and tomatoes.

balka Polish; conical yeast cake traditionally eaten for festivals, similar to Italian *panettone.

ballekes Belgian; croquettes of minced pork simmered in white wine or beer.

Balling A table of specific gravity of sugar solutions published by von Balling in 1843, giving the weight of cane sugar in 100 g of a solution for the specific gravity determined at 17.5 °C. It is used to calculate the percentage extract in *beer wort. The original table was corrected for slight inaccuracies by Plato in 1900, and extracts are referred to as percent Plato.

ball mill A vessel in which material is ground by rolling with heavy balls, used especially for hard materials.

ballottine A kind of galantine of meat, poultry, game, or fish, boned, stuffed, and rolled into a bundle; also small balls of meat or poultry.

balm A herb (*Melissa officinalis*) with hairy leaves and a lemon scent, therefore often known as lemon balm. Used for its flavour in fruit salads, sweet or savoury sauces, etc., as well as for preparation of herb teas. Claimed to have calming medicinal properties, and promoted at one time as an elixir of life and a cure for impotence; it is rich in tannins.

balmain bug A variety of *lobster found in Australia.

balsamic vinegar *See* vinegar.

balti Pakistani, Kashmiri; spiced meat or vegetable dishes cooked and served in a conical metal vessel, a karahi.

bambarra groundnut Also known as the Madagascar peanut or earth pea, *Voandseia subterranea*. It resembles the true *groundnut, but the seeds are low in oil. They are hard and require soaking or pounding before cooking.

bamboo shoots Thick, pointed young shoots of *Bambusa vulgaris* and *Phyllostachys pubescens* eaten in Eastern Asia. A 100-g portion is a *source of vitamin B_1; supplies 27 kcal (115 kJ).

bami (bahmi) Indonesian, Dutch; noodles with fried shredded vegetables, served with diced pork, chicken or prawns, topped with strips of omelette.

bamies, bamya *See* okra.

banana Fruit of the genus *Musa*; cultivated kinds are sterile hybrids, and so cannot be given species names. Dessert bananas have a high sugar content (17–19%) and are eaten raw; *plantains (sometimes known as green bananas) have a higher starch and lower sugar content and are picked when too hard to be eaten raw.

One medium banana (100 g) is a good *source of vitamin A; a source of vitamins B$_6$ and C, and copper; contains 0.3 g of fat of which 33% is saturated; provides 3 g of dietary fibre; supplies 86 kcal (360 kJ). The sodium content is low (1.2 mg/100 g) so bananas are used in *low-sodium diets.

banana, baking American name for *plantain.

banana, false The fruit of *Ensete ventricosum*, related to the banana. The fruits are small and, unlike bananas, contain seeds. The rhizome and inner tissue of the stem are eaten after cooking, and form a major part of the diet in southern Ethiopia.

banana figs Bananas that have been split longitudinally and sun-dried without treating with *sulphur dioxide. The product is dark in colour and sticky.

Banbury cake Flat oval cake of flaky pastry filled with dried fruit; originated in Banbury, Oxfordshire, England.

B and B Mixture of equal parts of *brandy and *Benedictine; also an abbreviation for accommodation offering bed and breakfast.

bangers Colloquial English term for *sausages. When served with mashed potatoes, the dish is known as bangers and mash.

banian days Days on which no meat was served; named after Banian (Hindu) merchants who abstained from eating meat. An obsolete term for 'days of short commons'.

bànitsa Bulgarian; tarts made from *phyllo pastry, filled with nuts and cream, cheese, or spinach.

bannock A flat round cake made from oat, rye, or barley meal and baked on a hearth or griddle. Pitcaithly bannock is a type of almond *shortbread containing *caraway seeds and chopped peel.

Bantu beer See beer.

bap Traditionally a soft, white, flat, flour-coated Scottish breakfast roll. Now also used for any relatively large soft-crusted roll, made from white, brown, or wholemeal flour.

bara brith See barm brack.

barak pálinka Hungarian; dry apricot *brandy.

bara lawr See laver.

Barbados cherry See cherry, West Indian.

Barbados sugar See sugar.

barbecue Originally Caribbean (native American) name for a wooden frame used to smoke and dry meat over a slow, smoky fire; the whole animal was placed on a spit over burning coals. Now outdoor cooking of meat, sausages, etc., on a charcoal or gas fire; also the fire on which they are cooked.

barbecue sauce Chopped onions fried in butter, made into a sauce with tomato paste and seasoned with sugar, vinegar, mustard, and *Worcestershire sauce, served with barbecued meat and sausages.

barbera A *grape variety widely used for *wine making, although not one of the classic varieties; makes the dark fruity and often sharp red wines of northern Italy.

barberry Fruits of *Berberis* spp.

barberry fig *See* prickly pear.

Barcelona nut Spanish variety of *hazel nut. A 30-g portion is a rich *source of copper; contains 19 g of fat of which 7% is saturated; provides 3 g of dietary fibre; supplies 190 kcal (800 kJ).

barding To cover the breast of a bird with slices of fat before roasting, to prevent the flesh from drying. *See also* larding.

barium A metal of no known metabolic function, and hence not a dietary essential. Barium sulphate is opaque to X-rays and a suspension is used (a barium meal) to allow examination of the shape and movements of the stomach for diagnostic purposes, and as a barium enema for X-ray investigation of the lower intestinal tract.

barley Grain of *Hordeum vulgare*, one of the hardiest of the *cereals; mainly used for brewing beer. The whole grain with only the outer husk removed (pot, Scotch, or hulled barley) requires several hours' cooking; the commercial product is usually pearl barley where most of the husk and germ is removed. Barley flour is ground pearl barley; barley flakes are the flattened grain. A 150-g portion of cooked pearl barley (50 g dry cereal) is a *source of niacin, vitamin B_6, folate, zinc, copper, and iron; provides 9 g of dietary fibre; supplies 180 kcal (750 kJ).

barleycorn An obsolete measure of length; the size of a single grain of barley; $^1/_3$ inch (0.85 cm).

barley, malted *See* malt.

barley sugar *Sugar confectionery made by melting and cooling sugar, originally made by boiling with a decoction of barley.

barley water A drink made by boiling pearl barley with water, commonly flavoured with orange or lemon.

barley wine Fermented malted barley, stronger than *beer (8–10% *alcohol by volume), bottled under pressure, so sparkling.

Barlow's disease Infantile *scurvy, also known as Moeller's disease and Cheadle's disease.

barm An alternative name for *yeast or leaven, or the froth on fermenting malt liquor. Spon (short for spontaneous) or virgin barm is made by allowing wild yeast to fall into sugar medium and multiply.

barm brack Irish; yeast cake made with butter, egg, buttermilk, and dried fruit, flavoured with caraway seed. Similar Welsh cake is bara brith.

Barmene Trade name for *yeast extract, prepared from autolysed brewer's yeast, plus vegetable juices, used for flavouring.

baron of beef The pair of sirloins of *beef, left uncut at the bone.

barquette Small boat-shaped pastry cases, used for savoury or sweet mixtures.

barrel A standard barrel contains 36 gallons. (36 imperial gallons (UK) = 163.6 L; 36 US gallons = 113.7 L.)

basal metabolic rate (BMR) The *energy cost of maintaining the metabolic integrity of the body, nerve and muscle tone, respiration and circulation. It depends on the amount of metabolically active body tissue, and hence can be calculated from body weight, using different factors for males and females, and at different ages. For children the BMR also includes the energy cost of growth. Experimentally, BMR is measured as the heat output from the body, or the rate of oxygen consumption, under strictly standardized conditions, 12–14 hours after the last meal, completely at rest (but not asleep) and at an environmental temperature of 26–30 °C, to ensure thermal neutrality. Measurement of metabolic rate under less rigorously controlled conditions gives the resting metabolic rate (RMR).

For people with a sedentary lifestyle and relatively low physical activity, BMR accounts for about 70% of total energy expenditure. The energy costs of different activities are generally expressed as the physical activity ratio, the ratio of energy expenditure in the activity to BMR.

base See alkali.

Basedow's disease See thyrotoxicosis.

base formers See acid foods.

basic foods See acid foods.

basil An aromatic herb Ocimum basilicum and O. minimum; other members of the genus Ocimum are also used as seasoning.

basmati Long-grain Indian variety of rice; much prized for its delicate flavour (the name means 'fragrant' in Hindi).

baste To ladle hot fat (or other liquid) over meat, poultry, etc., at intervals while it is baking or roasting, in order to improve the texture, flavour, and appearance.

batata See potato, sweet.

Bath bun A small English cake made from milk-based yeast dough, with dried fruit and a topping of sugar crystals, attributed to Dr W. Oliver of Bath (18th century).

Bath chap The cheek and jawbones of the pig, salted and smoked. Originated in Bath.

Bath cheese A small English *cheese, made from cow's milk with the subsequent addition of cream.

Bath Oliver A biscuit made with yeast, attributed to Dr W. Oliver of Bath (18th century).

Battenberg cake A two-coloured sponge cake, baked in an oblong tin, usually covered with almond paste; named in honour of the marriage of Queen Victoria's granddaughter to Prince Louis of Battenberg, 1884.

batter Thick liquid mixture of flour, milk, and eggs, used to coat fish before frying, fried alone to make pancakes or griddle cakes, or baked to make Yorkshire pudding.

Bauernschmaus Austrian; pork loin chops, bacon, and sausages cooked in beer with *sauerkraut, grated raw potato, and seasoning.

bavarois(e) 1 A hot drink made from eggs, milk, and tea, sweetened and flavoured with a liqueur; seventeenth-century Bavarian.
   2 French; (crème bavarois) a cold dessert made from egg custard with gelatine and cream.
   3 *Hollandaise sauce with *crayfish garnish.

bay (bay leaf) A herb, the leaf of the Mediterranean sweet bay tree (Lauris nobilis) with a strong characteristic flavour. Rarely used alone, but an important component of *bouquet garni, and used with other herbs in *marinades, pickles, stews, and stuffing.

Bay lobster Or Moreton Bay bug, a variety of sand lobster found in Australia.

bdelygmia An extreme loathing for food.

bean, adzuki Also known as aduki or feijoa bean, the seed of the Asian adzuki plant Phaseolus (Vigna) angularis. Sweet tasting, the basis of Cantonese red bean paste used to fill *dim sum. Also ground to a flour and used in bread, pastry, and sweets or eaten after sprouting as *bean sprouts. Like all *pulses contains *lectins. A 100-g portion is a *source of protein, iron, zinc, vitamin B_1, and niacin; provides 5 g of *dietary fibre; supplies 125 kcal (525 kJ).

bean, black-eyed Also known as black-eyed pea or cow pea, Vigna sinensis; creamy white bean with a black mark on one edge.

bean, borlotti Italian variety of Phaseolus vulgaris, haricot or common bean. See bean, haricot.

bean, broad Also known as fava or horse bean, Vicia faba. A 75-g portion is a good *source of copper; a source of niacin, folate, and vitamin C; contains 0.5 g of fat of which 16% is saturated; provides 3 g of dietary fibre; supplies 35 kcal (145 kJ). See also favism.

bean, butter Several large varieties of Phaseolus vulgaris, also known as Lima, curry, Madagascar, and sugar bean. A 100-g cooked portion is a *source of protein, copper, iron; provides 5 g of dietary fibre; supplies 80 kcal (335 kJ).

bean curd See tofu.

bean, French Unripe seeds and pods of Phaseolus vulgaris; ripe seeds are haricot beans. A 100-g portion is a rich *source of folate; a source of vitamin A (as carotene) and copper; provides 3 g of dietary fibre; supplies 7 kcal (30 kJ).

bean, haricot Ripe seed of Phaseolus vulgaris (the unripe seed is the *French bean). Also known as navy, string, pinto, or snap bean. A 100-g portion of dried haricot beans is a good *source of copper; a source of protein, vitamin B_1, and iron; contains 0.5 g of fat of which 20% is saturated; provides 7 g of dietary fibre; supplies 100 kcal (420 kJ).

bean, Lima See bean, butter.

bean, mung Whole or split seed of Vigna radiata (Phaseolus aureus, P. radiatus), green gram. A 150-g portion is a rich source of folate, copper, and selenium; a good *source of vitamin B_6, iron, and zinc; a source of protein and vitamin B_1; provides 3 g of dietary fibre; supplies 90 kcal (380 kJ). *See also* bean sprouts.

bean, red kidney Ripe seed of *Phaseolus vulgaris*. A 100-g portion of dried raw beans is a rich *source of protein, vitamin B_1, folate, iron, copper, and selenium; a good source of vitamin B_6 and zinc; a source of vitamin B_2, niacin, and calcium; contains 1.7 g of fat of which 11% is saturated; provides 25 g of dietary fibre; supplies 280 kcal (1180 kJ). Like all *pulses contains toxic *lectins; uncooked or partially cooked beans cause vomiting, diarrhoea, and serious damage to the intestinal mucosa. The lectins are inactivated by boiling for about 10 min., but not by cooking below boiling point.

bean, runner *Phaseolus multiflorus*. A 100-g portion is a rich *source of folate; contains 0.2 g of fat of which 50% is saturated; provides 3 g of dietary fibre; supplies 20 kcal (85 kJ).

beans Seeds of the family *leguminosae*, eaten as food. *See also* lectins; legumes.

beans, baked Usually mature haricot beans, small variety of *Phaseolus vulgaris*, cooked in sauce; often canned with tomato sauce and starch with added sugar (or sweetener) and salt. A 225-g portion (small can) is a good *source of protein; a source of vitamin B_1, niacin, calcium, and iron; contains about 700 mg of sodium; 8 g of dietary fibre; supplies 160 kcal (670 kJ).

bean, soya *See* soya bean.

bean sprouts Any of a number of peas, beans, and seeds which can be germinated and the sprouts eaten raw or cooked. The sprouting causes the synthesis of vitamin C. One of the commonest sprouts is that of the mung bean, but *alfalfa and adzuki beans are also used. An 80-g portion is a good *source of folate; provides 2.4 g of dietary fibre; supplies 7 kcal (30 kJ).

bean, string Either runner beans or French beans which have a climbing habit rather than growing as small bushes. The name derives from the method of growing them up strings.

béarnaise sauce A thick French *sauce made with egg yolk, butter, wine vinegar or white wine, and chopped *shallots, named after Béarn in SW France.

beat 1 To agitate an ingredient or a mixture by vigorously turning it over and over with an upward motion, in order to introduce air, using a spoon, fork, whisk, or electric mixer.
   2 Raw meat is beaten by hitting it briskly all over the surface to break down the fibres and make it more tender when cooked.

Beaujolais Red *wine from the Beaujolais region of France, made from Gamay grapes. Beaujolais nouveau (*primeur* in French) is the new season's wine, drunk young. It is 'officially' available on 18 November.

béchamel sauce Also known as white *sauce. One of the basic French sauces, made with milk, butter, and flour. Named after Louis de Béchamel, of the court of Louis XIV of France.

bêche-de-mer The sea slug, *Stichopus japonicus*, an occasional food in many parts of the world; also called trepang.

beechwood sugar *See* xylose.

beef Flesh of the ox (*Bos taurus*); flesh from young calves is *veal. A 150-g portion of most cuts is a rich *source of protein, niacin, iron, copper, and vitamin B_{12}; a good source of vitamin B_2 and copper; a source of vitamins B_1, B_6, and selenium; contains 20–30 g of fat of which half is *saturated (lean part is 5% fat); supplies 350–500 kcal (1470–2100 kJ). (French: *bœuf*; German: *Rindfleisch*.)

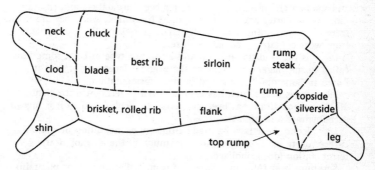

FIGURE 1.

beefalo A cross between the domestic cow (*Bos taurus*) and the buffalo (*Bubalus* spp.) which can be fattened on range grass rather than requiring cereal and protein supplements.

beef bourgignon *See* bourgignonne, à la.

beefburger *See* hamburger.

beef, corned *See* corned beef.

beef, cow Meat from cows at the end of their lives as milk producers.

beef olives Thin strips of beef filled with savoury stuffing, braised in stock.

beef, pressed (Salt beef); boned brisket beef that has been salted, cooked, and pressed. Known as *corned beef in USA.

beefsteak fungus Large edible fungus (*Fistulina hepatica*) with a stringy, meat-like texture and deep red juice. *See* mushrooms.

beef stroganoff Thin strips of beef, fried and served in a sour cream and mushroom sauce.

beef tea An extract of stewing beef, formerly used for invalids, since the extractives stimulate the appetite. *See also* meat extract.

beer *Alcoholic beverage made by the fermentation of *cereals; traditionally barley, but also maize, rice, and sorghum. The first step is the malting of barley: it is allowed to sprout, when the *enzyme *amylase hydrolyses some of the starch to dextrins and maltose. The sprouted (malted) barley is dried, then extracted with hot water (the process of mashing) to produce wort. After the addition of *hops for flavour, the wort is allowed to ferment. Two types of *yeast are used in brewing: top fermenting yeasts which float on the surface of the wort and bottom or deep fermenters. Most traditional British beers (ale, bitter, stout, and porter) are brewed with top fermenting yeasts.

UK beers, brown ale, and stout: around 3% alcohol by volume, 2-4 % carbohydrate, 75-110 kcal (315-460 kJ) per 300 mL (half pint). Strong ale is 6.6% alcohol, 6% carbohydrate, 210 kcal (880 kJ) per 300 mL (half pint). Ale is a light-coloured beer, relatively high in alcohol content, and moderately heavily hopped. Bitter beers are darker and contain more hops. Porter and stout are almost black in colour; they are made from wort containing some partly charred malt; milk stout is made from wort containing added *lactose.

Lager is the traditional mainland European type of beer, sometimes called Pilsner lager or Pils, since the original lager was brewed in Pilsen in Bohemia. It is brewed by deep fermentation.

Lite beer is beer which has been allowed to ferment until virtually all the carbohydrate has been converted to alcohol and so it is low in carbohydrate and high in alcohol.

Low alcohol beer may be made either by fermentation of a low carbohydrate wort, or by removal of much of the alcohol after fermentation (de-alcoholized beer).

Sorghum beer (African, made also from millet, maize, or plantain) is a thick sour beverage consumed while still fermenting. Also known by numerous local names, kaffir beer, bouza, pombé, bantu beer. 3-8% alcohol, 3-10% carbohydrate, a rich source of vitamin B_1 per 300 mL portion.

beerenauslese *See* wine classification, Germany.

bees' royal jelly *See* royal jelly.

beestings The first milk given by the cow after calving, the colostrum, rich in immunoglobulins.

beet, common red *See* beetroot.

beet, leaf, sea kale, silver, spinach, or white leaf *See* Swiss chard.

beetroot The root of *Beta vulgaris*, eaten cooked or pickled. Known simply as beet in North America. The violet-red pigment, betanin, is used as a food colour (E-162). One small beetroot (40 g) is a good *source of folate; provides 1.6 g of dietary fibre; supplies 18 kcal (75 kJ).

beet sugar *See* sugar; sugar beet.

beeturia Excretion of red-coloured urine after eating *beetroot, due to excretion of the pigment betanin. It occurs, not consistently, in about one person in eight.

bee wine Wine produced by the usual fermentation of sugar, but using yeast in the form of a clump of yeast and lactic bacteria; the clump rises and falls with the bubbles of carbon dioxide formed during fermentation, hence the name 'bee'.

beignets French; *fritters, especially deep fried *choux pastry.

belching *See* eructation.

belegte brote German; open sandwiches.

belle hélène 1 garnish of mushrooms stuffed with cooked tomatoes or green peas.
   2 Pears poached in vanilla-flavoured syrup, served in vanilla ice cream with a chocolate sauce.

bell pepper *See* pepper.

beluga Russian name for the white sturgeon (*Acipenser huro*), whose roe forms the most prized *caviar.

Bemax Trade name for a wheat germ preparation. A 30-g portion is a rich *source of vitamins B_1 and E, folate, copper, and zinc; a good source of iron; a source of protein, vitamins B_2, B_6, and niacin; provides 5 g of dietary fibre; contains 2.4 g of fat; supplies 120 kcal (500 kJ).

Benedictine A French *liqueur invented in about 1510 by the monks of the Benedictine Abbey of Fécamp in France. The Abbey was closed, and the recipe lost after the French Revolution, then rediscovered about 1863. It is based on double-distilled *brandy, flavoured with some 75 herbs and spices; it contains 40% (by volume) alcohol and 30% sugar; 300 kcal (1.3 MJ)/100 mL. *See also* B and B.

Benedict-Roth spirometer *See* respirometer.

benniseed *See* sesame.

bentonite *See* fuller's earth.

benzoates Salts of *benzoic acid.

benzoic acid A preservative normally used as the sodium, potassium, or calcium salts and their derivatives (E-210–E-219), especially in acid foods such as pickles and sauces. It occurs naturally in a number of fruits, including *cranberries, *prunes, *greengages, and *cloudberries, and in *cinnamon. Cloudberries contain so much benzoic acid that they can be stored for long periods of time without any precautions being taken against bacterial or fungal spoilage. Benzoic acid and its derivatives are excreted from the body conjugated with the *amino acids glycine (hippuric acid) and alanine. Because of this, benzoic acid is sometimes used in the treatment of *argininaemia, *argininosuccinic aciduria, and *citrullinaemia, permitting excretion of nitrogenous waste from the body as these conjugates.

beolas Jewish; fritters made from matzo meal, flour, and eggs.

bercy *Sauce made from white wine, light stock, shallots, and herbs.

bergamot 1 A pear-shaped orange, *Citrus bergamia*, grown mainly in Calabria, Italy, for its peel oil;
   2 An ornamental herb, *Monarda didyma*, the dried leaves of which were used to make Oswego tea;
   3 A type of *pear, *Pyrus persica*.

beriberi The result of severe and prolonged deficiency of *vitamin B_1, still a problem in parts of South East Asia where the diet is high in carbohydrate (polished *rice) and poor in vitamin B_1. In developed countries vitamin B$_1$ deficiency is associated with alcohol abuse; while it may result in beriberi, more commonly the result is central nervous system damage, the *Wernicke-Korsakoff syndrome. In beriberi there is degeneration of peripheral nerves, starting in the hands and feet and ascending the arms and legs, with a loss of sensation and deep muscle pain. There is also enlargement of the heart, which may lead to *oedema (wet beriberi), and death results from heart failure. Fatal heart failure may develop without the nerve damage being apparent (Shoshin or sudden beriberi). The name is derived from the Bahasa-Malay word for sheep, to describe the curious sheep-like gait adopted by sufferers.

berry Botanical term for fleshy juicy fruits with one or more seeds not having a stone e.g. grape, gooseberry, tomato, banana, blackcurrant, cranberry.

bessan Indian; *chick-pea flour.

best before *See* date-marking.

beta-carotene (β-carotene) *See* carotene.

betanin The violet-red pigment of *beetroot.

betel Leaf of the creeper *Piper betel*, which is chewed in some parts of the world for its stimulating effect, due to the presence of the *alkaloids arecoline and guvacoline. The leaves are chewed with the nuts of the areca palm, *Arecha catechu*, which is therefore often called the betel palm, and the nut is called betel nut. The Indian delicacy *pan* is based on betel leaf and areca nut, together with aromatic spices and herbs.

beurre, au Cooked or served with butter.

beurre manié Butter with an equal amount of flour blended in, used for thickening sauces.

beurre noir *See* butter, black.

bezoar A hard ball of undigested food, sometimes together with hair, which forms in the stomach or intestine and can cause obstruction. Foods with a high content of indigestible *pectin, such as orange pith, can form bezoars if swallowed without chewing. The name is derived from the Arabic meaning 'protection against poison', since bezoars were formerly believed to have protective properties.

BHA *See* butylated hydroxyanisole.

bhaji 1 Chinese spinach (*Amaranthus gangeticus*), also known as *callaloo.
  2 Also bhajia, Indian; vegetable fritters, normally made with gram (lentil) flour.

bhindi *See* okra.

bhoona Indian term for frying. Sukha bhoona is a simple sauté. Dumned bhoona is a pot roast, or steam-fried dish; marinated meat is seared, moistened, and cooked in a tightly closed vessel in the oven. Ard bhoona is a dry pot roast; the meat is seared then cooked in a tightly closed vessel in the oven with butter but no water.

BHT *See* butylated hydroxytoluene.

bhujia Indian; vegetable dishes, highly spiced. In the final stage of cooking they are fried in *ghee which has been heated with onions, chillies, garlic, and ginger.

bianco Italian; white wines.

BIBRA The British Industrial Biological Research Association.

bicarbonate of soda *See* sodium bicarbonate.

BIE *See* bio-electrical impedance.

bienmesabe Caribbean (Puerto Rico); custard made with coconut milk and eggs.

bierplinse German; batter made with dark beer, used for sweet or savoury fritters.

biersuppe German soup made from light beer, thickened with potato flour and flavoured with cinnamon and lemon peel.

biffins Apples that have been peeled, partly baked, then pressed and dried.

bifidus factor A carbohydrate in human milk which contains nitrogen and stimulates the growth of *Lactobacillus bifidus* in the intestine. In turn, this organism lowers the *pH of the intestinal contents and suppresses the growth of *E. coli* and other pathogenic *bacteria. *See also* lactulose.

bigarade (bigaradier) *See* orange, bitter.

bigarade, à la With orange or orange sauce.

bigos Polish; casserole of *sauerkraut, cooked meat, game, sausages, ham, etc., with vodka and wine.

bilberry The berry of wild shrubs of the genus *Vaccinium*, not generally cultivated. Variously known as whortleberry, blaeberry, whinberry, huckleberry. A 110-g portion is a rich *source of vitamin C; a source of copper; provides 7.7 g of dietary fibre; supplies 60 kcal (250 kJ).

bile Fluid produced by the liver and stored in the gall bladder before secretion into the small intestine (duodenum) via the bile duct. It contains the *bile salts, which function in the emulsification and hence digestion of fats, bile pigments (bilirubin and biliverdin, which are the result of breakdown of the haemoglobin of red blood cells) and *cholesterol. It is alkaline, and hence neutralizes the *acid from the stomach as the food reaches the small intestine. Relatively large amounts of *vitamin B_{12} and *folic acid are secreted in the bile and then reabsorbed from the small intestine. Most of the cholesterol and bile salts are also reabsorbed from the small intestine. *See also* gastrointestinal tract.

bile salts (bile acids) Salts of cholic and deoxycholic acid and their glycine and taurine conjugates, secreted in the *bile; they assist the digestion of fats by emulsifying them.

bilirubin, biliverdin The *bile pigments, formed by the degradation of *haemoglobin.

biltong South African; strips of dried meat, salted, spiced, and dried in air for 10–14 days.

bind To add liquid, fat, or egg to a mixture to hold it together. *See also* panada.

binge–purge syndrome A feature of the eating disorder *bulimia nervosa, characterized by the ingestion of excessive amounts of food and the excessive use of *laxatives.

bioassay Biological assay; measurement of biologically active compounds (e.g. vitamins and essential amino acids) by their ability to support growth of micro-organisms or animals.

biocides Chemicals used to kill unwanted organisms: herbicides, insecticides, fungicides.

biocytin The main form of the *vitamin *biotin in most foods, bound to the *amino acid *lysine.

bio-electrical impedance (BIE) A method of measuring the proportion of fat in the body by the difference in the resistance to passage of an electric current between fat and lean tissue.

bioflavonoids *See* flavonoids.

biological oxygen demand (BOD) A way of assessing bacterial contamination of water, milk, etc. by micro-organisms which take up oxygen for their metabolism.

Biological Value (BV) A measure of *protein quality.

biopterin The *coenzyme for a number of enzymes, including phenylalanine, tyrosine, and tryptophan hydroxylases. Not a dietary requirement, since it can readily be synthesized in the body. Rare patients with a variant form of *phenylketonuria cannot synthesize biopterin, and have to receive supplements.

bios A name given to a factor in cell-free extract of yeast which was essential for the growth of yeast, by Wildiers in 1901. Three components were subsequently identified: *inositol, β-alanine and *biotin. Of these, only biotin is a *vitamin and essential for human beings.

biotin A *vitamin, sometimes known as vitamin H, required for the synthesis of fatty acids and glucose, among other reactions. Biotin is widely distributed in foods such as liver, kidney, egg yolk, yeast, vegetables, grains, and nuts; dietary deficiency is unknown. There is no evidence on which to base *reference intakes other than to state that current average intakes (between 15–70 µg/day) are obviously more than adequate to prevent deficiency.

The protein, avidin, in raw egg-white binds biotin strongly, preventing its absorption, and individuals who consume abnormally large amounts of uncooked egg (several dozen eggs per week) have been reported to show biotin deficiency. Avidin is *denatured on cooking, and does not combine with biotin; indeed cooked egg is a rich *source of available biotin.

biphenyl *See* diphenyl.

birch beer A non-alcoholic carbonated beverage flavoured with oil of wintergreen or oils of sweet birch and *sassafras.

bird's nest soup Chinese; made from the dried gelatinous coating of the nest of various species of southern Asian swifts with chicken broth, ham, egg white, and spring onion.

biriani (biryani) Indian; highly spiced rice dish flavoured with saffron and layered with meat. *See also* pilau.

birnbrot Swiss; bread with filling of dried pears and other dried fruits.

biscuit A baked flour confectionery dried down to low moisture content. The name is derived from the Latin *bis coctus*, meaning cooked twice. A 100-g portion provides 400–500 kcal (1680–2100 kJ). Known as cookie in the USA, where 'biscuit' means a small cake-like bun.

Five chocolate fingers (30 g) provide 0.6 g of dietary fibre and 8 g of fat of which 60% is saturated; supplies 160 kcal (670 kJ). Four cream crackers (30 g) provide 1.2 g of dietary fibre and 5 g of fat; supplies 135 kcal (570 kJ). Two plain digestive biscuits (30 g) provide 1.5 g of dietary fibre and are a *source of copper; provide 6 g of fat of which 45% is saturated; supply 145 kcal (610 kJ). Four semi-sweet biscuits (30 g) provide 1 g of dietary fibre and 5 g of fat of which 50% is saturated; supply 140 kcal (590 kJ). One piece of *shortbread (30 g) provides 1 g of dietary fibre and 8 g of fat of which two-thirds is saturated; supplies 155 kcal (650 kJ). Four filled wafer biscuits (30 g) provide 0.6 g of dietary fibre and 9 g of fat of which 40% is saturated; supplies 165 kcal (695 kJ). Four water biscuits (30 g) provide 1 g of dietary fibre and 4 g of fat of which 20% is saturated; supplies 140 kcal (590 kJ).

biscuit check The development of splitting and cracking in *biscuits immediately after baking.

bishop A medieval beverage of hot spiced and sweetened wine (commonly *port).

Biskoids Trade name for *saccharin.

Bismarck herring Pickled and spiced whole *herring.

bisque Thick rich soup, generally made from *fish or *shellfish stock.

bitki Polish, Russian; meatballs made from raw minced beef with fried onions, grilled or fried.

Bitot's spots Irregularly shaped foam-like plaques on the conjunctiva of the eye, characteristically seen in *vitamin A deficiency, but not considered to be a diagnostic sign without other evidence of deficiency.

bitter Traditional British *beer with a bitter flavour due to its content of *hops.

bitterballen Dutch; fried meatballs flavoured with Worcestershire sauce and nutmeg.

bitterness One of the five senses of *taste.

bitters Extracts of herbs, spices, roots, and bark, steeped in, or distilled with, *spirits. Originally prepared for medicinal use (tinctures or alcoholic extracts of the natural products); now used mainly to flavour spirits and cocktails, or as aperitifs. *See also* Angostura; wine, aperitif.

biuret test A chemical test for proteins (actually for the presence of peptide bonds) which depends on the formation of a violet colour when copper sulphate reacts with a peptide bond in alkaline solution.

bixin A *carotenoid pigment found in the seeds of the tropical plant *Bixa orellana*; the crude extract is the colouring agent *annatto (E-160).

blackberry Berry of the bramble, *Rubus fruticosus*. A 100-g portion is a good *source of vitamin C (a source when stewed); a source of folate and copper; provides 7.5 g of dietary fibre; supplies 25 kcal (105 kJ).

black bun See Scotch bun.

black butter See butter, black.

blackcock See grouse.

black cumin Seeds of *Nigella sativa*, used as a spice; unrelated to *cumin.

blackcurrant Fruit of the bush *Ribes nigra*, of special interest because of its high vitamin C content (150–230 mg/100g). The British National Fruit Collection has 120 varieties. A 100-g portion is a rich *source of vitamin C; a source of iron and copper; provides 9 g of dietary fibre; supplies 35 kcal (145 kJ).

black-eyed bean (pea) See bean, black-eyed.

black forest gâteau (German: *Schwartzwalder Kirschtorte*.) Chocolate sponge with whipped cream and cherries, decorated with chocolate curlicues.

black forest mushroom Or shiitake, *Lentinula (Lentinus) edodes*, see mushrooms.

black fungus Or wood-ears, edible wild fungus, *Auricularia polytricha*; see mushrooms.

black jack See caramel.

black PN A black food colour (E-151), also known as brilliant black BN.

black pudding (French: *boudin noir*; German: *Blutwurst*.) Also known as blood pudding. Traditional European dish made with sheep or pig blood and suet, originally together with oatmeal, liver and herbs, stuffed into membrane casings shaped like a horseshoe. Although it is already cooked, it is usually sliced and fried. In Germany and France it is made without cereal. A 100-g portion is an exceptionally rich *source of iron; a rich source of protein; a good source of niacin and copper; a source of vitamin B_1; contains 22 g of fat of which 40% is saturated; supplies 300 kcal (1260 kJ).

blackthorn See sloe.

black tongue disease A sign of *niacin deficiency in dogs, the canine equivalent of *pellagra, historically important in the isolation of the *vitamin.

black velvet Mixture of equal parts of sparkling wine and stout (traditionally Guinness stout).

blaeberry See bilberry.

blanc, au Cooked in a white stock or served with a white *sauce.

blanc de blancs White *wine made from white grapes. By contrast, blanc de noirs is white wine made from black grapes; but the skin is removed before fermentation begins.

blanching A partial precooking by plunging the food into hot water (82–95 °C) for $^1/_2$–5 min. Fruits and vegetables are blanched before canning, dehydrating, or freezing, to soften the texture, shrink the food or remove air, destroy *enzymes that may cause spoilage when frozen, and remove undesirable flavours. Blanching is also performed to remove excess salt from preserved meat, and to aid the removal of skin, e.g. from almonds and tomatoes. There can be a loss of 10–20% of the sugars, salts, and protein, as well as some of the vitamins B_1, B_2 and niacin, and up to one third of the vitamin C.

blancmange powder Usually a cornflour base with added flavour and colour, mixed with hot milk to make a dessert.

blanco Spanish; white wines.

bland diet A diet that is non-irritating, does not over-stimulate the digestive tract and is soothing to the intestines; generally avoiding alcohol, strong tea or coffee, pickles, spices, and high intake of *dietary fibre.

blanquette White stew of chicken, veal, lamb, or sweetbreads, with a rich cream sauce.

blätterteig German; puff pastry (literally 'leaf dough').

blawn fish Scottish (Orkney); fresh fish, rubbed with salt and hung in a windy passage for a day, then grilled.

bleach figure (for flour) A measure of the extent of bleaching of the flour from the relative paleness of the extracted (yellow) pigments.

bleaching The removal or destruction of colour. In the context of food it usually refers to the bleaching of flour. It also refers to the bleaching of oils, a stage in the purification by which dispersed impurities and natural colouring materials are removed by activated or *fuller's earth. *See also* ageing.

bleeding bread A bacterial infection with *Bacillus prodigiosus*, which stains the bread bright red. Under warm and damp conditions the infection can appear overnight, and contamination of the shewbread in churches has led to accusations and riots against religious minorities over the centuries.

bleu, au Fish such as trout, cooked immediately after they are caught, by simmering in white wine with herbs, or in water containing salt and vinegar.

blewits Edible wild fungus, *Tricholoma* (*Lepista*) *saevum*, also known as bluetail; also wood blewits, *T. nudum*, *see* mushrooms.

blind, baking *See* baking blind.

blind staggers Acute *vitamin B_1 deficiency in horses and other animals, caused by eating bracken, which contains *thiaminase, which destroys the vitamin.

blinis Russian; small yeast pancakes made from buckwheat flour, served with salt herring, smoked salmon, or caviar, and sour cream.

blintzes Middle European (and especially Jewish); pancakes, stuffed with either curd cheese (and then served with soured cream) or minced meat.

bloaters Salted, cold-smoked *herrings.

blood Various *blood cells suspended in plasma; carries nutrients and oxygen to tissues, and removes waste metabolic products from the tissues. Oxygenated blood travels from the lungs in arteries, while deoxygenated blood returns to the lungs in veins; in the tissues the blood from the arteries enters smaller vessels, the arterioles, then capillaries, which then drain into venules, then the veins. See also blood plasma.

blood cells Three main types of cell are present in blood: erythrocytes or red cells, *leucocytes or white cells, and platelets. Red blood cells carry the red colouring matter of the blood, the protein *haemoglobin, which is responsible for the transport of oxygen from the lungs to tissues, and of carbon dioxide from tissues to the lungs. White blood cells are generally concerned with protection against invading micro-organisms, and platelets with the ability of the blood to coagulate, and so prevent excessive blood loss through bleeding. Platelets are also involved in the inappropriate formation of blood clots in the blood vessels, *thrombosis.

blood clotting The process by which the soluble protein fibrinogen in *blood plasma is converted to insoluble fibrin, thus preventing blood loss through cuts, etc. *Vitamin K is required and deficiency is characterized by excessive bleeding.

Thrombosis is the inappropriate formation of blood clots in the blood vessels, and can be a cause of serious illness and death when blood vessels are blocked. Antagonists of vitamin K, including Warfarin, are commonly used to reduce the ability of blood to clot in patients at risk of thrombosis.

blood plasma The liquid component of blood, accounting for about half the total volume of the blood. Plasma is a solution of nutrients and various proteins, mainly albumin and various globulins, including the immunoglobulins which are responsible for much of the body's defence against infection, as well as some *adverse reactions to foods. When blood has clotted (see blood clotting), the resultant fluid is known as serum. See also lipids, plasma.

blood pressure See hypertension.

blood sausage See black pudding.

blood serum See blood plasma.

blood sugar *Glucose; normal concentration is about 5 mmol (90 mg)/L, and is maintained in the fasting state by mobilization of tissue reserves of *glycogen and synthesis from *amino acids. Only in prolonged starvation does it fall below about 3.5 mmol (60 mg)/L. If it falls to 2 mmol (35 mg)/L there is loss of consciousness (hypoglycaemic coma). See also hypoglycaemia.

After a meal the concentration of glucose rises, but this rise is limited by the hormone *insulin, which is secreted by the pancreas to stimulate the uptake of glucose into tissues. *Diabetes mellitus is the result of failure of the insulin mechanism.

blood volume The average blood volume is 5.3 L (78 mL/kg body weight, 9 pints) in males and 3.8 L (56 mL/kg body weight, 6.5 pints) in females.

bloom Fat bloom is the whitish appearance on the surface of chocolate which sometimes occurs in storage. It is due either to a change in the form of the fat at the surface or to fat diffusing outwards and being deposited as crystals on the surface. Sugar bloom is due to the deposition of sugar crystals on the surface, but is less common than fat bloom.

Bloom gelometer An instrument for measuring the strength of jellies, and also for any test of firmness, e.g. the staleness of bread.

blueberry Fruit of *Vaccinium corymbosum* (the high-bush blueberry) or *V. augustifolium* (low-bush blueberry) grown mainly in north America.

blue cheese *See* cheese, blue.

bluetail *See* blewits.

blush wine Californian term for rosé *wines.

BMI *See* body mass index.

BMR *See* basal metabolic rate.

boar, wild Meat of *Sus scrofa*. Hunted in parts of Europe, farmed on small scale in UK. A 150-g portion is a rich *source of protein; contains 4.5 g of fat of which one third is saturated; and supplies 160 kcal (670 kJ).

bobby veal *Veal from calves younger than 3 months.

bocadillo Spanish; a sandwich made by slicing a long crusty loaf or roll lengthways.

bocal French; wide-mouthed glass jar used for bottling or pickling fruit and vegetables.

BOD *See* biological oxygen demand.

bodega Spanish; winery or wine cellar.

body-building food A term used indiscriminately, but generally referring to proteins. The Code of Practice in advertising suggests that no claim should be made for the body-building properties of a food unless a reasonable (unspecified) amount of protein is present in a normal portion.

body fluid *See* water balance.

body mass index (BMI) An index of fatness and obesity. The weight (in kg) divided by the square of height (in m). The acceptable (desirable) range is 20–25. Above 25 is *overweight, and above 30 is *obesity. BMI below the lower end of the acceptable range indicates undernutrition and wasting. Also called Quetelet's index. *See also* weight, ideal; Appendix VII.

body surface area Heat loss from the body is related to surface area and *basal metabolic rate and energy expenditure are sometimes expressed per unit body surface area. It is commonly calculated according to the formulae of:

Du Bois: area (cm^2) = 71.84 × $weight^{0.425}(kg)$ × $height^{0.725}(cm)$

Meeh: area (cm^2) = 11.9 × $weight^{2/3}(kg)$.

The surface area of adults is about 18,000 cm^2 (men) or 16,000 cm^2 (women).

bog butter Norsemen, Finns, Scots and Irish used to bury firkins of butter in bogs to ripen and develop a strong flavour.

bog myrtle A wild plant (*Myrica gale*) with a strong resinous flavour. The leaves and seeds are used to flavour soups and stews.

boiled sweets Sugar and water boiled at such a high temperature (150–166 °C) that practically no water remains and a vitreous mass is formed on cooling.

bole *See* Armenian bole

boletus Edible wild *mushroom, *Boletus edulis* or *B. granulatus*, also known as the yellow mushroom or cep (French: *cèpe*).

boller Danish, Norwegian; dumplings.

bologna Italian smoked pork and veal *sausage, also known as polony.

Bombay duck Fish found in Indian waters, *Harpodon nehereus* or *Saurus ophiodon*, eaten either fresh or after salting and curing. The name is a corruption of the local name of the fish, bombil.

Bombay halva Indian dessert made from semolina, almonds and pistachio nuts. *See also* halva.

Bombay mix *See* chevda.

bomb calorimeter *See* calorimeter.

bombe A mould with a tight-fitting lid, used to shape ice cream and sometimes fruit. Bombe glacée is a hemispherical frozen dessert made from two separate layers of different ice creams.

bombil *See* Bombay duck.

bommerlunder A German schnapps; *see* aquavit.

Bonal *See* wines, aperitif.

bonbon General term for *sugar confectionery.

bondiola Italian (Parma); cured shoulder of pork.

bondon French (Normandy); soft cheese shaped in the form of a bun.

bone Bones consist of an organic matrix composed of *collagen and other proteins and crystalline mineral, mainly hydroxyapatite (calcium phosphate and calcium hydroxide), together with magnesium phosphate, fluorides, and sulphates. *See also* calcium.

bone broth Prepared by prolonged boiling of bones to break down the *collagen and extract it as *gelatine. Of little nutritive value, since it consists of 2–4% gelatine, with little calcium. *See also* stock.

bone charcoal Charcoal produced by heating pieces of bone sufficiently to burn off the organic matter, leaving the carbon deposited on a framework of calcium carbonate. It is used to purify solutions because it will absorb colouring matter and other impurities. Also known as animal charcoal.

bone-meal Prepared from degreased bones and used as a supplement in both animal and human foods as a source of calcium and phosphate. Also used as a plant fertilizer as a slowly released source of phosphate.

boniatillo Caribbean (Cuba); creamed dessert made from sweet potato and eggs.

bonnag Manx; soda bread.

bonne-bouche Small savoury appetizers.

bonne femme Cooked in a simple or 'housewifely' style, with a garnish of fresh vegetables or herbs, usually including mushrooms. Applied especially to fish dishes and cream soups.

Bontrae Trade name for *textured vegetable protein prepared by spinning or extrusion.

boonchi Caribbean name for yard-long beans or asparagus beans, *Vigna sesquipedalis*.

boquerones Spanish; fresh anchovies, floured and joined together by making a small incision at the tail of one and slipping the tails of 3 or 4 others through. Fried in the shape of a fan.

boracic acid *See* boric acid.

borage A herb, *Borago officinalis*. The flowers and leaves have a cucumber-like flavour and are used to flavour drinks.

borax The sodium salt of *boric acid.

borborygmos (Plural borborygmi); audible abdominal sound produced by excessive intestinal motility.

Bordeaux Red and white wines produced in the Bordeaux region of France; red Bordeaux wines are called claret in the UK.

Bordeaux mustard *See* mustard.

bordelaise, à la Dish with a wine sauce and ceps (*boletus mushrooms), or a garnish of artichokes and potatoes.

bordure, en Dish with a border of cooked vegetables.

borecole *See* kale.

börek Turkish; fried or baked *phyllo pastry with a savoury filling, generally cheese. The Greek equivalent is bourekia.

boric acid Chemically H_3BO_4, derived from the element *boron, boric acid has been used in the past as a preservative in bacon and margarine, but boron accumulates in the body. It was formerly used as an anti-infective agent and eye-wash (boracic acid) but there was a high incidence of toxic reactions.

Borneo tallow *See* vegetable butters.

boron An element, known to be essential for plant growth, but not known to have any function in human beings or animals. Suggested to modify the actions and metabolism of *oestrogens, and sometimes used in preparations to alleviate the pre-menstrual syndrome, although there is little evidence of efficacy; toxic in excess. Occurs mainly as salts of *boric acid.

borscht (also borsch, borshch) Russian, Polish; beetroot soup, served hot or cold.

Boston brown bread An American spiced pudding, steamed in the can.

botargo A relish or dip prepared from fish roe (usually mullet or *tuna); *see also* taramasalata.

boti kabab Indian; small pieces of meat, marinated and cooked rapidly under intense heat, basted with butter or *ghee.

bottle The traditional wine bottle holds 700, 720, or 750 mL of wine, depending on the variety; within the EU wine bottles are being standardized at 700 mL.

A two-bottle size is a magnum; four-bottle is a Jeroboam or double magnum, six is a Methuselah, twelve a Salmanzar, and twenty is a Nebuchadnezzar.

bottle feeding *See* infant formula.

bottle house An old English term for a manufacturer of glass containers (bottles and jars) as distinct from tableware.

bottlers' sugar *See* sugar.

botulinum cook The degree of heat required to ensure destruction of (virtually) all spores of *Clostridium botulinum*, the causative organism of *botulism, which are the most resistant of bacterial spores.

botulism A rare form of food poisoning caused by the extremely potent neurotoxins produced by *Clostridium botulinum*. At least seven different toxins have been identified; they can be inactivated by heating at 80 °C for 10 min., but in foods are more resistant to heat. Although rare, it is often fatal unless the antitoxin is given.

The name is derived from *botulus*, for sausage, since the disease was originally associated with sausages in Germany. A wide range of foods have been involved, including meat, fish, milk, fruits, and vegetables which have been incorrectly preserved or treated, so that competing micro-organisms have been destroyed; spores of *C. botulinum* are extremely resistant to heat, and dangerous amounts of toxins can accumulate in contaminated foods without any apparent spoilage.

boucanning A Caribbean process by which meat was preserved by sun-drying and smoking while resting on a wooden grid known as a boucan.

bouchée Small open pastry case (vol au vent) filled with chopped meat, game, or fish, served hot with a thick sauce.

bouchet *See* cabernet franc.

bouillabaisse French; fish stew or soup flavoured with saffron, spices, and herbs; speciality of the Mediterranean region. So named because it is repeatedly boiled. *See also* bourride.

bouillon A plain, unclarified beef or veal broth; also used synonymously with *stock.

boula boula American (originally Seychelles); *turtle soup mixed with puréed fresh green peas.

boulangère, à la Originally French for something baked in the oven. Nowadays means potatoes and onions cooked with meat in stock.

bouquet garni A small bundle of parsley, thyme, marjoram, and bay leaves, tied together with cotton and added to the dish being cooked. Now also the same mixture of herbs in a porous paper sack. Also known as a faggot.

bourbon American *whiskey made by distilling fermented *maize mash. Sour mash bourbon is made from mash that has yeast left in it from a previous fermentation.

bourbonal Ethylvanillin, *see* vanilla.

bourekia *See* börek.

bourgeoise, à la Family style dish, homely but appetizing cookery. Also means garnished with carrots, onions, and diced lean bacon.

bourguignonne, à la Also à la bourgogne; dish with a garnish incorporating mushrooms, onions, and grilled bacon and cooked in or served with red wine sauce.

Bournvita Trade name for a preparation of malt, milk, sugar, cocoa, eggs, and flavouring, to make a beverage when mixed with milk.

bourride French (Marseilles region); fish soup similar to *bouillabaisse but without saffron, flavoured with aïoli (garlic mayonnaise).

bouza *See* beer.

bovine somatotropin (BST) The natural growth hormone of cattle; biosynthetic BST is used in some dairy herds to increase milk production.

bovine spongiform encephalopathy *See* BSE.

Bovril Trade name for a preparation of *meat extract, hydrolysed beef, beef powder and yeast extract, used as a beverage, a flavouring agent, and for spreading on bread. A 10-g portion is a good *source of vitamin B_2 and a source of niacin.

boysenberry Similar to *loganberry.

bozbash Russian; mutton soup.

brachyose *See* isomaltose.

bracken Young unopened leaves (fronds) of bracken (*Pteridium* spp.), eaten as a vegetable and regarded as a delicacy in the Far East. Known as fiddleheads in Canada. They contain an antagonist of vitamin B_1; cattle and horses eating large amounts suffer from *blind staggers due to acute vitamin B_1 deficiency; also contain a number of known or suspected *carcinogens.

bradycardia An unusually slow heartbeat, less than 60 beats/min. Such a low rate may be normal in trained athletes.

bradyphagia Eating very slowly.

brain Traditionally the brains of sheep and calves are stewed and eaten; probably not advisable because of the risk of transmitting the agents responsible for various degenerative brain diseases, including scrapie and bovine spongiform encephalopathy (*BSE).

brain sugar Obsolete name for *galactose.

braise A method of cooking in a closed container, with very little liquid, normally in an oven.

bramble Wild *blackberry.

bran The outer layers of cereal grain, which are largely removed when the grain is milled (i.e. in the preparation of white flour or white rice). The germ is discarded at the same time, and there is a considerable loss of iron and other minerals, and particularly of the B vitamins, as well as of dietary fibre. A 30-g portion of wheat bran is a rich *source of niacin, iron, and zinc; a good source of vitamin B_1; a source of vitamin B_2; provides 12 g of dietary fibre; supplies 70 kcal (295 kJ). *See also* flour, extraction rate; wheatfeed.

branched-chain amino acids *See* amino acids.

branco Portuguese; white wines.

brandade Southern French dish of salt cod flavoured with garlic.

brander Scottish name for gridiron or grill.

brandy A *spirit distilled from wine, and containing 37–44% (most usually 40%) alcohol by volume. The name is derived from the German *brandtwein*, meaning burnt wine, corrupted to brandy wine. Most wine-producing countries also make brandy.

The age of brandy is generally designated as 3-star (3–5 years old before bottling); VSOP (very special old pale, aged 4–10 or more years, the name indicating that it has not been heavily coloured with caramel); Napoleon (premium blend aged 6–20 years); XO, Extraordinary Old (Extra or Grand Reserve, possibly 50 years old). *Cognac and *Armagnac are brandies made in defined regions of France.

Fruit brandies are either distilled from fruit wines (e.g. plum and apple brandies) or are prepared by soaking fruit in brandy (e.g. cherry and apricot brandies). *See also* eau de vie; marc.

brandy butter Hard sauce made from butter, caster sugar, and *brandy, traditionally served with Christmas pudding and mince pies.

brandy sauce English; sauce made from egg yolk, cream, sugar, and *brandy, traditionally served with Christmas pudding.

brandy snaps Crisp toffee-like biscuits made from flour, butter, syrup, and powdered ginger, baked, then rolled into cylinders while still warm and pliable.

Bran Plus Trade name for untreated wheat bran with germ.

Brassica Genus of vegetables that includes broccoli, Brussels sprouts, cabbage, cauliflower, kale, kohl rabi, mustard, and swedes.

bratwurst German; pork *sausage with many regional specialist varieties; may be served boiled, grilled, or fried.

brawn Made from pig meat, particularly the head, boiled with peppercorns and herbs, minced and pressed into a mould. Mock brawn (head cheese) differs in that other meat by-products are used. A 150-g portion is a rich *source of protein; a good source of niacin and iron; contains 18 g of fat; supplies 230 kcal (960 kJ).

Brazil nuts From wild trees of *Bertholletia excelsa*. A 60-g portion (eighteen nuts) is an exceptionally rich *source of selenium; a rich source of vitamins B$_1$ and E; a good source of protein, niacin, and calcium; a source of iron; contains 40 g of fat of which 25% is *saturated and 40% mono-unsaturated; provides 5.5 g of dietary fibre; supplies 400 kcal (1680 kJ).

bread Baked dough made from cereal flour, usually wheat, although rye, barley, and other cereals are also used. Normally leavened by fermentation of the dough with yeast, or addition of sodium bicarbonate. Soda bread is an Irish speciality, made with whey or buttermilk, and leavened with *sodium bicarbonate and acid in place of yeast, although yeast may also be used.

Unleavened bread is flat bread made by baking dough which has not been leavened with yeast or baking powder. *Matzo is baked to a crisp texture, while *pitta and *chapattis have a softer texture.

Aerated bread was made from dough containing water saturated with carbon dioxide under pressure, rather than being leavened with yeast. The aim was to produce an aerated loaf without the loss of carbohydrate involved in a yeast fermentation (7% of the total ingredients). The resultant loaf was insipid in flavour and the method went out of use.

Wholemeal bread is baked with 100% extraction flour, i.e. containing the whole of the cereal grain. White bread is made from 72% extraction flour. Brown bread is made with flour of extraction rate intermediate between that of white bread (72%) and wholemeal (100%). A loaf may not legally be described as brown unless it contains at least 0.6% *fibre on a dry weight basis. Black bread is a coarse wholemeal wheat or rye bread leavened with sourdough (*sauerteig*).

The white loaf in the UK has added iron, vitamin B$_1$, and niacin, but not to the level of wholemeal bread, and white but not wholemeal is enriched with calcium. Some bakers also enrich white bread with *folate. In some countries *riboflavin but not calcium is added.

Four slices of brown bread (120 g) are a rich *source of folate; a good source of protein, vitamin B$_1$, iron, and copper; a source of calcium and zinc; contain 3.3 g of fat of which 18% is saturated; provide 10.5 g of dietary fibre; supply 350 kcal (1470 kJ).

Four slices of white bread (120 g) are a rich *source of copper and selenium; a good source of protein, vitamin B$_1$, and folate; a source of calcium and iron; contain 2.6 g of fat of which 23% is saturated; provide 4.5 g of dietary fibre; supply 370 kcal (1550 kJ).

Four slices of wholemeal bread (140 g) are a rich *source of vitamin B$_1$, copper, and selenium; a good source of protein, folate, and iron; a source of zinc; contain 4.1 g of fat of which 18% is saturated; provide 11.3 g of dietary fibre; supply 340 kcal (1430 kJ).

Rye bread is baked wholly or partially with rye flour, of varying extraction rate, so that it can vary from very light to grey or black. It is commonly a sourdough bread and may contain caraway seeds. A 100-g portion (4 slices from a small loaf) is a good *source of vitamin B$_1$ and niacin; a source of protein, calcium, and iron; contains 4.5 g of dietary fibre; supplies 220 kcal (925 kJ).

Sourdough bread is commonly wholemeal wheat or rye bread, but may also be white bread, that has been leavened with sourdough (*sauerteig*); dough that has been left to ferment overnight, and contains a mixture of fermenting micro-organisms, including peptonizing bacteria that turn the dough to a more plastic state, yeast, and lactic or acetic bacteria that produce the sour flavour.

There is a wide variety of different types of bread, with loaves baked in different shapes, or with various additions to the dough. For batch bread, the moulded pieces of dough touch each other in the oven, so that when baked and separated only the top and bottom of the loaf have crusts. Traditional French bread is made with soft-wheat flour, and has a more open texture and crisp crust. It is generally baked as a *baguette, a long thin loaf. It does not keep well, and is traditionally purchased three times a day. Focaccia is Italian; white bread made with olive oil (9%) and herbs; ciabatta (also Italian) is a flat white bread with large holes, made with olive oil (5%); literally 'old slipper'. Bank holiday bread is made with extra fat to soften the crumb so that it will last over a long (Bank holiday) weekend.

Cornell bread was originally developed at Cornell University, with increased nutritional value from the addition of 6% soya flour and 8% skim milk solids. Lactein bread has added milk, usually about 6% milk solids (3–4% milk solids are often added to the ordinary loaf in the USA).

See also flour, extraction rate; quickbreads; Chorleywood bread process.

breadfruit Large spherical, starchy fruit of the tree *Artocarpus communis* or *A. incisa* (fig family). Staple though seasonal food in the Caribbean, eaten roasted whole when ripe, or boiled in pieces when green. A 200-g portion is a rich *source of vitamin C; a source of iron and vitamin B_1; supplies 220 kcal (925 kJ).

bread sauce Thick white sauce made from bread and milk in which an onion has been boiled; a traditional accompaniment to poultry.

breadspreads General term for fats used to spread on bread, including *butter, *margarine, and low-fat spreads that may not legally be called margarine.

bread, starch-reduced Bread is normally 9–10% protein and about 50% starch; if the starch is reduced, either by washing some of it out of the dough or by adding extra protein, the bread is referred to as starch-reduced, and is often claimed to be of value in *slimming and *diabetic diets. Legally, the name 'starch-reduced bread' may be applied only to bread containing less than 50% carbohydrate, and any claims for its value as a slimming aid are strictly controlled.

breadstick *See* grissini.

breakfast cereal (breakfast food) Legally defined as any food obtained by the swelling, roasting, grinding, rolling, or flaking of any cereal. Products are described under their individual names.

break middlings *See* dunst.

break rolls *See* milling.

breast-feeding *See* lactation, nutritional needs.

breathing Of red *wine, opening the bottle some time before serving to allow oxidation and development of the full mature flavour.

Bredsoy Trade name for an unheated (i.e. enzyme active) full-fat *soya flour.

bresaola Italian; thinly sliced dried salted beef.

bretonne, à la Dish with a garnish of haricot beans or bean purée.

bretonne sauce used with eggs and fish, made with onions or leeks and white wine.

bretzels *See* pretzels.

brewers' grains Cereal residue from brewing, containing about 25% protein; used as animal feed.

brewing The process of making *beer.

brie Soft white cheese originally from the Brie region of France, made from cows' milk and moulded into a flat disc; it has a white rind, is ripened for 3–4 weeks, and deteriorates rapidly. A 30-g portion is a rich *source of vitamin B$_{12}$, a source of protein and vitamin A, contains 8 g of fat of which 70% is saturated, 200 mg sodium, and 160 mg calcium; supplies 100 kcal (400 kJ).

Brillat-Savarin A French gourmet (1755–1826) whose name is given to a *consommé, *baba, and several other dishes.

brilliant acid green BS *See* green S.

brimstone *See* sulphur.

brine Salt solutions of varying concentrations used in *pickling. 'Fresh' brine may have added nitrite; 'live' brine contains micro-organisms that convert nitrate to nitrite (pickling salts).

brining The process of soaking vegetables in *brine before pickling in vinegar, in order to remove some of the water, and retain a crisp texture. Dry brining is when the vegetables are covered with dry salt, rather than immersed in a salt solution.

brioche French; sweet bread or yeast cake, sometimes containing currants and candied fruit, sometimes filled with chocolate (*pain au chocolat*).

brioli Corsican; chestnut meal, prepared in the same way as *polenta.

brisket The meat covering the breast bone of the animal. *See* beef.

brislings Young sprats, *Clupea sprattus*. A 100-g portion is an extremely rich *source of vitamin D and a rich source of vitamin A.

British wine *See* wine, British.

Brix A table of specific gravity based on the *Balling tables, calculated in grams of cane sugar in 100 g of solution at 20 °C; degree Brix = % sugar. It is used to refer to the concentration of sugar syrups used in canned fruits.

broa Portuguese; yellow bread made from maize and wheat flour, with egg.

broasting A cooking method in which the food is deep fried under pressure, which is quicker than without pressure, and the food absorbs less fat.

broccoli, Chinese (Chinese kale) *Brassica oleracea* var. *alboglabra*; similar to *calabrese and purple sprouting *broccoli.

broccoli, sprouting Member of the cabbage family, *Brassica oleracea Italica* group with purple and white clusters of flower buds (which turn green when boiled) with smaller heads than *calabrese. (Italian *broccoli* means 'little shoots'.) A 100-g portion, boiled, is a rich *source of vitamin C; a source of vitamin A (500 µg carotene); provides 3 g of dietary fibre; supplies 25 kcal (105 kJ).

broche, en Also en brochette; roasted or grilled on a spit or skewer.

broiler *See* chicken.

broiling Cooking by direct heat over a flame, as in a barbecue; American term for grilling. Pan broiling is cooking through hot dry metal over direct heat.

bromatology The science of foods, from the Greek *broma*, food.

bromelains *Enzymes in the *pineapple and related plants of the family Bromelidaceae, which hydrolyse proteins. They are available as by-products from commercial pineapple production, usually from the stems, and are used to tenderize meat, to treat sausage casings, and to *chill-proof beer. Similar enzymes are found in figs (*ficin) and pawpaw (*papain).

brominated oils Oils from a variety of sources, including peach and apricot kernels, olive and soya oils which have been reacted with *bromine. They are used to help to stabilize emulsions of flavouring substances in soft drinks. Also known as weighting oils.

bromine An element, chemically related to *iodine, *chlorine, and *fluorine, not known to have any function in the body, and not a dietary essential.

brooklime A wild plant (*Veronica beccabunga*) that grows in very wet marshy conditions. The large, round, fleshy leaves can be added to salads.

broonie Orkney; gingerbread made with oatmeal.

brose A Scottish dish made by pouring boiling water onto oatmeal or barley meal; fish, meat, and vegetables may be added.

broth Thick soup.

broussiko Greek sweet fortified wine from the Cyclades.

brown adipose tissue (brown fat) Metabolically highly active adipose tissue, which is involved in heat production to maintain body temperature, as opposed to white *adipose tissue, which is storage fat and has a relatively low rate of metabolic activity.

brown betty American; pudding made from apple and breadcrumbs; similar to apple charlotte.

brown colours Three brown colours are used in foods: Brown FK (E-154), synthetic, which is used to colour *kippers; Chocolate-brown HT (E-155), synthetic, and *caramel (E-150).

brown fat *See* brown adipose tissue.

brownie American cake made with chocolate.

browning, gravy *See* gravy browning.

browning, non-enzymic *See* Maillard reaction.

browning reactions Chemical reactions in foods which result in the formation of a brown colour. *See* Maillard reaction; phenol oxidases.

brugnon Hybrid fruit, a cross between plum and peach. Resembles nectarine, and name sometimes used in France for nectarines.

brûlé Literally 'burnt'; food grilled or otherwise heated sufficiently to give it a good brown colour. *See also* crème brûlée.

brunoise Mixture of diced or shredded vegetables used as base for a soup, sauce, or garnish.

bruschetta Italian; toasted bread moistened with olive oil (and optionally also garlic).

Brussels sprouts Leaf buds of *Brassica oleracea gemmiferra*. Nine sprouts (90 g) are a rich *source of folate and vitamin C; a source of vitamin B_6; provide 2.7 g of dietary fibre; supply 16 kcal (65 kJ).

brut Dry wines. *See* wine, sweetness.

BS 5750 British Standard of excellence in quality management; originally an engineering standard but applicable to food companies, hospitals, etc.; incorporates the EU equivalent ISO 9002.

BSE Bovine spongiform encephalopathy; a degenerative disease of the *brain, transmitted between animals by feeding slaughter-house waste from infected animals. Commonly known as 'mad cow disease'. The infective agent is believed to be a *prion. It is not known whether it can be transmitted to human beings, but similar infectious agents cause scrapie in sheep and Kreutzfeld-Jacob disease (and possibly other dementias) in human beings.

BST *See* bovine somatotropin.

bual *See* Madeira wines.

bubble and squeak English; originally cold boiled beef fried with cooked potatoes and cabbage (the name comes from the sound made as it cooks, or, it is said, from the gasps of those eating it). More commonly a fried mixture of left-over cabbage and potatoes. Colcannon is a similar Irish dish.

buckling A hot-smoked *herring (the *kipper is cold-smoked).

buck rarebit *See* Welsh rarebit.

buck's fizz Sparkling wine mixed with orange juice; known in the USA as a mimosa.

buckwheat A cereal, the grains of *Fagopyrum esculentum* and other species, also known as Saracen corn, and, when cooked, as kasha

(Russian). It is unsuitable for bread making, and is eaten as the cooked grain, a porridge, or baked into pancakes. A 100-g portion is a good *source of protein, niacin, and vitamin B₁; a source of vitamin B₂; supplies 350 kcal (1470 kJ).

budino Italian name for (usually cooked) puddings, often containing cheese, fruit, or nuts.

buffalo currant Two varieties of N. American currant: *Ribes odoratum*, which has a distinctive smell, and *R. aureum*, the golden or Missouri currant.

buffers Substances that prevent a change in the *pH when *acid or *alkali is added. Salts of weak acids and bases are buffers and are commonly used to control the acidity of foods. Amino acids and proteins also act as buffers. The pH of blood (acid-base balance) is maintained by physiological buffers including phosphates, bicarbonate, and proteins.

bulgur The oldest processed food known. Prepared precooked wheat, originally from the Middle East. Wheat is soaked, cooked, and dried, then lightly milled to remove the outer bran and cracked. It is eaten in soups and cooked with meat (when it is known as kibbe). Also called ala, burghul, cracked wheat, and American rice.

bulimia nervosa An *eating disorder, characterized by powerful and intractable urges to overeat, followed by self-induced vomiting and the excessive use of purgatives. It is mainly a problem of women aged between 15 and 30, and is considered by many to be a variant of *anorexia nervosa.

buljol Caribbean; salad of salt cod, chilli, tomato, and avocado.

bulking agents Non-nutritive substances (commonly *non-starch polysaccharides) added to foods to increase the bulk and hence sense of *satiety, especially in foods designed for weight reduction.

bulk sweeteners *See* sugar alcohols.

bullace Fruit of the wild damson, *Prunus insititia*; similar to *sloe (*P. spinosa*), and very acidic.

bullnose pepper *See* pepper.

bullock's heart *See* custard apple.

bull's eye Cushion-shaped, mint-flavoured boiled sweet, with dark and light stripes.

bully beef The name given by troops during the First World War to *corned beef (canned salted beef).

bulrush A wild plant common in ponds and marshes (correctly the false bulrush or common reedmace, *Typha latifola*). The young sprouts and shoots can be eaten in salads, the pollen is used as a flavouring, and the roots and unripe flower heads may be boiled as a vegetable.

bun Sweetened bread roll; correctly made with yeast dough, although sometimes applied to small cakes made with baking powder, or to cream buns, which are made with choux pastry. Also applied to the rolls used for hamburgers (burger buns).

buni Coffee beans left in the field to dry; generally hard and of poor quality.

bunt *See* smut.

burger *See* hamburger.

burghul *See* bulgur.

Burgundy Red and white wines produced in the Burgundy region of France (Bourgogne).

burnet Salad burnet, a wild plant (*Poterium sanguisorba*) growing in grassland on chalky soil. The leaves have the flavour of cucumber, and can be used to flavour fruit *wines, vinegar, and butter, and are used in salads. Also called pimpernel.

burning foot syndrome Nutritional melalgia (neuralgic pain); severe aching, throbbing, and burning pain in the feet, associated with nerve damage, observed in severely under-nourished prisoners of war in the Far East. It results from long periods on a diet poor in protein and B *vitamins, and may (doubtfully) be due specifically to a deficiency of *pantothenic acid.

busa *See* milk, fermented.

bushel A traditional dry measure of capacity, equivalent to 80 lb of distilled water at 17 °C with a barometer reading of 30 inches, i.e. 8 imperial gallons (36.4 L); used as a measure of corn, potatoes, etc. The American (Winchester) bushel is 3% larger.

The weight of a bushel varies with the product: wheat 27 kg, maize and rye 25 kg, barley 22 kg, paddy rice 20 kg, oats 14.5 kg.

butifarra Spanish (Catalan and Mallorquin); spiced pork sausage containing pine nuts, almonds, cumin seed, and cinnamon. Butifarrones are smaller.

butt A cask for beer or wine, containing 108 imperial gallons (491 L).

butter Made from separated *cream by churning (sweet cream butter); legally not less than 80% fat (and not more than 16% water) of which around 60% is *saturated, a small proportion (3%) polyunsaturated, the rest being mono-unsaturated. Lactic butter, which is preferred in some countries, is made by first ripening the cream with a bacterial culture to produce lactic acid and increase the flavour (due to diacetyl). This is normally unsalted or up to 0.5% salt added. Sweet cream butter may be salted up to 2%. Butter supplies 72 kcal (300 kJ) per g; a 40-g portion (as spread on 4 slices of bread) is a rich *source of vitamin A and contains 32 g of fat, of which two-thirds is saturated; supplies 300 kcal (1260 kJ).

Clarified butter is butter fat, prepared by heating butter and separating the fat from the water. It does not become *rancid as rapidly as butter. Also known as ghee or ghrt (India) and samna (Egypt). Process or renovated butter has been melted and rechurned with the addition of milk, cream, or water. Drawn butter is melted butter used as a dressing for cooked vegetables. Devilled butter is mixed with lemon juice, cayenne and black pepper, and curry powder. Ravigote butter is creamed with chopped fresh aromatic herbs (tarragon, parsley, chives, chervil), usually served with grilled meat. Green butter is mixed with chopped herbs and other seasonings to produce a savoury spread. Black butter is browned by heating, then vinegar, salt, pepper, or other seasonings are added.

butterine *See* margarine.

buttermilk The residue left after churning butter, 0.1–2% fat, with the other constituents of milk proportionally increased. It is slightly acidic, with a distinctive flavour due to the presence of *diacetyl and other substances. Usually made by adding lactic bacteria to skim milk; 90–92% water, 4% lactose with acidic flavour from lactic acid, it is similar to skim *milk in composition. Dried buttermilk is used in bakery products and ice cream.

butter, Mowrah *See* vegetable butters.

butternockerln *See* knödeln.

butterscotch *See* toffee.

butter, vegetable *See* vegetable butters.

butter, whey (serum butter) Butter made from the small amount of fat left in *whey; it has a slightly different *fatty acid composition from ordinary butter.

butylated hydroxyanisole (BHA) An *antioxidant (E-320) used in fats and fatty foods; stable to heating, and so is useful in baked products.

butylated hydroxytoluene (BHT) An *antioxidant (E-321) used in fats and fatty foods.

butyric acid A short-chain saturated *fatty acid containing four carbon atoms. It occurs as the triglyceride in 5–6% of butter fat, and in small amounts in other fats and oils.

BV Biological Value, a measure of *protein quality.

Byrrh *See* wines, aperitif.

CA Controlled atmosphere. *See* gas storage, controlled.

cabbage Leaves of *Brassica oleracea capitata*. A 100-g portion (boiled) is a rich *source of vitamin C; a good source of folate; a source of vitamin B_1; provides 2 g of dietary fibre; supplies 15 kcal (65 kJ). *See also* collard; sauerkraut; savoy; spring greens.

cabbage, Chinese Name given to two oriental vegetables: *Brassica pekinensis* (pe-tsai, Pekin cabbage, snow cabbage), pale green compact head resembling lettuce, and *B. chinensis* (pak choi, Chinese greens, Chinese chard), loose bunch of dark green leaves and thick stalks; a 50-g portion is an exceptionally rich *source of vitamin C; a rich source of *folate; a source of vitamin A (as carotene); supplies 15 kcal (65 kJ).

cabbie-claw Scottish (Shetland); fresh codling, salted and hung in the open air for 1–2 days, then simmered with horseradish. The name derives from the Shetland dialect name for young *cod, kabbilow (from the German *Kabbeljau*).

cabello de angel *See* angel's hair.

cabernet franc A *grape variety widely used for *wine making, although not one of the classic varieties. Also known as bouchet.

cabernet sauvignon One of the 9 'classic' *grape varieties used for *wine making, used for some of the great red wines of Bordeaux, and widely grown throughout the world.

cabinet pudding Moulded pudding made from bread and butter or sponge cake, with custard; sometimes glacé cherries and egg are added.

cacao butter *See* cocoa butter.

cacciatora, alla Italian; in the hunter's style, generally game or poultry with onions, herbs, and tomatoes in a wine sauce.

cacciatore Small Italian *salami.

cacen-gri Welsh; soda scones made with currants and *buttermilk.

cachelos Spanish (Galician) dish of potatoes, cabbage, ham, and chorizo (spiced sausage).

cachexia The condition of extreme emaciation and wasting seen in patients with advanced diseases such as cancer and AIDS. Due to both an inadequate intake of food and the effects of the disease in increasing *metabolic rate (hypermetabolism) and the breakdown of tissue protein.

cachou Small scented tablets for sweetening the breath.

cadmium A mineral of no known function in the body, and therefore not a dietary essential. It accumulates in the body throughout life, reaching a total body content of 20–30 mg (200–300 µmol). It is toxic, and cadmium poisoning is a recognized industrial disease. In Japan cadmium poisoning has been implicated in itai-itai disease, a severe and sometimes fatal loss of calcium from the bones, as the disease occurred in an area where rice was grown on land irrigated with contaminated waste water. Accidental contamination of drinking water with cadmium salts also leads to kidney damage, and enough cadmium can leach out from cooking vessels with cadmium glaze to pose a hazard.

caecum The first part of the large intestine, separated from the small intestine by the ileo-colic sphincter. It is small in carnivorous animals and very large in herbivores, since it is involved in the digestion of cellulose. In omnivorous animals, including man, it is of intermediate size. *See also* gastro-intestinal tract.

caffeine An *alkaloid (chemically trimethylxanthine) found in coffee and tea, and also known as theine. It raises blood pressure, stimulates the kidneys, and temporarily averts the feeling of fatigue or tiredness, so has a stimulant action. It can also be a cause of insomnia in some people, and decaffeinated coffee and tea are commonly available.

Coffee beans contain about 1% caffeine, and the beverage contains about 70 mg/100 mL. Tea contains 1.5–2.5% caffeine, about 50–60 mg/100 mL of the beverage. Cola drinks contain 12–18 mg/100 mL. *See also* coffee, decaffeinated; theobromine; xanthine.

caffeol A volatile oil in coffee beans, giving the characteristic flavour and aroma.

cafiroleta Caribbean (Cuba); dessert made from *boniatillo (creamed sweet potato) and *coquimol (coconut milk custard).

cake Baked from flour with added fat (butter or margarine), sugar, and eggs. Plain cakes are made by rubbing the fat and sugar into the flour, with no egg; sponge cakes by whipping with or without fat; rich cakes contain dried fruit.

A 100-g portion of typical rich fruit cake is a *source of calcium and iron; contains 10 g of fat of which one-third is saturated and one-quarter polyunsaturated; supplies 340 kcal (1430 kJ). A 100-g portion of sponge made without added fat ('fatless sponge') is a good source of protein; a source of vitamin B_2, niacin, and iron; contains 6 g of fat; supplies 300 kcal (1260 kJ).

calabasa West Indian or green pumpkin, with yellow flesh.

calabash *See* gourd.

calabrese An annual plant (*Brassica oleracea italica*), a variety of *broccoli which yields a crop in the same year as it is sown. Also called American, Italian, or green sprouting broccoli. A 75-g portion is a rich *source of vitamin A (as carotene), folate, and vitamin C; provides 3 g of dietary fibre; supplies 25 kcal (105 kJ).

calamary Spanish: *calamares*; Italian: *calamari*. Mediterranean squid (*Lodogo vulgaris*).

calamondin A *citrus fruit resembling a small tangerine, with a delicate pulp and a lime-like flavour.

calas 1 American (New Orleans) rice fritters.
2 *Akkra.

calcidiol The 25-hydroxy-derivative of *vitamin D, also known as 25-hydroxycholecalciferol, the main storage and circulating form of the vitamin in the body.

calciferol Used at one time as a name for ercalciol (ergocalciferol or vitamin D$_2$), made by the ultra-violet irradiation of ergosterol. Also used as a general term to include both *vitamers of *vitamin D (vitamins D$_2$ and D$_3$).

calciol The official name for cholecalciferol, the naturally occurring form of *vitamin D (vitamin D$_3$).

calcionetta Italian; dessert made from fried ravioli filled with spiced sweetened chestnut purée.

calcitriol The 1,25-dihydroxy-derivative of *vitamin D, also known as 1,25-dihydroxycholecalciferol; the active metabolite of the vitamin in the body.

calcium The major inorganic component of bones and teeth; the total body content of an adult is about 1–1.5 kg (15–38 mol). The small amounts in blood plasma (2.1–2.6 mmol/L, 85–105 mg/L) and in tissues play a vital role in the excitability of nerve tissue, the control of muscle contraction and the integration and regulation of metabolic processes.

The absorption of calcium from the intestinal tract requires *vitamin D, and together with parathyroid hormone, vitamin D also controls the body's calcium balance, mobilizing it from the bones to maintain the plasma concentration within a very narrow range. An unacceptably high plasma concentration of calcium is *hypercalcaemia.

The RNI (*see* reference intakes) for calcium is 800 (women) to 1000 (men) mg/day, with a considerable increase in pregnancy and lactation. Although a net loss of calcium from bones occurs as a normal part of the ageing process, and may lead to *osteoporosis, there is no evidence that higher intakes of calcium in later life will affect this process.

The richest *sources of calcium are milk and cheese; in some countries it is added to flour. Other rich sources include: haggis, canned pilchards and sardines, spinach, sprats, tripe.

calcium acid phosphate Also known as monocalcium phosphate and acid calcium phosphate or ACP, Ca(H$_2$PO$_4$)$_2$. Used as the acid ingredient of *baking powder and self-raising *flour, since it reacts with bicarbonate to liberate carbon dioxide. Calcium phosphates are permitted food additives (E-341).

calculi (calculus) Stones formed in tissues such as the gall bladder (biliary calculus or *gallstone), kidney (renal calculus), or ureters. Renal calculi may consist of *uric acid and its salts (especially in *gout) or of *oxalic acid salts. Oxalate calculi may be of metabolic or dietary origin and people at metabolic risk of forming oxalate renal calculi are advised to avoid dietary sources of *oxalic acid and its precursors. Rarely, renal calculi may consist of the amino acid *cystine.

caldereta Spanish; stewed fish or meat, named from the *caldera* or cauldron in which it is cooked.

caldo Portuguese, Spanish; broth.

Calfos Trade name for a prepared *bone meal (i.e. calcium phosphate) used as a source of calcium and phosphate in foods.

calf's foot jelly Stock made by boiling calves' feet in water; it sets to a stiff jelly on cooling; largely water, so of little nutritional value.

calipash The gelatinous green fat attached to the upper shell (carapace) of the *turtle; the yellow fat attached to the lower shell is calipee.

calipee *See* calipash.

calisay Spanish (Catalan); liqueur made from chinchona (cinchona) bark, aged in oak casks.

callaloo (calaloo, calilu, calalou, callau) Caribbean name for leaves of both *taro and Chinese spinach (*Amaranthus gangeticus*), and for the soup made from them.

calorie A unit of *energy used to express the energy yield of foods and energy expenditure by the body. One calorie (cal) is the amount of heat required to raise the temperature of 1 g of water through 1 °C (from 14.5–15.5 °C). Nutritionally the kilocalorie (1000 calories) is used (the amount of heat required to raise the temperature of 1 kg of water through 1 °C), and is abbreviated as either kcal or Cal to avoid confusion with the cal.

The calorie is not an SI unit, and correctly the Joule is used as the unit of energy, although kcal are widely used. 1 kcal = 4.18 kJ; 1 kJ = 0.24 kcal.

See also energy; energy conversion factors.

calories, empty A term used to describe foods that provide energy but little, if any, of the nutrients.

calorimeter (bomb calorimeter) An instrument for measuring the amount of oxidizable energy in a substance, by burning it in oxygen and measuring the heat produced. The energy yield of a foodstuff in the body is equal to that obtained in a bomb calorimeter only when the metabolic end-products are the same as those obtained by combustion. Thus, proteins liberate 5.65 kcal (23.64 kJ)/g in a calorimeter, when the nitrogen is oxidized to the dioxide, but only 4.4 kcal (18.4 kJ)/g in the body, when the nitrogen is excreted as urea (which has a heat of combustion equal to the 'missing' 1.25 kcal (5.23 kJ)). *See also* energy conversion factors.

calorimetry The measurement of energy expenditure by the body. Direct calorimetry is the direct measurement of heat output from the body, as an index of energy expenditure, and hence energy requirements. The subject is placed inside a small, thermally insulated room, and the heat produced is measured. Few such difficult studies have been performed, and only a limited range of activities can be studied under these confined conditions.

Indirect calorimetry is a means of estimating energy expenditure indirectly, rather than by direct measurement of heat production. There are two methods in use: (1) Measurement of the rate of oxygen consumption, using a *spirometer, permits calculation of energy expenditure. Most studies of the energy cost of activities have been performed by this method. (2) Estimation of the total production of carbon dioxide over a period of 7–10 days, after consumption of dual isotopically labelled water (i.e. water labelled with both ^2H and ^{18}O). *See also* isotopes.

Calphos Trade name for a prepared *bone-meal used as a source of calcium and phosphate in foods.

caltrops *See* chestnut, water.

calvados French; apple brandy made by distillation of *cider. Appellation contrôllée calvados is from the Calvados region in Normandy, and is double distilled.

calzone Italian (especially of Naples); crescent-shaped turnover of leavened dough, filled with ham and cheese; may be fried or baked. Sometimes called pizza calzone.

camash *See* quamash.

Cambridge sauce English; substitute for mayonnaise, made with oil, vinegar, and pounded yolk of hard-boiled eggs, flavoured with capers, anchovies, and herbs. *See also* salad dressing.

Camembert A major soft, French *cheese made from cows' milk, originating from Auge, Normandy, France. Covered with a white mould (*Penicillium candidum* or *P. camembertii*) which participates in the ripening process; deteriorates after a few days.
Commonly in the UK it contains 50% water and 25% fat (= '50% fat in dry matter'); a 30-g portion is a rich *source of vitamin B_{12}, a source of protein, vitamins A, B_2, and niacin, contains 8 g of fat, 100 mg of calcium and 200 mg of sodium; supplies 90 kcal (370 kJ). Also made with '30% fat in dry matter' (= 13% of total), '40', '45' and '60% fat in dry matter' (= 18% of total).

camomile Either of two herbs, *Anthemis nobilis* or *Matricaria recutica*. The essential oil is used to flavour *liqueurs; camomile tea is a *tisane prepared by infusion of the dried flower heads, and the whole herb can be used to make a herb beer.

Campari Italian; bitter aperitif wine.

Campden process The preservation of food by the addition of sodium bisulphite (E-222), which liberates sulphur dioxide. Also known as cold preservation, since it replaces heat *sterilization.

Campden tablets Tablets of sodium bisulphite (E-222), used for sterilization of bottles and other containers and in the preservation of foods (the *Campden process).

Campylobacter A genus of pathogenic organisms which are the most commonly reported cause of gastro-enteritis in the UK, although it is not known what proportion of cases are foodborne. Campylobacteriosis has been associated with the consumption of undercooked meats, milk that has been inadequately pasteurized or contaminated by birds, and contaminated water. *Helicobacter pyloris* was formerly classified as a *campylobacter*.

camu-camu Fruit of the Peruvian bush *Myrciaria paraensis*; burgundy red in colour, weighing 6–14 g and about 3 cm in diameter; contains 3000 mg vitamin C/100 g pulp.

canapés Small rectangular slices of bread, toasted or fried, spread with meat or fish pâté; originally served as an accompaniment to winged game, and spread with forcemeat made from the entrails of the birds. The name derives from the French *canapé*, 'sofa', since these were traditionally eaten in the drawing room, before dinner was served in the dining room.

canbra oil Oil extracted from selected strains of *rapeseed containing not more than 2% *erucic acid.

cancer A wide variety of diseases characterized by uncontrolled growth of tissue. Dietary factors may be involved in the initiation of some forms of cancer, and a high-fat diet has been especially implicated. There is some evidence that *antioxidant nutrients such as *carotene, *vitamins C and E, and the mineral *selenium may be protective. *See also* carcinogen.
   Patients with advanced cancer are frequently malnourished, the condition of *cachexia.

Canderel Trade name for tablets of the *sweetener *aspartame.

candied peel Preserved fruit peel, commonly of *citrus fruits, used in confectionery and cake making. It is prepared by softening the peel, then boiling with sugar syrup.

candy 1 Crystallized sugar made by repeated boiling and slow evaporation.
   2 USA; a general term for *sugar confectionery.
   See also toffee.

candy doctor *See* sugar doctor.

cane sugar *Sucrose extracted from the sugar cane *Saccharum officinarum*; identical with sucrose prepared from any other source, such as sugar beet. *See* sugar.

canihua Seeds of *Chenopodium pallidicaule*, grown in the Peruvian Andes; nutritionally similar to cereals.

cannelloni *See* pasta.

canners' sugar *See* sugar.

canning The process of preserving food by sterilization and cooking in a sealed metal can, which destroys bacteria and protects from recontamination. If foods are sterilized and cooked in glass jars which are then closed with hermetically sealed lids, the process is known as bottling. Canned foods are sometimes known as tinned foods, because the cans are sometimes made using tin-plated steel. More commonly now they are made of lacquered steel or aluminium. In aseptic canning, foods are pre-sterilized at a very high temperature (150–175 °C) for a few seconds, and then sealed into cans under sterile (aseptic) conditions. The flavour, colour, and retention of vitamins are superior with this short-time, high-temperature process than with conventional canning.

canola A variety of *rape which is low in glucosinolates.

cantaloup *See* melon.

canthaxanthin A red *carotenoid pigment which is not a precursor of
*vitamin A. It is used as a food colour (E-161g), and can be added to
the diet of broiler *chickens to colour the skin and shanks, and to the
diet of farmed *trout to produce the same bright colour as is seen in
wild trout. These colours are normally derived from carotenoids in
natural foodstuffs. Canthaxanthin is also used to maintain the colour
of flamingos kept in captivity.

Cape gooseberry Fruit of the Chinese lantern *Physalis peruviana*, *P.
pubescens*, or *P. edulis*; herbaceous perennial resembling small cherry,
surrounded by dry, bladder-like calyx, also known as golden berry,
Peruvian cherry, and ground tomato. A 100-g portion is a rich *source
of vitamin C and a source of vitamin A (as carotene); supplies 70 kcal
(295 kJ).

caper Unopened flower buds of the subtropical shrub *Capparis spinosa* or
C. inermis with a peppery flavour; commonly used in pickles and
sauces. Unripe seeds of the nasturtium (*Tropaeolum majus*) can be
pickled and used as a substitute.

capercaillie (capercailzie) A large *game bird (*Tetrao urogallus*), also
known as wood grouse or cock of the wood.

capillary fragility A measure of the resistance to rupture of the small
blood vessels (capillaries), which would lead to leakage of red blood
cells into tissue spaces. Deficiency of *vitamin C can lead to increased
capillary fragility. There is some evidence that the *flavonoids reduce
capillary fragility, at least when given intravenously, and they may
have a clinical use. Although flavonoids have been called *vitamin P,
there is no evidence that they are a dietary essential, nor indeed that
they can be absorbed from the intestinal tract.

capon A castrated cockerel (male chicken), which has a faster rate of
growth, and more tender flesh, than the cockerel. Surgery has
generally been replaced by chemical caponization, the implantation of
pellets of female sex hormone.

caponata Sicilian; fried aubergine, in a tomato sauce containing capers,
olives, celery, and anchovy, garnished with slices of tuna, crawfish, etc.

cappelletti Italian; small hat-shaped pasta envelopes stuffed with
minced meat, etc.; a variant of *ravioli.

cappucino Italian; coffee with a head of frothy milk or whipped cream.

capric acid One of the medium-chain *fatty acids, containing ten
carbon atoms, found in the *triglycerides of coconut oil and in goat
and cow butter.

caproic acid One of the short-chain *fatty acids, containing six carbon
atoms, found in the *triglycerides of coconut oil and goat and cow
butter.

caprylic acid One of the medium-chain *fatty acids, containing eight
carbon atoms, found in the *triglycerides of goat and cow butter,
coconut oil, and human fat.

capsicum *See* pepper.

carambola Or star fruit, long (8–12 cm) ribbed fruit of *Averrhoa carambola* and *A. bilimbi*; a 50-g portion is a rich *source of vitamin C.

caramel Brown material formed by heating carbohydrates in the presence of acid or alkali; also known as burnt sugar. It can be manufactured from various sugars, starches, and starch hydrolysates and is used as a flavour and colour (E-150) in a wide variety of foods: soft drinks, alcoholic beverages, baked goods, sauces, canned meats, and stews.

caramel cream A dessert made either by gently heating eggs in milk and allowing to cool (egg *custard) or by using *cornflour and milk, topped with a caramel sauce. Also known as crème caramel and (in Spain) as flán.

caramels Sweets similar to *toffee but boiled at a lower temperature; may be soft or hard.

caraway Dried ripe fruit of *Carum carvi*, an aromatic spice, used to flavour the liqueur *kümmel, some types of *aquavit, on bread and rolls, and in *seed cake.

carbohydrate Carbohydrates are the major source of metabolic energy, the sugars and starches. Chemically they are composed of carbon, hydrogen, and oxygen in the ratio $C_n : H_{2n} : O_n$. The basic carbohydrates are the *monosaccharide *sugars, of which glucose, fructose, and galactose are the most important nutritionally.

Disaccharides are composed of two monosaccharides: nutritionally the important disaccharides are sucrose (a dimer of glucose + fructose), lactose (a dimer of glucose + galactose) and maltose (a dimer of two glucose units).

A number of oligosaccharides occur in foods, consisting of 3–5 monosaccharide units; in general these are not digested, and should be considered among the *unavailable carbohydrates.

Larger polymers of carbohydrates are known as polysaccharides or complex carbohydrates. Nutritionally two classes of polysaccharides can be distinguished: (1) starches, which are polymers of glucose units, either as a straight chain (amylose) or with a branched structure (amylopectin) and are digested; and (2) a variety of other polysaccharides which are collectively known as *non-starch polysaccharides (NSP), and are not digested by human digestive enzymes.

The reserve of carbohydrate in liver and muscles is glycogen, a glucose polymer with the same branched structure as the amylopectin form of starch.

Carbohydrates form the major part of the diet, providing between 50 and 70% of the energy intake, largely from starch and sucrose. The metabolic energy yield of carbohydrates is 4 kcal (17 kJ)/g. More precisely, monosaccharides yield 3.74 kcal (15.7 kJ), disaccharides 3.95 kcal (16.6 kJ), and starch 4.18 kcal (17.6 kJ)/g. *Glycerol is a 3-carbon sugar alcohol, and classified as a carbohydrate; it yields 4.32 kcal (18.1 kJ)/g.

See also sugar; sugar alcohols.

carbohydrate by difference It is relatively difficult to determine the various carbohydrates present in foods, and an approximation is often made by subtracting the measured *protein, *fat, *ash, and water from the total weight. The figure can be corrected by subtracting the (measured) *dietary fibre. Carbohydrate by difference is the sum of: nutritionally available carbohydrates (dextrins, starches, and sugars); nutritionally unavailable carbohydrate (pentosans, pectins, hemicelluloses, and cellulose) and non-carbohydrates such as organic acids and *lignins.

carbohydrate, complex *See* carbohydrate.

carbohydrate loading Practice of some endurance athletes (e.g. marathon runners) in training for a major event; it consists of exercising to exhaustion, so depleting muscle *glycogen, then eating a large carbohydrate-rich meal so as to replenish glycogen reserves with a higher than normal proportion of straight-chain glycogen.

carbohydrate metabolism *See* glucose metabolism.

carbohydrate, unavailable A general term for those carbohydrates present in foods that are not digested, and are therefore excluded from calculations of energy intake, although they may be fermented by intestinal bacteria and yield some energy. The term includes both indigestible oligosaccharides and the various *non-starch polysaccharides. *See also* fatty acids, volatile; starch, resistant.

carbon dioxide, available *See* baking powder; flour, self-raising.

carbon dioxide storage *See* gas storage.

carbonnade Stewed or braised meat, often with beer in the sauce; originally the French term for meat grilled over hot coals.

γ-carboxyglutamate A derivative of the *amino acid glutamate which is found in *prothrombin and other enzymes involved in *blood clotting. Its formation requires *vitamin K. It also occurs in the protein osteocalcin in *bone, where it has a function in ensuring the correct crystallization of bone mineral. Again its formation is dependent on vitamin K.

carboxymethylcellulose *See* cellulose derivatives.

carboxypeptidase An *enzyme secreted in the pancreatic juice which is involved in the *digestion of proteins.

carcinogen A substance that can induce cancer; carcinogenesis is the process of induction of cancer.

carciofi Italian; tender globe *artichokes, eaten whole.

cardamom The seeds and dried, nearly ripe, fruit of *Elettaria cardamomum*, a member of the ginger family. An aromatic spice used as a flavouring in sausages, bakery goods, *sugar confectionery, and whole in mixed pickling spice. It is widely used in Indian cooking (the Hindi name is elaichi), and as one of the ingredients of *curry powder. Arabic coffee (similar to Turkish *coffee) is flavoured with ground cardamom seeds.

cardinal, à la Dish with a scarlet effect, as when a fish dish is served with a *coral or lobster sauce dusted with paprika or cayenne.

cardoon Leafy vegetable (*Cynara cardunculus*); both the fleshy root and the ribs and stems of the inner (blanched) leaves are eaten. Sometimes called chard, although distinct from true *chard or spinach beet.

caries Dental decay caused by attack on the tooth enamel by acids produced by bacteria that are normally present in the mouth. Sugars in the mouth promote bacterial growth and acid production; *sucrose specifically promotes *plaque-forming bacteria, which cause the most damage. A moderately high intake of *fluoride increases the resistance of tooth enamel to acid attack. *See also* tooth-friendly sweets.

carignan A *grape variety widely used for *wine making, although not one of the classic varieties. Probably the commonest grape of France, a prolific cropper producing uninspiring wines.

cariogenic Causing tooth decay (*caries) by stimulating the growth of acid-forming bacteria on the teeth. The term is applied to sucrose and other fermentable carbohydrates.

carmine Brilliant red colour derived from *cochineal (E-120).

carminic acid *See* cochineal.

carmoisine A red colour, also known as azorubine, synthetic azo-dye, E-122.

carnatz Rumanian; croquettes of seasoned minced beef and pork, served with a tomato sauce.

carnitine A derivative of the *amino acid *lysine, required for the transport of fatty acids into *mitochondria for oxidation. There is no evidence that it is a dietary essential for human beings, since it can readily be formed from lysine in the body, although there is some evidence that increased intake may enhance the work capacity of muscles. It is a dietary essential for some insects, and was at one time called vitamin B_T.

carnosine A dipeptide, β-alanyl-histidine, found in the muscle of most animals. Its function is not known.

carob Seeds and pod of the tree *Ceratonia siliqua*, also known as locust bean and St John's bread. It contains a sweet pulp which is rich in sugar and gums, as well as containing 21% protein and 1.5% fat. It is used as animal feed, to make confectionery (as a substitute for chocolate), and is used for the preparation of *carob gum.

carob gum The *gum extracted from the *carob, used as an emulsifier and stabilizer (E-410) as well as in cosmetics and as a size for textiles. Also known as locust bean gum.

caroline French: small choux pastry filled with purée of meat or pâté.

Carophyll Trade name for apo-8-carotenal, a *carotene derivative.

carotene The red and orange pigments of many plants, obvious in carrots, red palm oil, and yellow maize, but masked by *chlorophyll in leaves. Three main types of carotene in foods are important as precursors of *vitamin A: α-, β- and γ-carotene, which are also used as food colours (E-160a). Plant foods contain a considerable number of other carotenes, most of which are not precursors of vitamin A.

Carotene is mostly converted into vitamin A (*retinol) in the wall of the intestine, but some is absorbed unchanged. 6 μg of β-carotene, and 12 μg of other provitamin A carotenoids, are nutritionally equivalent to 1 μg of preformed *vitamin A. About 30% of the vitamin A in Western diets, and considerably more in diets in less-developed countries, comes from carotene.

In addition to their role as precursors of vitamin A, carotenes (and especially β-carotene) are believed to be important as *antioxidant nutrients, and there is evidence that high intakes of carotene provide protection against both *ischaemic heart disease and some forms of cancer. There is no evidence on which to base *reference intakes of carotene other than as a precursor of vitamin A.

carotenoids A general term for the wide variety of red and yellow compounds chemically related to *carotene that are found in plant foods, some of which are precursors of *vitamin A, and hence known as provitamin A carotenoids.

carp Freshwater *fish, *Cyprinus carpio*.

carpaccio Italian; thinly sliced raw beef fillet, served as an antipasto or hors d'œuvre.

carpal tunnel syndrome Painful disorder of wrist and hand due to compression of the median nerve in the carpal tunnel. Claimed to be relieved by high intakes of *vitamin B$_6$, some 50–100 times the *reference intake, but there is little evidence. *See also* tenosynovitis; vitamin B$_6$ toxicity.

carrageen Edible seaweeds, *Chondrus crispus*, also known as Iberian moss or Irish sea moss, and *Gigartina stellata*; stewed in milk to make a jelly or blancmange. A source of *carrageenan.

carrageenan A *polysaccharide extracted from red algae, especially *Chondrus crispus* (Irish moss) and *Gigartina stellata*. One of the plant *gums, it binds water to form a gel, increases viscosity, and reacts with proteins to form emulsions. It is used as an emulsifier and stabilizer in milk drinks, processed cheese, low-energy foods, etc. (E-407).

carrot The root of *Daucus carota*, commonly used as a vegetable. A 100-g portion is a rich *source of vitamin A (5–10 mg carotene); provides 2.5 g of dietary fibre and supplies 35 kcal (145 kJ).

carte, à la Meal chosen from a list of foods and dishes available rather than from a set menu or meal (*table d'hôte).

cartilage The hard connective tissue of the body, composed mainly of *collagen, together with chondromucoid (a protein combined with chondroitin sulphate) and chondroalbuminoid (a protein similar to *elastin). New *bone growth consists of cartilage on which calcium salts are deposited as it develops.

Cartose Trade name for a steam hydrolysate of maize starch, used as a carbohydrate modifier in milk preparations for *infant feeding. It consists of a mixture of *dextrin, *maltose, and *glucose.

carubinose *See* mannose.

carvie Scottish name for *caraway.

casein About 75% of the proteins of milk are classified as caseins; a group of 12–15 different proteins. Often used as a protein supplement, since the casein fraction from milk is more than 90% protein.

caseinogen An obsolete name for the form in which *casein is present in solution in milk; when it was precipitated it was then called casein.

cashew nut Fruit of the tropical tree *Anacardium occidentale*, generally eaten roasted and salted. The nut hangs from the true fruit, a large fleshy but sour apple-like fruit, which is very rich in vitamin C. A 30-g portion of roasted salted nuts (30 nuts) is a *source of protein, niacin, iron, and zinc; contains 15 g of fat, of which 20% is saturated and 60% mono-unsaturated; provides 180 kcal (755 kJ).

Casilan Trade name for a *casein preparation used as a protein concentrate.

cassareep Caribbean; boiled-down juice squeezed from grated *cassava root, flavoured with cinnamon, cloves, and brown sugar; used as a base for sauces. It can also be fermented with *molasses.

cassata Italian; ice cream made in a mould with layers of diced fruit, nuts, and macaroons. Cassata Siciliana is sponge cake containing layers of ricotta cheese, grated chocolate, and crystallized fruit.

cassava (manioc) The tuber of the tropical plant *Manihot utilissima*. It is the dietary staple in many tropical countries, although it is an extremely poor source of protein; the plant grows well even in poor soil, and is extremely hardy, withstanding considerable drought. It is one of the most prolific crops, yielding, e.g. in Nigeria, 13 million kcal/acre, compared with *yam, 9 million, and *sorghum or *maize, 1 million. A 150-g portion is a rich *source of vitamin C; a source of iron and vitamin B_1; supplies 150 kcal (600 kJ).

   Cassava root contains cyanide, and before it can be eaten it must be grated and left in the open to allow the cyanide to evaporate. The leaves can be eaten as a vegetable, and the tuber is the source of *tapioca. *See also* cassareep.

casserole Lidded container designed for slow cooking of meat or fish and vegetables in the oven; also the food so cooked.

cassia The inner bark of a tree grown in the Far East (*Cinnamomium cassia*), used as a flavouring, similar to *cinnamon.

cassina A tea-like beverage made from cured leaves of a holly bush, *Ilex cassine*, containing 1–1.6% *caffeine and 8% *tannin.

cassis (crème de cassis) Extract of *blackcurrants (French: *cassis*); about 15% alcohol by volume, sweetened with sugar. Mixed with about 10 parts of white wine to make kir, or with sparkling wine to make kir royale.

cassolette Individual dish containing a single portion of a savoury mixture; sometimes lined with potato or puff pastry.

cassoulet French; stew of haricot beans with assorted meats. The name is derived from the earthenware vessel in which it is cooked, a *cassole d'Issel*.

castagnacci Corsican; fritters made from chestnut flour.

castor oil Oil from the seeds of the castor oil plant, *Ricinus* spp. The oil itself is not irritating, but in the small intestine it is hydrolysed by *lipase to release ricinoleic acid, which is irritant to the intestinal mucosa and therefore acts as a purgative. The seeds also contain the toxic *lectin, ricin.

caster sugar *See* sugar.

catabolism Those pathways of *metabolism concerned with the breakdown and oxidation of fuels and hence provision of metabolic energy. People who are undernourished or suffering from *cachexia are sometimes said to be in a catabolic state, in that they are catabolizing their body tissues, without replacing them.

catadromous fish Fish that live in fresh water and go to sea to spawn, such as eels.

catalane, à la Dish with a garnish of aubergine and rice.

catalase An *enzyme that splits hydrogen peroxide to yield oxygen and water; an important part of the body's *antioxidant defences.

catalyst An agent that participates in a chemical reaction, speeding the rate, but itself remains unchanged. Catalysts are used, for example, in the *hydrogenation of vegetable oils. *Enzymes and *coenzymes are biological catalysts.

catchup *See* ketchup.

catechin tannins *See* tannins.

cathartic *See* laxative.

cathepsins (Also kathepsins); a group of intracellular enzymes in animal tissues which hydrolyse proteins. They are involved in the normal turnover of tissue protein, and the softening of meat when *game is hung.

cation Chemical term for a positively charged *ion.

catmint The wild catmint (*Nepeta cataria*) is distinct from the cultivated catmint (*Nepeta* spp.) of gardens; both have a minty smell which is liked by cats. The leaves are used to prepare *herb teas and may be added to stews; young shoots can be eaten raw in salads.

catsup *See* ketchup.

caudle Hot spiced wine, *mulled wine.

caul Membrane enclosing the foetus; that from sheep or pig used to cover meat while roasting.

cauliflower The edible flower of *Brassica olearacea botrytis*, normally creamy-white in colour, although some cultivars have green or purple flowers. Horticulturally, varieties that mature in summer and autumn are called cauliflower, and those that mature in winter *broccoli, but commonly both are called cauliflower. A 90-g portion is a rich *source of vitamin C; a good source of folate; a source of vitamin B_6; provides 1.8 g of dietary fibre and supplies 8 kcal (33 kJ).

cava Spanish; sparkling wines made by the méthode champenoise. *See also* champagne.

caveached fish *See* escabeche.

caviar(e) The salted hard *roe of the sturgeon, *Acipenser* spp.; three main types, sevruga, asetra (ocietre), and beluga, the prime variety. A 50-g portion is a rich *source of protein and iron; a source of calcium; contains 1 g of sodium, 10 g of fat; supplies 170 kcal (715 kJ). *See also* beluga.

    Mock caviare (also known as German, Danish, or Norwegian caviare) is the salted hard roe of the lumpfish (*Cyclopterus lumpus*).

cayenne pepper *See* pepper.

cecil Old name for fried meat balls.

Celacol Trade name for methyl, hydroxyethyl, and other *cellulose derivatives.

celeriac A variety of *celery with a thick root which is eaten grated in salads or cooked as a vegetable, *Apium graveolens* var. *rapaceum*, also known as turnip-rooted or knob celery. A 40-g portion provides 1.2 g of dietary fibre and supplies 5 kcal (21 kJ).

celery Edible stems of *Apium graveolens* var. *dulce*. A 100-g portion (2 sticks) is a *source of vitamin C; provides 2 g of dietary fibre; supplies 8 kcal (34 kJ). *See also* celeriac.

celery pepper Milled black pepper mixed with ground celery seed, used as a flavouring in salads and cooking.

celery salt A mixture of ground celery seed and salt, used as a condiment.

celiac disease *See* coeliac disease.

cellobiose A disaccharide composed of 2 glucose units linked by a 1,4-β linkage, which is not hydrolysed by mammalian digestive enzymes (as distinct from the 1,4-α linkage of maltose). It is a product of the hydrolysis of *cellulose.

Cellofas Trade name for derivatives of *cellulose: Cellofas A is methylethylcellulose, Cellofas B is sodium carboxymethylcellulose.

Cellophane Trade name for the first of the transparent, non-porous films, made from wood pulp (*cellulose) (1925). Still widely used for wrapping foods and other commodities.

cellulase An *enzyme that hydrolyses *cellulose to its constituent monosaccharide (glucose) and disaccharide (cellobiose) units. It is present in the digestive juices of some wood-boring insects and in various micro-organisms, but not in mammals.

cellulose A *polysaccharide of *glucose units which is not hydrolysed by mammalian digestive enzymes. It is the main component of plant cell walls, but does not occur in animal tissues. It is digested by the bacterial *enzyme *cellulase, and hence only *ruminants and animals that have a large *caecum have an adequate population of intestinal bacteria to permit them to digest cellulose to any significant extent. There is little digestion of cellulose in the human large intestine; nevertheless, it serves a valuable purpose in providing bulk to the intestinal contents, and is one of the major components of *dietary fibre or *non-starch polysaccharides. *See also* cellulose, microcrystalline.

cellulose derivatives A number of chemically modified forms of cellulose are used in food processing for their special properties, including: (1) Carboxymethylcellulose (E-466), which is prepared from the pure cellulose of cotton or wood. It absorbs up to fifty times its own weight of water to form a stable colloidal mass. It is used, together with stabilizers, as a whipping agent, in ice-cream, confectionery, jellies, etc., and as an inert filler in 'slimming aids'. (2) Methylcellulose (E-461), which differs from carboxymethylcellulose (and other *gums) since its viscosity increases rather than decreases with increasing temperature. Hence it is soluble in cold water and forms a gel on heating. It is used as a thickener and emulsifier, and in foods formulated to be low in *gluten. (3) Other cellulose derivatives used as emulsifiers and stabilizers are hydroxypropylcellulose (E-463), hydroxypropyl-methylcellulose (E-464), and ethyl-methylcellulose (E-465).

cellulose, microcrystalline Partially hydrolysed *cellulose used as a filler in slimming and other foods (E-460).

celtuce Stem lettuce, *Lactuca sativa*; enlarged stem eaten raw or cooked, with a flavour between celery and lettuce; the leaves are not palatable.

centrifuge A machine that exerts a force many thousand times that of gravity, by spinning. Commonly used to clarify liquids by settling the heavier solids in a few minutes, a process that might take several days under gravity. Liquids of different density can also be separated by centrifugation, e.g. cream from milk.

cep French: *cèpe*; edible wild fungus, *Boletus edulis*, also known as boletus. *See* mushrooms.

cephalins *See* kephalins.

cephalopods Cuttlefish (*Sepia officinalis*), *squid, *octopus.

Ceplapro A protein-rich baby food (18–20% protein) in a granular form, made from degerminated maize flour, wheat, defatted soya flour, and skim milk powder, with added vitamins and minerals (US).

cerasuolo Italian; rosé wines (also chiaretto or rosato).

cereal Any grain or edible seed of the grass family which may be used as food; e.g. *wheat, *rice, *oats, *barley, *rye, *maize, and *millet. Collectively known as corn in the UK, although in the USA corn is specifically maize. Cereals provide the largest single foodstuff in almost all diets; in some less-developed countries up to 90% of the total diet may be cereal, and in the UK *bread and *flour provide 25–30% of the total energy and protein of the average diet. *See also* flour, extraction rate.

cereal coffee Beverages prepared from roasted cereal grains.

cereals, breakfast *See* breakfast cereals.

cerebrose Obsolete name for *galactose.

cerebrosides Complex lipids, containing the carbohydrate *galactose, which is important in nerve membranes and the myelin sheath of nerves.

cerebrovascular accident (CVA) *See* stroke.

cerelose A commercial preparation of *glucose containing about 9% water.

ceruloplasmin A copper-containing protein in *blood plasma, the main circulating form of *copper in the body.

cervelat *See* sausage.

cestode Alternative name for *tapeworm.

CF *See* citrovorum factor.

chafing dish Metal dish on a trivet over a spirit lamp (or sometimes a bottled gas flame), used for heating or cooking at the table.

chalasia Abnormal relaxation of the cardiac sphincter muscle of the stomach so that gastric contents reflux into the oesophagus, leading to regurgitation.

challa *See* cholla.

chalva *See* halva.

chamak *See* tarka.

chambré Red wines brought to room temperature (15–18 °C, 59–65 °F) before serving.

champagne Sparkling wine from the Champagne region of north-eastern France, made by a second fermentation in the bottle. Sparkling wines from other regions, even when made in the same way, cannot legally be called champagne, but are known as being made by the méthode champenoise.

champignon French; button *mushrooms, *champignons de Paris*.

chanakhi Russian (Georgian); mutton casserole with potatoes, onions, green beans, tomatoes, aubergines, and peppers.

chanfaina Spanish; stew made from the *offal of goat or kid, cooked together with the head and feet, with artichokes, chard, lettuce, and peas.

channa *See* chick peas.

chanterelle Edible wild fungus, *Cantharellus cibarius*, *see* mushrooms.

chantilly, à la Dessert including or accompanied by sweetened, vanilla-flavoured whipped cream.

chao shao roast pork Chinese (Cantonese); strips of pork marinated then roasted.

chapatti (chapati, chupatti) Indian; unleavened whole-grain wheat or millet bread, baked on an ungreased griddle. Phulka are small chapattis; roti are chapattis prepared with maize flour. Two chapattis (60 g) are a *source of vitamin B_1 and copper; provide 4.2 g of dietary fibre; if made with added fat contain 8 g of fat; supply 210 kcal (880 kJ); if made without added fat contain 0.6 g of fat; supply 130 kcal (545 kJ).

chapon Crust of bread rubbed with garlic and added to salad for flavour, then removed.

chaptalization Addition of sugar to grape must during fermentation to increase the alcohol content of the final *wine.

charcoal Finely divided carbon, obtained by heating bones (*bone charcoal) or wood in a closed retort to carbonize the organic matter. Used to purify solutions because it will absorb colouring matter and other impurities; wood charcoal is commonly used as a fuel for *barbecues.

charcuterie French; pork butchery; shop where various cold meats are sold, also the meats.

chardonnay One of the nine 'classic' *grape varieties used for *wine making, widely grown throughout the world. Chardonnay wines are among the white wines best adapted to maturing in oak barrels.

charlotte Dessert made from stewed fruit encased in, or layered alternately with, bread or cake crumbs, e.g. apple charlotte. In charlotte russe there is a cream mixture in the centre, surrounded by cake.

charollais Breed of cattle noted for the quality and leanness of the meat.

charqui (charki) South American (especially Brazilian); dried meat, normally prepared from beef, but may also be made from sheep, llama, and alpaca in Peru. Strips of meat cut lengthways and pressed after salting, then air-dried. The final form is flat, thin, flaky sheets, so differing from the long strips of *biltong. Also called jerky.

Chartreuse 1 A *liqueur invented in 1605 and still made by the Carthusian monks, named for the great charterhouse (*la grande Chartreuse*) which is the mother house of the order, near Grenoble in southern France. It is reputed to contain more than 200 ingredients. There are three varieties: green Chartreuse is 55%, yellow 43% and white 30% *alcohol.
  2 A dish turned out of a mould; more usually fruit enclosed in jelly.

chasnidarh Indian; sweet-sour foods.

chasseur, à la In the hunter's style; dish with a garnish of mushrooms cooked with shallots and white wine. Chasseur sauce is a highly seasoned sauce based on white wine, with mushrooms and shallots, served with meat or game.

Chastek paralysis Acute deficiency of vitamin B_1 in foxes and mink fed on diets high in raw fish, which contains *thiaminase.

chateaubriand thick steak cut from *beef fillet. Named originally in 1822 in honour of the Comte de Chateaubriand.

château salad French-Canadian; cooked frogs' legs with shredded lettuce and watercress, garnished with hard-boiled egg and lemon.

chaudfroid Sauce used to coat meat, fish, or poultry to be served cold.

chausson French; turnover; pastry folded over jam or fruit before baking.

chayote Tropical squash (originally Mexican), *Sechium edule*; prickly skin and a single edible seed. Also called cho-cho or christophene.

CHD Coronary heart disease, *see* heart disease.

cheddar Hard *cheese dating from sixteenth century prepared by a particular method (*cheddaring); originally from the Cheddar area of Somerset, England; matured for several months or even years. Red Cheddar is coloured with *annatto; fat-reduced versions are now made. A 30-g portion is a rich *source of vitamin B_{12}, a source of protein, niacin, and vitamin A; contains 10 g of fat, 200 mg of calcium, 200 mg of sodium; supplies 120 kcal (500 kJ).

cheddaring In the manufacture of *cheese, after coagulation of the milk, heating of the curd, and draining, the curds are piled along the floor of the vat, where they consolidate to a rubbery sheet of curd. This is the cheddaring process; for cheeses with a more crumbly texture the curd is not allowed to settle so densely.

cheese Prepared from the curd precipitated from milk by *rennet (containing the *enzyme *chymosin or rennin), purified chymosin, or lactic acid. Cheeses other than cottage and cream cheeses are cured by being left to mature with salt, under various conditions that produce the characteristic flavour of each type of cheese. Although most cheeses are made from cow's milk, goat's milk and sometimes ewe's milk can be used to make speciality cheeses. These are generally soft cheeses.

There are numerous variants (over 400) including more than 100 from England and Wales alone (nine major regional cheeses: Caerphilly, Derby, Double *Gloucester, *Cheddar, Lancashire, Red Leicester, *Stilton, and Wensleydale). Some varieties are regional specialities, and legally may only be made in a defined geographical area; others are defined by the process rather than the region of production. The strength of flavour of cheese increases as it ages; mild or mellow cheeses are younger, and less strongly flavoured, than mature or extra-mature cheeses.

Cheeses differ in their water and fat content and hence their nutrient and energy content, ranging from 50–80% water in soft cheeses (*mozarella, *quark, boursin, *cottage) to less than 20% in hard cheese (*Parmesan, *Emmental, *Gruyère, *Cheddar) with semi-hard cheeses around 40% water (Caerphilly, *Gouda, *Edam, Stilton). They retain much of the calcium of the milk and many contain a relatively large amount of sodium from the added salt. Blue-veined cheeses (Gorgonzola, *Stilton, Roquefort, etc.) derive the colour (and flavour) from the growth of the mould *Penicillium roquefortii*, during ripening. Holes (e.g. in Gouda, Gruyère) arise during ripening from gases produced by bacteria.

Traditionally, hard cheeses must contain not less than 40% fat on a dry weight basis, and the fat must be milk fat. However, a number of low-fat variants of traditional hard cheeses, and vegetarian cheeses, are now made. A 40-g portion of hard cheese is a rich *source of vitamin B_{12} and calcium; a good source of protein and vitamin A; a source of vitamin B_2, iodine, and selenium; depending on type contains 9–16 g of fat of which 64–69% is saturated; provides 120–190 kcal (500–800 kJ).

Cottage cheese is soft, uncured, white cheese made from pasteurized skim milk (or milk powder) by lactic acid starter (with or without added rennet), heated, washed, and drained (salt may be added). Contains more than 80% water. Also known as pot cheese, Schmierkäse and, in the USA, as Dutch cheese. A 50-g portion is a *source of protein and supplies 50 kcal (210 kJ).

Baker's or hoop cheese is made in the same way as cottage cheese, but the curd is not washed, and it is drained in bags, giving it a finer grain. It contains more water and acid than cottage cheese.

Cream cheese is unripened soft cheese made from cream with varying fat content (20–25% fat or 50–55% fat); at 50% fat a 100-g portion is a rich *source of vitamins B_{12} and A and supplies 440 kcal (1800 kJ).

Processed cheese is made by milling various hard cheeses with emulsifying salts (phosphates and citrates), whey, and water, and pasteurizing to extend the shelf life of the cheese. Typically 40% water, a 30-g portion contains 5 g of protein and 8 g of fat, and provides 100 kcal (410 kJ). A soft version with 50% water is used as a spread.

Feta is Greek and general Balkan; white, soft, crumbly, salted cheese made from goat's or ewe's milk.

Swiss cheese is an American name for any hard cheese that contains relatively large bubbles of air, such as the Swiss Emmentaler and Gruyère cheeses.

cheese analogues Cheese-like products made from *casein or *soya and vegetable fat.

cheese, Austrian Classified according to butterfat content as percentage of dry weight as: *doppelfett* (double cream) 65%, *überfett* (extra cream) 55%, *vollfett* (full cream) 45%, *dreiviertelfett* 35%, *halbfett* 25%, *viertelfett* 15%, and *mager* under 15% fat.

cheesecake A flan or tart filled with curd or cream cheese. Traditional Middle-European cheesecake is baked; most cheesecakes now sold are uncooked, set with gelatine, and topped with fruit.

cheese, vegetarian Cheese in which animal *rennet has not been used to precipitate the curd. Precipitation is achieved using lactic acid alone, or a plant *enzyme or biosynthetic *chymosin. Truly vegetarian cheese is made from vegetable protein rather than milk.

cheese, whey Made from *whey by heat coagulation of the proteins (lactalbumin and lactoglobulin).

cheilosis Cracking of the edges of the lips, one of the clinical signs of *vitamin B_2 (riboflavin) deficiency.

chelating agents Chemicals that combine with metal ions and remove them from their sphere of action, hence also called sequestrants. They are used in food manufacture to remove traces of metal ions which might otherwise cause foods to deteriorate and clinically to reduce absorption of a mineral, or to increase its excretion; e.g. citrates, tartrates, phosphates, various calcium salts, and *EDTA.

Chelsea bun A yeast bun that originated in Chelsea, London, in the eighteenth century.

chemical caponization *See* capon.

chemical ice Ice containing a preservative, e.g. a solution of *antibiotics or other chemicals; used to preserve fish.

chemical score A measure of *protein quality based on chemical analysis. *See* amino acid, limiting.

chenin blanc One of the nine 'classic' *grape varieties used for *wine making; the great white grape of the middle Loire valley.

chenopods Seeds of two species of *Chenopodium* eaten in the Peruvian Andes: *C. quinoa* (*quinoa) and *C. pallidicaule* (*canihua). Other species of Chenopodium have been considered for poultry feed, including Russian thistle, summer cypress, and garden orache.

cherimoya *See* custard apple.

cherry Fruits of *Prunus* spp.; a 100-g portion (ten cherries weighed without stones) is a *source of vitamin C; provides 2 g of dietary fibre; supplies 50 kcal (210 kJ).

cherry, ground Fruit of *Physalis pruinosa*, similar to *Cape gooseberry (*Physalis peruviana*). Grows wild, and can be eaten raw but is more usually boiled or made into a preserve; also called strawberry tomato or dwarf Cape gooseberry.

cherry, maraschino Cherries preserved in maraschino (cherry *liqueur).

cherry, morello A sour cherry (*Prunus cerasus*) that cannot be eaten uncooked; used for cooking and making *liqueurs and jams.

cherry, Peruvian *See* Cape gooseberry.

cherry, Surinam *See* pitanga.

cherry, West Indian The fruit of a small bush native to the tropical and sub-tropical regions of America, *Malpighia punicifolia*. It is the richest known source of vitamin C; the edible portion of the ripe fruit contains 1000 mg, and the green fruit 3000 mg/100 g. Also known as Barbados or Antilles cherry, acerola.

chervil 1 A herb, *Anthriscus cerefolium*, with parsley-like leaves, used in the fresh green state as a garnish and fresh or dried to flavour salads and soups.
  2 The turnip-rooted chervil, *Chaerophyllum bulbosum*, a hardy biennial vegetable cultivated for its roots.

chervil, sweet *See* sweet cicely.

Cheshire cheese Oldest English *cheese dating from Roman Britain; crumbly, may be pale yellow, blue-veined, or coloured orange with *annatto; matured 2–6 weeks; approx. 30% water, 24% protein, 30% fat. Cheshire cat is an old English measure of cheese.

chest sweetbread The thymus of an animal, as distinct from the gut sweetbread (sometimes called simply sweetbread), which is the *pancreas.

chestnut 1 Spanish or sweet chestnut from trees of *Castanea* spp. Unlike other common nuts it contains very little fat, being largely starch and water. Seven nuts (75 g) provide 5.3 g of dietary fibre and are a good *source of copper; a source of vitamins B_1 and B_6; contain 2 g of fat of which 18% is saturated; supply 135 kcal (570 kJ).

2 Water chestnut, seeds of *Trapa natans*, also called caltrops or sinharanut; eaten raw or roasted.

3 Chinese water chestnut, also called matai or waternut; tuber of the sedge, *Eleocharis tuberosa* or *dulcis*; white flesh in a black, horned shell.

chestnut mushroom *See* mushrooms.

chevda (chewda) A dry and highly spiced mixture of deep-fried rice, *dahl, *chickpeas, and small pieces of chickpea batter, with peanuts and raisins, seasoned with sugar and salt, a common North Indian snack food, also known as Bombay mix.

chewing gum Based on *chicle with sugar or other sweetener, balsam of Tolu and various flavours.

chiao-tzu *See* wuntun.

chicharrones Caribbean; fried pork *crackling.

chicken Domestic fowl, *Gallus domesticus* (French: *poule*; German: *Hühn*). A 150-g portion is a rich *source of protein and niacin; a good source of copper and selenium; a source of iron and vitamins B_1, B_2, and B_6. There are differences between the white (breast) and dark (leg) meat, the former being lower in fat but also lower in iron and vitamin B_2. Of a 150-g portion of boiled chicken, the white meat supplies 0.9 mg of iron, 0.09 mg of vitamin B_1, 0.18 mg of vitamin B_2, 7.5 g of fat of which one-third is saturated; the dark meat supplies 3.8 mg of iron, 0.1 mg of vitamin B_1, 0.4 mg of vitamin B_2, 15 g of fat of which one-third is saturated.

Poussin or spring chicken is a young bird, 4–6 weeks old, weighing 250–300 g.

chicken cordon bleu Boned breast of chicken stuffed with cheese and ham, coated in batter and breadcrumbs, and baked.

chicken Kiev Boned breast of chicken stuffed with garlic butter, coated in batter and breadcrumbs, and baked.

chicken Marengo *See* Marengo.

chicken Maryland Chicken fried in breadcrumbs or batter, served with fruit fritters.

chicken, mountain *See* crapaud.

chickling pea or vetch *Lathyris sativus*, *see* lathyrism.

chickpea Also known as garbanzo; seeds of *Cicer arietinum*, widely used in Mediterranean and Middle-Eastern stews and casseroles. Puréed chickpea is the basis of *humus and deep-fried balls of chickpea batter are *felafel. A 90-g portion is a rich *source of copper; a good source of folate; a source of protein, vitamin A, and iron; contains 3 g of fat of which 6% is saturated; provides 4.5 g of dietary fibre; supplies 130 kcal (545 kJ).

chicle The partially evaporated milky latex of the evergreen sapodilla tree (*Achra sapota*); it contains gutta (which has elastic properties) and resin, together with carbohydrates, waxes, and tannins. The same tree also produces the *sapodilla plum.

chicory Witloof or Belgian chicory (Belgian endive in the USA), *Cichorium intybus*; looks like a dandelion; the root is harvested and grown in the dark to produce bullet-shaped heads of young white leaves (chicons). Also called succory; red variety is radicchio. The leaves are eaten as a salad or braised as a vegetable and the bitter root, dried and partly caramelized, is often added to coffee as a diluent to cheapen the product. A 50-g portion of chicons supplies 1 g of dietary fibre, a little vitamin C, and 5 kcal (20 kJ).

chiffonade Shredded green vegetables.

chilled foods Perishable products stored at temperatures between 0 and 7 ˚C.

chill haze *See* haze.

chilli (chili) *See* pepper.

chilli (chili) sauce Piquant sauce made from tomatoes, with spices, onions, garlic, sugar, vinegar, and salt. Similar to tomato ketchup but containing more cayenne, onion, and garlic.

chilli con carne Minced beef stewed with onion, chilli, and red kidney beans; originally Mexican and south-western USA.

chillproofing A treatment to prevent the development of haziness or cloudiness due to precipitation of proteins when beer is chilled. Treatments include the addition of *tannins to precipitate proteins, materials such as *bentonite to adsorb them and proteolytic *enzymes to hydrolyse them.

china Italian; bitter aperitif wines containing *quinine.

chincona Spanish; bitter aperitif wines containing *quinine.

chine A joint of meat containing the whole or part of the backbone of the animal. *See also* chining.

Chinese cabbage (Chinese leaves) *See* cabbage, Chinese.

Chinese cherry *See* lychee.

Chinese eggs Known as pidan, houeidan, and dsaoudan, depending on variations in the method of preparation. Prepared by covering fresh duck eggs with a mixture of caustic soda, burnt straw ash, and slaked lime, then storing for several months (they are sometimes referred to as 'hundred year old eggs'). The white and yolk coagulate and become discoloured, with partial decomposition of the protein and *phospholipids.

Chinese gooseberry *See* kiwi fruit.

Chinese Restaurant Syndrome Flushing, palpitations, numbness associated at one time with the consumption of *monosodium glutamate, and then with *histamine, but the cause of these symptoms after eating various foods is not known.

Chinese water chestnut *See* chestnut.

chining To sever the rib bones from the backbone by sawing through the ribs close to the spine. *See also* chine.

chino Spanish; small conical strainer used to sieve chopped vegetables to make *gazpacho.

chipolata Small *sausage.

chips Chipped potatoes; pieces of potato deep fried in fat or oil. Known in French as *pommes frites* or just *frites*; in the USA *potato crisps are known as chips, and chips are called French fries or just fries. A 200-g portion is a rich *source of vitamins C and B$_1$; a source of protein, niacin, and iron; fat content depends on the size of the chip and the process: commonly about 25 g, but can be 40 g in fine-cut chips and as little as 8 g in frozen, oven-baked chips. Degree of saturation of the fat depends on the frying oil: 10% in blended oils, and up to 60% in dripping. A 200-g portion with an average of 25 g of fat supplies 500 kcal (2100 kJ); with 40 g of fat, supplies 700 kcal (2900 kJ); low-fat, oven-baked supplies 300 kcal (1260 kJ). *See also* crisps.

chiretto Italian; rosé wines (also cerasuolo or rosato).

chirga Indian; skinned chicken rubbed with cayenne, paprika, and lime juice, coated with a sauce of ginger, onion, and pimiento in yoghurt, then roasted, basting with *ghee. It has a red colour.

chitin The organic matrix of the hard parts of the exoskeleton of insects and crustaceans, and present in small amounts in mushrooms. It is an insoluble and indigestible *non-starch polysaccharide, similar to *cellulose, but composed of N-acetylglucosamine units rather than glucose. Partial deacetylation results in the formation of chitosans, which are used as protein-flocculating agents.

chitosans *See* chitin.

chitterlings The (usually fried) small intestine of ox, calf, or pig.

chive Small member of the onion family (*Allium schoenoprasum*); the leaves are used as a garnish or dried as a herb; mild onion flavour.

chlorella *See* algae.

chlorine An element found in biological tissues as the chloride *ion; the body contains about 100 g (3 mol) of chloride and the average diet contains 6–7 g (0.17–0.2 mol), mainly as sodium chloride (ordinary salt). Free chlorine is used as a sterilizing agent, e.g. for drinking water.

chlorine dioxide A bread improver, *see* ageing.

chlorophyll The green pigment of plant materials which is responsible for the trapping of light energy for photosynthesis, the formation of carbohydrates from carbon dioxide and water. Both α- and β-chlorophylls occur in leaves, together with the *carotenoids xanthophyll and carotene. Chlorophyll has no nutritional value, although it does contain *magnesium as part of its molecule, and although it is used in breath-fresheners and toothpaste, there is no evidence that it has any useful action.

chlorophyllide The green colour found in the water after cooking some vegetables; it is a water-soluble derivative of *chlorophyll formed by either enzymic action (chlorophyllase in the vegetables) or alkaline hydrolysis.

chlortetracycline An *antibiotic.

cho-cho *See* chayote.

chocolate Made from cocoa nibs (husked, fermented, and roasted *cocoa beans) by refining and the addition of sugar, *cocoa butter, flavouring, *lecithin, and, for milk chocolate, milk solids. It may also contain vegetable oils other than cocoa butter. A 100-g portion of milk chocolate is a rich *source of copper; a good source of calcium; a source of protein, vitamin B_2, iron, and selenium; contains 30 g of fat of which 60% is saturated and 30% mono-unsaturated; supplies 540 kcal (2270 kJ). A 100-g portion of plain chocolate is a rich *source of copper; a source of protein and iron; fat and energy as for milk chocolate.

chocolate, drinking Partially solubilized cocoa powder for preparation of a chocolate-flavoured milk drink, containing about 75% sucrose.

cholagogue A substance that stimulates the secretion of *bile from the gall bladder into the duodenum.

cholecalciferol *See* vitamin D.

cholelithiasis *See* gall stones.

cholent Traditional Jewish and Middle-European casserole of beans and beef, cooked extremely slowly (traditionally overnight beside the baker's oven).

cholesterol The principal sterol in animal tissues, an essential component of cell membranes and the precursor for the formation of the *steroid hormones. It is transported in the plasma *lipoproteins. Not a dietary essential, since it is synthesized in the body. Eggs contain about 450 mg, milk 14 mg, cheese 70–120 mg, brain 2.2 g, liver and kidney 300–600 mg, poultry 70–100 mg, and fish 50–60 mg/100 g.

An elevated plasma concentration of cholesterol is a risk factor for *atherosclerosis. The synthesis of cholesterol in the body is increased by a high intake of *saturated fats, but apart from people with a rare genetic defect in the regulation of cholesterol synthesis, a high dietary intake of cholesterol does not affect the plasma concentration, since there is normally strict control over the rate of synthesis. *See also* hypercholesterolaemia; hyperlipidaemia; HMG CoA reductase inhibitors; lipids, plasma.

cholestyramine Drug used to treat *hyperlipidaemia by complexing *bile salts in the intestinal lumen and increasing their excretion, so increasing the metabolic clearance of *cholesterol.

choline A derivative of the amino acid *serine, formed in the body; an important component of cell membranes. Phosphatidylcholine is also known as *lecithin, and preparations of mixed phospholipids rich in phosphatidylcholine are generally called lecithin, although they also contain other phospholipids; lecithin from *peanuts and *soya beans is widely used as an emulsifying agent (E-322). Choline released from membrane phospholipids is important for the formation of the neurotransmitter *acetylcholine, and choline is also important in the metabolism of methyl groups.

Choline is synthesized in the body, and it is a ubiquitous component of cell membranes and therefore occurs in all foods, so that dietary deficiency is unknown. Deficiency has been observed in patients on long-term total *parenteral nutrition, suggesting that the ability to synthesize choline is inadequate to meet requirements without some intake. There is no evidence on which to base estimates of requirements; the average intake is between 0.25–0.5 g/day.

cholla (challa) A loaf of white bread made in a twisted form by plaiting together a large and small piece of dough (the biblical beehive coil). The dough is made from white flour, enriched with eggs and a pinch of saffron, and the loaf is decorated with poppy seed. It is mentioned in the Bible, translated as 'loaves', and is traditionally used for benediction of the Jewish sabbath and festivals.

chondroitin A polysaccharide, classified as a mucopolysaccharide, a polymer of galactosamine and glucuronic acid. Chondroitin sulphate is a component of cartilage and the organic matrix of bone.

chondrometer An instrument used to determine the specific weight of wheat (kg/hectolitre). A wet English wheat may weigh 68 kg, and a dry American wheat 84 kg/hectolitre.

Chondrus crispus A seaweed, the source of *carrageenan.

chop A slice of mutton, lamb, or pork containing a part of the bone; commonly the rib, but also cut from the chump or tail end of the loin (chump chops) or neck (then called cutlets).

chopsuey Chinese dishes based on bean sprouts and shredded vegetables, cooked with shredded quick-fried meat, capped with a thin omelette. Not authentically Chinese, but an invention of Chinese restaurateurs in Western countries. Unlike true Chinese food, the flavours of a chopsuey are all mixed together; one translation is 'savoury mess'.

chorizo Spanish; coarse textured, red, spiced *sausage.

Chorleywood bread process A method of preparing dough for bread making by submitting it to intense mechanical working, so that, together with the aid of oxidizing agents, the need for bulk fermentation of the dough is eliminated. This is a so-called 'no-time' process and saves $1^{1}/_{2}$–2 hours in the process; permits use of an increased proportion of weaker flour, and produces a softer, finer loaf, which stales more slowly. Named after the British Baking Industries Research Association at Chorleywood.

choux (chou) pastry Light, airy pastry, invented by the French chef Carême, used in *éclairs and *profitéroles. The batter is pre-cooked in a saucepan, then baked. The name comes from the French for cabbage, *chou*, because of the characteristic shape of the cream-filled puffs.

chow-chow Chinese; preserve of ginger, orange peel and fruit in syrup, or a mixed vegetable pickle containing mustard and spices.

chowder Thick soup made from shellfish (especially clams) or other fish, with pork or bacon. Originally French, now mainly New England and Newfoundland.

chow mein Chinese; dishes based on fried noodles.

chrane Jewish and Middle-European condiment made from beetroot and horseradish.

christophene See chayote.

chromium A metallic element that is a dietary essential. It forms an organic complex with *nicotinic acid, known as the glucose tolerance factor, which facilitates the interaction of *insulin with receptors on cell surfaces. Deficiency results in impaired *glucose tolerance.

There is little evidence on which to base estimates of requirements; deficiency has been observed at intakes below 6 µg (0.12 µmol)/day, and the *safe and adequate level of intake is estimated at about 25 µg (0.5 µmol)/day. High intakes of inorganic chromium salts (in excess of 1–2 g/day) are associated with kidney and liver damage.

chromoproteins Proteins conjugated with a metal-containing group, such as the haem group of *haemoglobin, which contains iron.

chuck See beef.

chufa See tiger nut.

chump chop See chop.

chuño Traditional dried potato prepared in the highlands of Peru and Bolivia. The tubers are crushed, pressed, frozen during the night, then dried in the sunshine during the day, a process of freeze-drying.

chupatti See chapatti.

churros Spanish; sausage-shaped, deep-fried doughnuts, dusted with sugar.

chutney Pickled fruits or vegetables, normally spiced, used as a relish; of Indian origin.

chyle See lymph.

chylomicrons The droplets of unhydrolysed fat (triglycerides) absorbed from the small intestine into the lymphatic system, circulating in the *lymph and bloodstream. See also lipids, plasma.

chymase Alternative name for *chymosin.

chyme The partly digested mass of food as it exists in the stomach.

chymosin *Enzyme in the abomasum of calves and the stomach of human infants which clots milk by precipitation of the casein. There is no evidence that it plays any part in digestion in the adult. Also known as rennin; however, to avoid confusion with the kidney enzyme renin the name rennin should be replaced by chymosin. Biosynthetic chymosin is used in cheese making (vegetable *rennet). See also cheese.

chymotrypsin An *enzyme involved in the *digestion of proteins; secreted as the inactive precursor chymotrypsinogen in the pancreatic juice. It is activated by *trypsin, and is an *endopeptidase, with a different specificity from trypsin and *pepsin.

ciabatta See bread.

cibophobia Dislike of food.

cider, cyder An *alcoholic beverage; fermented *apple juice (in the UK may include not more than 25% *pear juice). Dry cider has 2.6% sugars, 3.8% alcohol, and 110 kcal (460 kJ) per 300 mL. Sweet cider has 4.3% sugars and supplies 125 kcal (525 kJ) per 300 mL. Vintage cider has 7.3% sugars, 10.5% alcohol, and supplies 300 kcal (1260 kJ) per 300 mL (half pint).

In the USA cider or fresh cider is the term used for unfermented apple juice; the fermented product is termed hard or fermented cider.

cieddu *See* milk, fermented.

ciguatera Poisoning from eating fish feeding in the region of coral reefs in the Caribbean and the Indian and Pacific Oceans. The species of fish are normally edible, and appear to derive the toxins, ciguatoxins, from their diet. Reported in seafarers' tales in the sixteenth century.

ciguatoxins The toxins responsible for *ciguatera.

cinnamon The aromatic bark of various species of the genus *Cinnamomum*; it is split from the shoots, cured, and dried. During drying the bark shrinks and curls into a cylinder or 'quill'. It is used as a flavour in meat products, bakery goods, and confectionery, and may be available either as the whole quill or powdered ready for use.

Ceylon or true cinnamon (*C. zeylican*) differs from other types and the oil contains mostly cinnamic aldehyde, together with some eugenol. Saigon cinnamon also contains cineol; Chinese cinnamon has no eugenol.

cinsaut A *grape variety widely used for *wine making, although not one of the classic varieties. The common bulk wine producing grape of southern France. In South Africa it has been crossed with the pinot noir to produce the pinotage grape.

cis- A chemical prefix sometimes found on food labels to designate the precise chemical form of polyunsaturated fatty acids (as in the phrase '*cis-cis* methylene interrupted'). This is used because some compounds can exist in two forms with the same chemical structure but with different shapes and so have different biological activities. The opposite conformation to *cis-* is the *trans-* form.

cissa An unnatural desire for foods; alternative words, cittosis, allotriophagy, and pica.

citral An important constituent of many essential oils, especially lemon. Used as the starting material for the synthesis of ionone (the synthetic perfume with an odour of violets), which is an intermediate in the chemical synthesis of *retinol.

citrange An American *citrus fruit resulting from a cross between the ordinary orange and the trifoliate orange, *Poncirus trifoliata*.

citric acid An organic *acid (chemically a tricarboxylic acid) which is widely distributed in plant and animal tissues; it is an important metabolic intermediate, and yields 2.47 kcal (10.9 kJ)/g. It is used as a flavouring and acidifying agent (E-330), and its salts (citrates) are used as acidity regulators (E-331, 332, 333). Commercially it is either prepared by the fermentation of sugars by the mould *Aspergillus niger* or extracted from citrus fruits (lemon juice contains 5–8% citric acid).

citrin A mixture of two flavonones found in citrus pith, hesperidin and eriodictin. A constituent of what is sometimes called *vitamin P.

citron The first of the *citrus fruits to become known to Europeans; *Citrus medica*; can be grown only in warm regions. The fruit has a very thick peel and solid, sweet, and acid-free pith with practically no juice. It is used for preparing *candied peel.

citronella Lemon-scented tropical grass *Cymbopogon nardus* used in salads and dressings; the essential oil is also used as an insect repellent.

citronin A flavonone *glycoside from the peel of immature Ponderosa lemons; *see* flavonoids.

citrovorum factor The name given to a growth factor for the micro-organism *Leuconostoc citrovorum*, now known to be one of the main forms of the vitamin *folic acid (chemically formyl-tetrahydropteroylglutamic acid).

citroxanthin A yellow *carotenoid pigment in orange peel which has vitamin A activity. Also known as mutachrome.

citrullinaemia A *genetic disease affecting the formation of urea, and hence the elimination of end-products of protein metabolism. The defect may be mild, or so severe that affected infants become comatose and may die after a moderately high intake of protein. Treatment is usually by restriction of protein intake and feeding supplements of the amino acid arginine. Sodium benzoate may be given to increase the excretion of nitrogenous waste as hippuric acid. *See also* benzoic acid.

citrulline An *amino acid formed as a metabolic intermediate, but not involved in proteins, and of no nutritional importance.

Citrus Genus of trees with fleshy, juicy fruits; there is considerable confusion over the names because of hybridization and mutations. Sweet orange *Citrus sinensis*; various cultivars including Valencia, Washington navel, Jaffa, Shamouti. Sour, bitter, or Seville orange, *C. aurantium*, is too bitter to eat and is used for marmalade. Lemon, *C. limon*. Lime, *C. aurantifolia*. Citron, *C. medica*, has white, white inner skin and is used mainly to make candied peel. Pomelo (shaddock), *C. grandis*, is the parent of the grapefruit. Grapefruit, *C. paradisi*, is a hybrid of pomelo and sweet orange. Tangerine, satsuma, mandarin, calamondin, naartje (S. Africa), are small citrus fruits with loose skins. Clementine, a hybrid of tangerine and bitter orange, is sometimes regarded as a variety of tangerine. Mineola is a hybrid of grapefruit and tangerine. Ortanique is a hybrid of orange and tangerine, unique to Jamaica. Citrange is a hybrid of citron and orange. Tangors are hybrids of tangerine and sweet orange (e.g. Variety Temple). Ugli fruit is a hybrid of grapefruit and tangerine. Tangelo is a hybrid of tangerine and pomelo. All are a rich *source of vitamin C and contain up to 10% sugars (glucose and fructose).

cittosis An unnatural desire for foods; alternative words are, cissa, allotriophagy, and pica.

clabbered milk Unpasteurized milk that has soured naturally, becoming thick and curdy. Clabber cheese is curd or cottage cheese.

clafoutis French; batter pudding with black cherries or other fruit.

claims, misleading descriptions There are no restrictions on the sales of foods so long as they are not harmful and do not transgress the regulations. What is controlled by law is any claim (on the label, leaflets, or in advertisements). It is illegal to claim that a food is capable of preventing, treating, or curing a disease unless it has a specific Product Licence under the Medicines Act. Misleading claims are illegal even if, strictly speaking, they are true.

clam bake American; beach picnic.

clam chowder *See* chowder.

clams (French: *rye*; German: *Steckmuschel*.) Several types of marine bivalve molluscs, including *scallop, large tropical clam, *Tridacna gigas*, quahog, *Mya arenaria*, and *Venus mercenaria*. A 100-g portion of clams is an exceptionally rich *source of vitamin B_{12}; a good source of protein and niacin; contains 120 mg of sodium; supplies 60 kcal (250 kJ).

clapshot Scottish (Orkney); mashed potato and turnip, seasoned with chives and bacon fat.

claret Name given in the UK to red wines from the Bordeaux region of France.

clarete Portuguese, Spanish; light red wines.

clarification The process of clearing a liquid of suspended particles. It may be carried out by filtration, *centrifugation, the addition of *enzymes to hydrolyse and solubilize particulate matter (proteolytic or pectolytic enzymes), or the addition of flocculating agents.

clarifixation A method of homogenizing milk in which the cream is separated, homogenized, and remixed with the milk in one machine (the clarifixator).

clarifying Of fats; freeing the fat of water so that it can be used for frying, pastry-making, etc. Clarified fats are less susceptible to *rancidity on storage; ghee is clarified butterfat. Also the process of filtering juices before making jellies, etc.

Clarke degrees Units of measurement of *water hardness.

clay A dried mineral clay under the names of sikor, mithi, pakhuri, and khatta, is sometimes used by Asians as a treatment for indigestion and as a vitamin supplement, but can be toxic since it contains varying amounts of arsenic and lead.

clementine A *citrus fruit, *Citrus nobilis* var. *deliciosa*; regarded by some as a variety of tangerine and by others as a cross between the tangerine and a wild North African orange.

clofibrate Drug used to treat *hyperlipidaemia by lowering specifically low density lipoproteins. *See also* lipids, plasma.

Clostridium A genus of bacteria, of which *C. botulinum* is responsible for *botulism, a rare but often fatal form of food poisoning. It is found widely distributed in soil; during growth on favourable food materials, the organism synthesizes an extremely potent neurotoxin which is released into the food when the cell dies. The spores are the most heat-resistant food-poisoning organism encountered and their thermal death time is used as a minimum standard for processing foods with *pH values higher than 4.5.

cloudberry An orange-yellow fruit resembling the raspberry in shape; *Rubus chamaemorus*, known as avron in Scotland, and baked-apple berry in Canada. It is an extremely rich natural source of *benzoic acid and will not ferment; it remains fresh for many months without preservation.

clove The dried aromatic flower buds of *Caryophyllus aromaticus*; mother of clove is the ripened fruit, which is inferior in flavour. Used as a flavour in meat products and baked goods.

club sandwich American; double-decker sandwich made with toast, turkey, lettuce, bacon, and mayonnaise.

club soda *See* soda water.

club steak American name for *entrecôte steak.

CMC Carboxymethylcellulose, *see* cellulose derivatives.

Co I, Co II Abbreviations of coenzymes I and II, now known as nicotinamide adenine dinucleotide (*NAD) and nicotinamide adenine dinucleotide phosphate (NADP), respectively.

CoA (Coenzyme A) *See* coenzymes.

coacervation The heat-reversible aggregation of the *amylopectin form of *starch, which is believed to be one of the mechanisms involved in the staling of bread.

coagulase The name given to an enzyme said to be present in milk and to account for the ability of milk to clot a solution of fibrinogen.

coagulation A process involving the denaturation of proteins, the loss of their native, soluble structure, so that they become insoluble; it may be effected by heat, strong acids and alkalis, metals, and various other chemical agents. Some proteins are coagulated by specific enzymic action. Coagulation occurs when, for example, an egg is cooked or flour dough is baked, and the action of *chymosin in cheese making is to coagulate the proteins of milk.

Denaturation is due to the breaking of hydrogen bonds which maintain the protein in its native structure. As the process continues, there is considerable unfolding of the protein, and interaction between adjacent molecules, forming aggregates which reach such a size that they precipitate, i.e. coagulate.

coagulation, blood The final stage in blood clotting is the precipitation of fibrils of insoluble fibrin, formed from the soluble plasma protein fibrinogen. This is an example of *coagulation caused by the action of an *enzyme; the enzyme responsible is prothrombin, which is normally inactive, but in response to injury is activated by a cascade of events. *Vitamin K is required for the synthesis of prothrombin, and clotting requires calcium ions. *See also* blood plasma.

coalfish, coley Saithe, *Pollachius virens; see* fish.

cobalamin *See* vitamin B_{12}.

cobalt A mineral whose main function is in *vitamin B_{12}, although there are some cobalt-dependent *enzymes. There is no evidence of cobalt deficiency in human beings, and no evidence on which to base estimates of requirements for inorganic cobalt. 'Pining disease' in cattle and sheep is due to cobalt deficiency (their intestinal micro-organisms synthesize vitamin B_{12}) and is a growth factor for chicks, turkeys, pigs, and rats. Cobalt salts are toxic in excess, causing degeneration of the heart muscle, and habitual intakes in excess of 300 mg/day are considered undesirable.

cobamide A derivative of *vitamin B_{12}.

cobbler 1 Sweetened cold drink made from fruit with wine or liqueur and ice.

    2 Meat or fruit dishes topped with scone rounds.

cob nut *See* hazel nut.

coburg cakes Small cakes containing syrup and flavoured with spices.

Coca Cola Trade name for a *cola drink. *See also* coca leaves.

coca leaves From the S. American plant, *Erythroxylon coca*; they contain the narcotic alkaloid cocaine, and are traditionally chewed by the natives of Peru as a stimulant. Originally the beverage *Coca Cola contained coca leaf extract, although this was removed from the formulation many years ago.

cocarboxylase An obsolete name for thiamin diphosphate, the metabolically active *coenzyme form of *vitamin B_1.

cocarcinogen A substance which, alone, does not cause the induction of cancer, but potentiates the action of a *carcinogen.

cochineal A water-soluble red colour obtained from the female conchilla, *Dactilopius coccus* (*Coccus cactus*), an insect found in Mexico, Central America, and the Caribbean; 1 kg of the colour is obtained from about 150 000 insects. Legally permitted in foods in most countries (E-120). Contains carminic acid (E-120). Cochineal red A is an alternative name for *Ponceau 4R (E-124), often used to replace cochineal. Carmine is produced from cochineal.

cock-a-leekie Scottish; soup made from leeks and chicken.

cockles (arkshell) Several types of marine bivalve molluscs of genus *Cardium*, often sold preserved in brine or vinegar. A 50-g portion is a rich *source of iron, iodine, and selenium; a source of protein and copper; contains 0.2 g of fat of which 33% is saturated; supplies 25 kcal (105 kJ).

cock of the wood *See* capercaillie.

cocktail Mixed alcoholic drink; there are many recipes based on a wide variety of spirits and liqueurs, with fruit juice, milk, or coconut milk, normally shaken with crushed ice.

cocoa Originally known as cacao, introduced into Europe from Mexico by the Spaniards in the early sixteenth century. The powder prepared from the seed embedded in the fruit of the cocoa plant, *Theobroma cacao*, also a milk drink prepared with cocoa powder. Used to prepare *chocolate. Contains the *alkaloid *theobromine; *caffeine is trimethylxanthine.

cocoa butter The fat from the cocoa bean, used in chocolate manufacture and in pharmaceuticals; it has a low sharp melting point, between 31 and 35 °C, so it melts in the mouth; mostly 2-oleopalmitostearin.

cocoa butter equivalents Vegetable fats (and various mixtures) with physical and chemical properties similar to those of cocoa butter; useful for the partial or complete replacement of cocoa butter, which is expensive. Examples are illipe and shea nut butter.

cocoa, Dutch Cocoa treated with a dilute solution of alkali (carbonate or bicarbonate) to improve its colour, flavour, and solubility. The process is known as 'Dutching'.

cocoa nibs Seeds of the fruit of the cocoa plant, *Theobroma cacao*, are left to ferment, which modifies the bitterness, and their colour darkens. They are then roasted and separated from the husks as two halves of the seed known as cocoa nibs. They contain about 50% fat, part of which is removed in the preparation of chocolate and cocoa for beverages.

cocolait A form of coconut 'milk' made by applying high pressure to coconuts and homogenizing the oil and water emulsion plus coconut water (coconut milk) obtained. Bottled and used (e.g. in the Philippines) in place of cow's milk.

coconut Fruit of the tropical palm, *Cocos nucifera*. The dried nut is copra which contains 60–65% coconut oil. The residue after extraction of the oil is used for animal feed. The hollow, unripe nut contains a watery liquid known as coconut milk, which is gradually absorbed as the fruit ripens. A 50-g portion is a rich *source of copper; contains 18 g of fat of which 90% is saturated; provides 7 g of dietary fibre; supplies 175 kcal (735 kJ).

coconut oil Semi-solid oil extracted from copra (dried *coconut), *Cocos nucifera*; contains 90% saturated fats.

cocotte, en Describes a dish cooked and served in a small casserole.

cocoyam New cocoyam is the West African name for *tannia; the old cocoyam is the West African name for *taro.

cod A white *fish, *Gaddus morrhua* and other species. The composition of all non-fatty fish, such as cod, hake, haddock, flatfish, is similar.

coddle To cook slowly in water kept just below boiling point.

Codes of Practice In the area of food production these refer to standards of procedure which cannot be covered by exact specifications and serve as agreed guidelines. They may originate from Government Departments, trade organizations, the Institute of Food Science and Technology, or individual companies.

Codex Alimentarius Originally Codex Alimentarius Europaeus; since 1961 part of the United Nations FAO/WHO Commission on Food Standards to simplify and integrate food standards for adoption internationally.

cod liver oil The oil from codfish liver; the classic source of vitamins A and D, used for its medicinal properties long before the vitamins were discovered. An average sample contains 120–1200 µg vitamin A and

1–10 μg vitamin D per gram. British Pharmacopoeia standard: minimum 180 μg vitamin A and 2 μg vitamin D per gram.

coeliac disease (celiac disease) Intolerance of the proteins of wheat, rye, and barley; specifically, the gliadin fraction of the protein *gluten. The villi of the small intestine are severely affected and absorption of food is poor. Stools are bulky and fermenting from unabsorbed carbohydrate, and contain a large amount of unabsorbed fat (steatorrhoea). As a result of the malabsorption, affected people are malnourished and children suffer from growth retardation. Treatment is by exclusion of wheat, rye, and barley proteins (the starches are tolerated); rice, oats, and maize are generally tolerated. Manufactured foods that are free from gluten, and hence suitable for consumption by people with coeliac disease are usually labelled as 'gluten-free'. Also known as gluten-induced enteropathy, and sometimes as non-tropical sprue.

coenzymes Organic compounds required for the activity of some *enzymes; most are derived from vitamins. Coenzymes that remain tightly bound to the enzyme at all times are sometimes known as prosthetic groups, non-protein components of the enzyme molecule. Other coenzymes act to transfer groups from one enzyme to another, e.g. *coenzyme A transfers acetyl groups between enzymes, *NAD transfers hydrogen between enzymes in oxidation and reduction reactions.

An enzyme that requires a tightly bound coenzyme is inactive in the absence of its coenzyme; this can be exploited to assess *vitamin B_1, B_2, and B_6 *nutritional status, by measuring the activity of enzymes that require coenzymes derived from these vitamins (*see* enzyme activation tests).

Coenzyme A (CoA) is derived from the *vitamin *pantothenic acid; it is required for the transfer and metabolism of acetyl groups (and other fatty acyl groups).

Coenzyme I and coenzyme II are obsolete names for nicotinamide adenine dinucleotide (*NAD) and nicotinamide adenine dinucleotide phosphate (NADP). Coenzyme Q is *ubiquinone; coenzyme R is the obsolete name for *biotin.

cœur à la crème *See* fromage à la crème.

coffee A beverage produced by roasting the beans from the berries of two principal types of shrub: *Coffea arabica* (arabica coffee) and *C. canephora* (robusta coffee). *Niacin is formed during the roasting process, and the coffee can contain 10–40 mg of niacin per 100 g, depending on the extent of roasting, thus making a significant contribution to average intakes of niacin.

Instant coffee is dried coffee extract which can be used to make a beverage by adding hot water or milk. It may be manufactured by *spray-drying or *freeze-drying. Coffee essence is an aqueous extract of roasted coffee; usually about 400 g of coffee/L.

Coffee contains *caffeine. Decaffeinated coffee is coffee beans (or instant coffee) from which the *caffeine has been extracted with solvent (e.g. methylene or ethylene chloride), carbon dioxide under pressure (supercritical CO_2), or water. Coffee decaffeinated by water extraction is sometimes labelled as 'naturally' decaffeinated.

coffee, Irish Sweetened coffee, laced with Irish whiskey and with cream floated on top. Originated in Chinatown in San Francisco. Many restaurants offer a range of related speciality coffees laced with spirits such as rum or brandy, or liqueurs such as Tia Maria.

coffee sugar *See* sugar.

coffee whitener *See* creamer, non-dairy.

cognac *Brandy made in the Charentes region of north-west France, around the town of Cognac, from special varieties of grape grown on shallow soil and claimed to be distilled only in pot, not continuous, stills. Sometimes used (incorrectly) as a general name for brandy. *See also* armagnac.

cointreau Orange-flavoured liqueur.

cola drinks *Carbonated drinks containing extract of cola bean, the seed of the tree *Cola acuminata*, and a variety of other flavouring ingredients. Cola seed contains *caffeine, and the drink contains 10–15 mg caffeine/100 mL; decaffeinated or caffeine-free varieties are also made.

colcannon 1 Irish; potato mashed with kale or cabbage, often fried (*see also* bubble and squeak).
  2 Scottish; cabbage, carrots, potatoes, and turnips mashed together.

colchicine An *alkaloid isolated from the meadow saffron, or autumn crocus (*Colchicum* spp.). It is an old remedy for *gout. It inhibits cell division, and is used in experimental horticulture to produce plants with abnormal numbers of genes.

cold preservation *See* Campden process.

cold-shortening (of meat) When the temperature of muscle is reduced below 10 ˚C while the *pH remains above 6–6.2 (early in the post-mortem conversion of glycogen to lactic acid) the muscle contracts in reaction to cold and, when cooked, the meat is tough.

cold sterilization *See* irradiation; sterilization, cold.

cold store bacteria *See* psychrophilic bacteria.

cole, coleseed *See* rape.

colectomy Surgical removal of all or part of the colon, to treat cancer or severe ulcerative *colitis.

coleslaw Salad made from finely shredded white cabbage dressed with cream or mayonnaise; other vegetables may be included.

colewort *See* collard.

coley, coalfish Saithe, *Pollachius virens*; *see* fish.

coliform bacteria A group of aerobic, lactose-fermenting bacteria, of which *Escherichia coli* is the most important member. Many coliforms are not harmful, but since they arise from faeces, they are useful as a test of faecal contamination, and particularly as a test for water pollution. Some strains of *E. coli* produce toxins, or are otherwise pathogenic, and are associated with *food poisoning.

colitis Inflammation of the large intestine, with pain, diarrhoea, and weight loss; there may be ulceration of the large intestine (ulcerative colitis). *See also* Crohn's disease; gastro-intestinal tract; irritable bowel syndrome.

collagen Insoluble protein in *connective tissue, bones, tendons, and skin of animals and fish; converted into the soluble protein, *gelatine, by moist heat.

collagen sugar An old name for *glycine.

collard (collard greens) American name for varieties of cabbage (*Brassica oleracea*) which do not form a compact head. Generally known in the UK as greens or spring greens.

collared Pickled or salted meat which is rolled, boiled with seasonings and served cold.

colloid Particles (the disperse phase) suspended in a second medium (the dispersion medium); can be solid, liquid, or gas suspended in a solid, liquid, or gas. Examples of gas-in-liquid colloids are beaten egg-white and whipped cream; of liquid-in-liquid colloids, emulsions such as milk and salad cream. *See also* emulsifying agents; stabilizers.

collop Scottish; originally a small boneless piece of meat (from the French *escalope*); now a savoury dish made from finely minced meat.

colocasia *See* taro.

cologel Alternative name for methylcellulose, *see* cellulose derivatives.

colon Also known as the large intestine or bowel, consisting of three anatomical regions: the ascending, the transverse, and the descending colon. The colon normally has a considerable population of bacteria, while it is rare to find a significant bacterial population in the small intestine. The colon terminates at the rectum, where faeces are compacted and stored before voiding. *See also* gastro-intestinal tract.

colon, spastic *See* irritable bowel syndrome.

colostomy Surgical creation of an artificial conduit on the abdominal wall for voiding of intestinal contents following surgical removal of much of the colon and/or rectum. *See also* gastro-intestinal tract.

colostrum The milk produced by mammals during the first few days after parturition; compared with mature human milk, human colostrum contains more protein (2 compared with 1.3 g/100 mL); slightly less lactose (6.6 compared with 7.2 g/100 mL), considerably less fat (2.6 compared with 4.1 g/100 mL), and overall slightly less energy (56 kcal (235 kJ)/100 mL compared with 69 kcal (290 kJ)). Colostrum is a valuable source of antibodies for the new-born infant. Animal colostrum is sometimes known as beestings.

colours Widely used in foods to increase their aesthetic appeal; may be natural, *nature-identical, or synthetic. Natural colours include carotenoids (yellow to orange-red in apricots, carrots, maize, tomatoes), some of which are vitamin precursors. *Chlorophylls are the green pigments in all leaves and stems. *Anthocyanins are the red, blue, and violet pigments in beetroots, raspberries, and red cabbage. *Flavones are yellow pigments in most leaves and flowers. There are twenty permitted synthetic colours (mainly azo dyes). *Caramel is used for both flavour and as a brown colour made by heating sugar.

In addition to all these there are various ingredients such as paprika, saffron, and turmeric that also provide colour. *See* Appendix VIII.

colza *See* rapeseed; colza oil is rapeseed oil.

COMA Committee on Medical Aspects of Food Policy; permanent Advisory Committee to the UK Department of Health.

combining diet *See* Hay diet.

comfrey Wild member of the *borage family, *Symphytum officinale*. Leaves may be cooked like spinach or fried in batter.

comminuted Finely divided; used with reference to minced meat products and fruit drinks made from crushed whole fruit including the peel.

Complan Trade name for a mixture of dried skim milk, arachis oil, casein, maltodextrins, sugar, and vitamins, used as a nutritional supplement.

complementation This term is used with respect to proteins when a relative deficiency of an *amino acid in one is compensated by a relative surplus from another protein consumed at the same time. The *protein quality is not the average of the separate values, but higher.

complex carbohydrate Polysaccharides, both *starch and *non-starch polysaccharides; *see* carbohydrate.

compôte Fruit stewed with sugar; a single fruit or a mixture, served hot or cold. Also sometimes used for a stew of small birds such as pigeons.

conalbumin One of the proteins of egg-white, comprising 12% of the total solids. It binds iron in a pink-coloured complex; this accounts for the pinkish colour resulting when eggs are stored in rusty containers.

con crianza Spanish; aged wines.

condé Dessert of creamed rice with fruit and red jam sauce. Also the name of a type of patisserie.

condiment Seasoning added to flavour foods, such as salt, or herbs and spices such as mustard, ginger, curry, pepper, etc. Although some are relatively rich in nutrients, they are generally used in such small quantities that they make a negligible contribution to the diet (*but see* curry).

conditioning of meat After slaughter, the muscle *glycogen is broken down to *lactic acid, and this acidity gradually improves the texture and keeping qualities of the meat. When all the changes have occurred, the meat is 'conditioned'. *See also* rigor mortis.

confectioner's custard Thick, sweet sauce based on *cornstarch, used as a filling for cakes and pastries.

confectioner's glucose *See* syrup.

confectionery *Sugar confectionery is sweets, candies, chocolates, etc.; flour confectionery is cakes, pastries, etc.

confit 1 French; Fruit or vegetables preserved in brandy, vinegar, or sugar.

2 Poultry meat or pork preserved in a vessel and covered with a layer of fat to exclude air.

congee Chinese soft rice soup or gruel; may be sweet or savoury. Commonly eaten for breakfast. *See also* congie.

congeners Flavour substances in alcoholic *spirits that distil over with the alcohol; chemically a mixture of higher alcohols and esters. Said to be responsible for many of the symptoms of *hangover after excessive consumption. *See also* fusel oil.

congie (congee) The water from cooking rice, which contains much of the thiamin and niacin from the rice; used as a drink.

congress tart Small pastry case filled with ground almonds, sugar, and egg.

congris Caribbean (Cuban); casseroled red beans served with rice.

connective tissue Consists of the protein *collagen which in fish is found between the muscle segments (myotomes); in meat it is spread through the muscle, uniting the muscle fibres into bundles and supporting the blood vessels (a kind of soft skeleton), and consists of both collagen and *elastin.

A high content of connective tissue results in tougher meat.

Collagen is insoluble; it is converted to soluble *gelatine by moist heat, so making the food more tender. Tough meat is softened to some extent by stewing, but roasting or frying has little effect. Elastin is unaffected by heating, and remains tough, elastic, and insoluble.

consommé A clear soup made from meat or meat extract.

constipation Difficulty in passing stools or infrequent passage of hard stools. In the absence of intestinal disease, frequently a result of a diet low in *non-starch polysaccharide, and treated by increasing the intake of fruits, vegetables, and especially wholegrain cereal products.

contaminants Undesirable compounds found in foods, the result of residues of agricultural chemicals (pesticides, fungicides, herbicides, fertilizers, etc.), through the manufacturing process or as a result of pollution. For many such compounds there are limits to the amount that may legally be present in the food. *See also* Acceptable Daily Intake.

controliran *See* wine classification, Bulgaria.

controlled atmosphere storage *See* gas storage, controlled.

convenience foods Processed foods in which a considerable amount of the preparation has already been carried out by the manufacturer, e.g. cooked meats, canned foods, baked foods, breakfast cereals, frozen foods.

convicine One of the toxins in broad beans, responsible for the acute haemolytic anaemia of *favism.

coo-coo Caribbean; a cooked side-dish of starchy vegetables such as breadfruit or corn meal with herbs and spices.

cook-chill A method of catering involving cooking followed by fast chilling and storage at −1 to +5 ˚C, giving a storage time of only a few days.

cooker, fireless *See* haybox cooking.

cook-freeze A method of catering involving cooking followed by rapid freezing and storage between −18 and −30 ˚C, giving a storage time of several months.

cookie *See* biscuit.

cooking Required to make food more palatable, more digestible, and safer. There is breakdown of the *connective tissue in meat, softening of the *cellulose in plant tissues, and proteins are denatured by heating, so increasing their digestibility. *See also:* boiling; broiling; coddling; devilled; fricassée; frying; grilling; roasting; sautéing; simmering; steaming; stewing.

cooking, loss of nutrients In general, water-soluble vitamins and minerals are lost in the cooking water, the amount depending on the surface area to volume ratio, i.e. greater losses take place from finely cut or minced foods. Fat-soluble vitamins are little affected except at frying temperatures. Proteins suffer reduction of available lysine when they are heated in the presence of reducing substances, and further loss under extreme conditions of temperature. Dry heat, as in baking, results in some loss of vitamin B_1 and available lysine. The most sensitive nutrient by far is vitamin C, with vitamin B_1 next. Average losses from cereals are: boiling, 40% vitamins B_1, B_2, B_6, niacin, biotin, and pantothenic acid; 50% total folate; baking, 5% niacin, 15% vitamin B_2; 25% vitamins B_1, B_6, and pantothenic acid; 50% folate; with biotin being stable. In meat, losses are approximately 20% of all the vitamins for roasting, frying, and grilling and 20–60% for stewing and boiling.

copper A dietary essential trace metal, which forms the *prosthetic group of a number of *enzymes. The *Reference Nutrient Intake is 1.2 mg/day. Toxic in excess, and it is recommended that not more than 2–10 mg/day should be consumed habitually. Rich *sources include: meat, poultry, game, fish and shellfish, avocado, nuts, pulses, bread, chocolate, beer, cider, coconut, mushrooms.

copra Dried *coconut 'meat' used for production of coconut oil for *margarine and soap manufacture.

coprophagy Eating of faeces. Since B vitamins are synthesized by intestinal bacteria, animals that eat their faeces can make use of these vitamins, which are not absorbed from the large intestine, the site of bacterial action.

Co Q *See* ubiquinone.

coquille, en Normally a seafood dish, served in the shell, or made to resemble a shell.

coquille St Jacques *See* scallop.

coquimol Caribbean (Cuba); custard made with coconut milk and eggs.

coracan *See* millet.

coral The ovaries of female *lobsters, used as the basis for sauces; red-coloured when cooked.

cordial, fruit Originally a fruit *liqueur, and still used in this sense in the USA; in the UK a cordial is now used to mean any fruit drink, usually a concentrate to be diluted. *See* soft drinks.

coriander *Coriandrum sativum* (a member of the parsley family); the leaf is used fresh or dried as a herb, and the dried ripe fruit (also called dhanyia) as a spice in meat products, bakery goods, tobacco, gin, and curry powder.

coring Removal of the pips and central membranes (the core) from apples, pears, etc.

corked Of wines, the development of an unpleasant flavour due to fungal contamination of the cork.

corm The thickened, underground base of the stem of plants, often called bulbs, as, for example, *taro and *onion.

corn Term used in the UK for wheat, in the USA for maize, and sometimes for oats in Scotland and Ireland, originally any grain. *See also* maize.

corned beef In the UK a canned product made from low-quality beef that has been partially extracted with hot water to make *meat extract. A 150-g portion is an exceptionally rich *source of protein, niacin, and iron; a good source of vitamin B_2; contains 18 g of fat of which half is saturated and supplies 330 kcal (1390 kJ). In the USA and elsewhere corned beef is pickled beef (in the UK this is called salt beef).

Cornell bread *See* bread.

cornflakes Breakfast cereal made from *maize, often enriched with vitamins. A 40-g portion of enriched cornflakes is a rich *source of vitamins B_2, B_6, B_{12}, niacin, and folate; a good source of vitamin B_1 and iron; provides 4.4 g of dietary fibre; supplies 145 kcal (610 kJ).

cornflour Purified starch from maize; in the USA called corn starch; used in custard, blancmange, and baking powders and for thickening sauces and gravies.

corn, flour Flour corn is a variety of *maize with large, soft grains and very friable endosperm, making it easy to grind to flour.

corn grits *See* hominy.

corn, Guinea, kaffir *See* sorghum.

Cornish pasty *See* pasty.

corn oil (maize oil) Extracted from maize germ, *Zea mays*; 13% saturates, 60% polyunsaturates.

corn pone Small corn (maize) cakes, a speciality of Alabama, USA.

corn salad Winter salad vegetable, *Valeriana olitoria*, also known as lamb's lettuce.

corn starch *See* cornflour.

corn starch hydrolysate, corn syrup *See* syrup.

corn sugar *See* glucose.

coronary heart disease *See* ischaemic heart disease.

coronary thrombosis *See* atherosclerosis.

corrinoids (corrins) The basic chemical structure of *vitamin B_{12} is the corrin ring; compounds with this structure, whether or not they have vitamin activity, are corrinoids.

cosecha Spanish; vintage of wine.

cos lettuce Long-leafed variety of *lettuce.

cossettes Thin chips of sugar beet shredded for hot-water extraction of the sugar.

costmary *See* alecost.

cottage loaf Traditional English loaf consisting of a large round base with a smaller round topknot of bread.

cottage pie *See* shepherd's pie.

cottonseed Seed of *Gossypium* spp.; of double use in the food field since the oil is valuable as cooking oil, or for margarine manufacture when hardened, and the protein residue is a valuable animal feed. The oil is 25% saturated and 50% polyunsaturated.

coulis Also cullis; originally the juices that run out of meat when it is cooked, now used to mean rich sauce or gravy made from meat juices, puréed shellfish, vegetables, or fruit. Most usually a sauce made from puréed and sieved fruit.

coupe Dessert of ice cream and fruit, a sundae.

courgette Variety of *marrow developed to be harvested when small; also known as Italian marrow, Italian squash, or zucchini.

Courlose Trade name for sodium carboxymethylcellulose. *See* cellulose derivatives.

court-bouillon Fish stock used in place of water to cook fish; may contain wine, vinegar, or milk.

couscous North African; millet flour or fine semolina, steamed until fluffy and usually served with mutton stew.

cow-heel Dish made from heel of ox or cow, stewed to a jelly; also known as neat's-foot.

cow manure factor *See* vitamin B_{12}.

cow pea See bean, black-eyed.

crab *Shellfish; *Cancer* and *Carcinus* spp.; king crab is *Limulus polyphemus*. A 100-g portion (500 g with shell) is a rich *source of protein, niacin, zinc, copper, and selenium; a good source of iron; a source of vitamins B_2 and B_6; contains 400 mg of sodium and 5 g of fat of which 13% is saturated; supplies 130 kcal (545 kJ).

crab apple Wild varieties of *apple (*Malus* spp.), normally very sour; used to make sweet-sour jelly as accompaniment to meat. Commonly grown as an ornamental plant, and to enhance fertilization of cultivated apple trees.

crab stick *See* seafood stick.

crackers Plain, thin biscuits such as water biscuits, cream crackers, and wholemeal crackers, made from wheat flour, fat, and bicarbonate as a raising agent. A 40-g portion (5 biscuits) contains 3–6 g of fat; provides 1–2 g of dietary fibre and 160–280 mg of sodium; supplies 170 kcal (715 kJ).

crackling Crisp rind of a joint of pork after baking or roasting.

cracknel 1 Plain biscuit made with paste which is boiled before baking so that it puffs up.
    2 Brittle *toffee filling for chocolates.

cran A traditional measure for herrings containing 37$^1/_2$ gallons (167 L) or about 800 fish.

cranberry The fleshy, acid fruit of *Vaccinium oxycoccus* or *V. macrocarpon*, resembling a cherry; commonly used to make cranberry sauce (a traditional American accompaniment to turkey) and for the preparation of juice. An 80-g portion is a *source of vitamin C and copper; provides 3.2 g of dietary fibre; supplies 15 kcal (60 kJ). A 300-mL portion of juice is a rich *source of vitamin C and copper; a good source of iron; supplies 150 kcal (630 kJ).

crapaud Large edible Caribbean frogs, also known as mountain chicken.

crawfish (French: *languste*; German: *Languste*.) Crustaceans (without claws) of the family *Palinuridae*, also called spiny lobster, rock lobster, sea crayfish. *See* lobster.

crayfish (French: *écrevisse*; German: *Krebs*.) Crustaceans; freshwater crayfish are members of the families *Astacidae*, *Parasticidae*, and *Austroastacidae*, sea crayfish (crawfish) of the family *Palinuridae*. *See* lobster.

crayfish, fresh water Families of *Astacidae*, *Parastacidae*, and *Austroastacidae*.

cream Fatty part of milk; 4% of ordinary milk, 4.8% of Channel Islands milk. Half cream is similar to 'top of the milk', 12% fat (30-mL portion supplies 45 kcal (190 kJ), and cannot be whipped or frozen; single cream, 18% fat (60 kcal, 250 kJ), will not whip and cannot be frozen unless included in a frozen dish; extra thick single cream is also 18% fat, but has been homogenized to a thick spoonable consistency; whipping cream, 34% fat (110 kcal, 460 kJ) will whip to double volume; double cream, 48% fat (135 kcal, 570 kJ) will whip and can be frozen; clotted, Devonshire, and Cornish cream contains 55% fat (150 kcal, 630 kJ). Of this fat, two-thirds is *saturated and 30% mono-unsaturated.
    Soured cream is made from single cream; *crème fraîche is soured double cream; 'extra thick double cream' is also 48% fat, but has been homogenized to be spoonable, and will not whip or freeze successfully.
    In the USA, light cream has 20–25% fat; heavy cream, 40% fat.

cream, artificial 1 An emulsion of vegetable oil, milk or milk powder, egg yolk, and sugar.
    2 An emulsion of water with methyl *cellulose, *monoglycerides, and other synthetic materials.

cream, bitty Cream on the surface of milk appears as particles of fat released from fat globules when the membrane is broken down by lecithinase from *Bacillus cereus*, the spores of which have resisted destruction during *pasteurization.

creamer, non-dairy Milk substitute used in tea and coffee (coffee whitener or creamer) made with glucose, fat, and emulsifying salts. A stable product dry or as liquid. May be made with *casein, in which case it is not technically (or by US law) non-dairy.

creaming Beating together fat and sugar to give a fluffy mixture, for making cakes with a high fat content. The creaming quality of a fat is its ability to take up air during mixing.

cream line index The cream line or layer usually forms about 6% of the total depth of milk. The cream line index is the ratio between the percentage cream layer and the percentage of fat in the milk; in ordinary bulk pasteurized milk it is about 1.7.

cream of tartar Potassium hydrogen tartrate, used with *sodium bicarbonate as *baking powder because it acts more slowly than *tartaric acid and gives a more prolonged evolution of carbon dioxide. This is tartrate baking powder. Also used to 'invert' *sugar in making boiled sweets.

cream, plastic A term used for a cream containing as much fat as butter (80–83%) but as a dispersal of fat in water, while butter is water in fat. Prepared by intense centrifugal treatment of cream; crumbly, not greasy, in texture; used for preparation of cream cheese and whipped cream.

cream sherry *See* sherry.

cream, sleepy Cream that will not churn to butter in the normal time.

cream, synthetic *See* cream, artificial.

creatine A derivative of the *amino acids glycine and arginine, important in muscle as a store of phosphate for resynthesis of *ATP during muscle contraction and work.

Meat extract contains a mixture of creatine and *creatinine derived from the creatine that was present in the fresh muscle. Creatine plus creatinine is used as an index of quality of commercial meat extract, and as a measure of meat extract present in manufactured products, such as soups.

creatinine Formed non-enzymically from *creatine (chemically the anhydride of creatine). Urinary excretion of creatinine is relatively constant from day to day, and reflects mainly the amount of muscle tissue in the body. Therefore the amounts of various components of urine are often expressed as unit/creatinine.

crécy, à la Dish made or garnished with carrots.

creeping sickness *Osteomalacia in livestock due to phosphate deficiency.

crème 1 Term used for cream, custards, and desserts. Crème brûlée is a cream and egg custard with sugar sprinkled on top and caramelized under a hot grill; a traditional speciality of Trinity College Cambridge and also known as burnt cream or Cambridge cream. Crème caramel is topped with caramel. Crème Chantilly is whipped cream sweetened and flavoured with *vanilla.

2 Various liqueurs, including: crème de bananes (banana); crème de cacao (chocolate); crème de café (coffee); crème de menthe (peppermint); crème de mûres (wild blackberries); crème de myrtilles (wild bilberries); crème de noix (green walnuts and honey); crème de violettes (violet petals).

crème fraîche French; double *cream that has been thickened and slightly soured by lactic fermentation.

cremet Milk curd made in the Dauphinois region of France.

créole The traditional cuisine of Louisiana and the French-speaking Caribbean; *see also* criolla.

créole, à la Usually a dish served on rice. In the case of savoury dishes, with a garnish or sauce of red peppers and tomatoes; for sweet dishes orange, banana, pineapple, or rum may be included.

créole sauce American; *espagnole sauce with onions, mushrooms, and peppers served with grilled steak.

crêpe French; a thin pancake. Crêpe suzette is made with orange-flavoured batter and served with a sauce flavoured with an orange liqueur.

crépinette French; small sausage-shaped cakes of minced meat wrapped in fat bacon or pig's *caul.

crescioni Italian; fried pastry squares filled with spinach chopped with shallots and raisins.

crespolini Italian; pancakes filled with spinach, cream cheese, and chicken liver, baked in *béchamel sauce.

cress Garden cress, pepper grass, *Lepidium sativum*. The seed leaves can be eaten raw with mustard seed leaves as mustard and cress or salad rape (*Brassica napus* var. *napus*) and cress. Can be grown on wet blotting paper. *See also* watercress.

cress, American or land *Barbarea verna*; the leaves have a peppery flavour. Unlike *watercress it can be grown in soil without running water.

Creta Praeparata Official British Pharmacopoeia name for prepared chalk, made by washing and drying naturally occurring calcium carbonate. The form in which calcium is added to flour (14 oz per 280 lb sack, or approximately 3g/kg).

cretinism Underactivity of the *thyroid gland (hypothyroidism) in children, resulting in poor growth and severe mental retardation. Hypothyroidism in adults is myxoedema. Commonly the result of a dietary deficiency of *iodine; may be congenital if the mother's iodine intake was severely inadequate during pregnancy.

crevettes *See* shrimps.

crimping 1 Slashing a large fish at intervals before cooking, to make it easier for the heat to penetrate the flesh.

2 Trimming cucumber or similar foods in such a way that the slices appear to be 'deckled'.

3 Decorating the double edge of a pie or tart or the edge of shortbread by pinching it at regular intervals with the fingers, giving a fluted effect.

criolla The traditional cuisine of the Spanish-speaking Caribbean and Latin America; derived from French, Spanish, African, and American cookery. *See also* créole.

crispbread Name given to a flour and water wafer, originally Swedish and made from rye flour, but may be made from wheat flour. It has a much lower water content than bread and some brands are richer in protein because of added wheat *gluten. Although popularly believed to be an aid in slimming, crispbreads provide more energy than the same weight of ordinary bread since they contain less water. Three pieces of crispbread (30 g) provide up to 3 g of dietary fibre and supply 100 kcal (420 kJ).

crisps *See* potato crisps.

cristal height A measure of leg length taken from the floor to the summit of the iliac crest. As a proportion of height it increases with age in children, and a reduced rate of increase indicates undernutrition. *See also* anthropometry.

crocin *See* saffron.

Crohn's disease Chronic inflammatory disease of the bowel, of unknown origin, treated with antibiotics to prevent infection and with anti-inflammatory agents. Sufferers may be malnourished as a result of both loss of appetite due to illness and also malabsorption. Also known as regional enteritis, since only some regions of the gut are affected. *See also* gastro-intestinal tract.

croissant French; flaky crescent-shaped rolls traditionally served hot for breakfast, made from a yeast dough with a high fat content. A 50-g croissant contains 10 g of fat of which 30% is saturated; supplies 180 kcal (750 kJ).

cropadeau Scottish; oatmeal dumpling with haddock liver in the middle.

croque-monsieur French; ham and cheese toasted sandwich. When topped with a fried egg it is called croque-madame.

croquette Finely chopped meat, fish, or vegetables, mixed with a rich sauce or *panada, shaped into balls or small cylinders, coated in egg and breadcrumbs and fried. The commonest filling is potato.

croustade Small case of fried bread, pastry, or duchesse potato used to serve a savoury mixture.

croûte, en Literally 'in a crust'; game, meat, or fish served in a pastry case or surrounded by slices of bread.

croûtons Small diced or shaped pieces of bread, fried in fat, and commonly used to garnish soup and salads.

crowdie Scottish; soft cheese made from buttermilk or soured milk curd, also a dish of buttermilk and oatmeal.

crowdies See milk, fermented.

Cruciferae Family of plants with flowers with four equal petals; most vegetables in this family belong to the genus *Brassica*.

crude fibre See fibre, crude.

crude protein See protein, crude.

crudités Raw vegetables, sliced or cut into small pieces or strips, served with a variety of dressings or dips, as an hors d'œuvre. (French *crudité*, 'rawness'.)

cruller American; deep-fried bun made from baking powder dough. Similar to a doughnut.

crumb Small particle of bread, cake, or biscuit, as broken off by rubbing.

crumble Flour, fat, and sugar (a rubbed-in plain cake mix) baked as a topping over fruit instead of pastry. For savoury crumble the sugar is omitted and cheese and seasoning are added.

crumb softeners Derivatives of *monoglycerides added to bread as emulsifiers to give a softer crumb and retard staling. There are several of these compounds which are combinations of different monoglycerides, E-430–436; also called polysorbates. See also superglycinerated fats.

crumpets See dough cakes.

crust The crisp outer part of a loaf of bread; also used for the sediment thrown off as wines mature.

crustacea Zoological class of hard-shelled marine arthropods (*shellfish) including *crabs, *crayfish, *lobster, *prawns, *scampi, *shrimps.

cryodesiccation See freeze-drying.

cryogenic freezing Freezing with extremely cold freezants such as liquid nitrogen or solid carbon dioxide.

Cryovac Trade name of thermoplastic resin wrapping film which can be heat-shrunk onto foods.

cryptoxanthin Yellow *carotenoid in a few foods such as yellow maize and the seeds of *Physalis, the Cape gooseberry. A hydroxylated derivative of carotene which is a source of *vitamin A in the body.

crystal boiling Chinese method of cooking; food is heated in a pan of boiling water, then removed from the heat and cooking continued by the retained heat.

CSM Corn-soya-milk; a protein-rich baby food (20% protein) made in the USA from 68% pre-cooked maize (corn), 25% defatted soya flour, and 5% skim milk powder, with added vitamins and calcium carbonate.

CTC machine A device consisting of two contra-rotating toothed rollers that rotate at different speeds and provide a crushing, tearing, and curling action: used in breaking up leaves of tea to form small particles.

cuaranta y tres Spanish; liqueur flavoured with herbs and spices; the name means 'forty-three'.

cubeb Grey pepper (*Piper cubeba*) native to South East Asia; pungent flavour akin to camphor.

Cubs Trade name for a breakfast cereal made from wheat.

cucumber Fruit of *Cucumis sativus*, a member of the *gourd family, eaten as a salad vegetable; it is 95% water; a 50-g portion provides 0.3 g of dietary fibre and supplies 5 kcal (20 kJ). *See also* gherkin.

cucurbit A term used for vegetables of the family *Cucurbitaceae*, or *gourds.

cuisson Cooking juices from meat, poultry, or fish.

cullis *See* coulis.

Cumberland sauce Sauce made from redcurrant jelly, orange, lemon, and port, served with ham, venison, and lamb.

cumin (cummin) Pungent herb, the crescent-shaped seed of *Cuminum cyminum* (parsley family); used in curry powder and for flavouring cordials. Black cumin is the seed of *Nigella sativa* (fennel flower) and sweet cumin is *anise (*Pimpinella anisum*).

cumquat *See* kumquat.

cup North American and Australian measure for ingredients in cooking; the standard American cup contains 250 mL (8 fl oz).

cup cake Small individual cake or bun, typically baked in a paper case and topped with icing. Also known as fairy cake.

curaçao A *liqueur made from the rind of Seville oranges and brandy or gin; 30% *alcohol, 30% sugar; 300 kcal (1260 kJ)/100 mL.

curcumin *See* turmeric.

curds Clotted protein formed when fresh milk is treated with *rennet; the fluid left is *whey.

curd tension A measure of the toughness of the curd formed from milk by the digestive enzymes, and used as an index of the digestibility of the milk.

curing of meat A method of preservation by treating with *salt and sodium nitrate (and nitrite), which serves to inhibit the growth of pathogenic organisms while salt-tolerant bacteria develop. During the *pickling process the nitrate is converted into nitrite, which combines with the muscle pigment, myoglobin, to form the red-coloured nitrosomyoglobin which is characteristic of pickled meat products.

curly kale *See* kale.

currants Fruit of *Ribes* spp.; white, red, and black. A 100-g portion of *red- or whitecurrants is a rich *source of vitamin C, and of *blackcurrants an exceptionally rich source; supplies 25 kcal (105 kJ).

currants, dried Made by drying the small seedless black grapes grown in and around Greece and in Australia; usually dried in bunches on the vine or after removal from the vine on supports. The name is derived from 'raisins of Corauntz' (Corinth). A 25-g portion provides

1.8 g of dietary fibre and is a good *source of copper; supplies 65 kcal (275 kJ). *See also* dried fruit; raisins; sultanas.

curry Name given by the British (it means 'sauce' in Tamil) to an Indian dish of stewed meat or vegetables. It is served with a pungent sauce whose components and pungency vary. *See also* curry powder; vindaloo.

curry plant (curry leaves) An aromatic herb, *Murraya koenigii*.

curry powder A mixture of turmeric with several spices including cardamom, cinnamon, cloves, coriander, cumin, and fenugreek, made pungent with mustard, chilli, and pepper. A 10-g portion can contain 7.5–10 mg of iron, but much of this is probably the result of contamination during the milling of the spices.

cushion The cut nearest the udder in lamb or beef.

custard Sweet sauce, traditionally made by cooking milk with eggs; more commonly using custard powder (coloured and flavoured *cornflour) and milk; a 100-g portion (sweetened) is a *source of calcium and vitamin B_2, and supplies 85 kcal (355 kJ). *See also* caramel cream; confectioner's custard.

custard apple The fruit of one of a number of species of tropical American trees of the family Anonaceae. Sour sop, *Anona muricata*, has white fibrous flesh and is less sweet than the others; the fruit may weigh up to 4 kg (8 lb). The sweet sop (*A. squamosa*) is also known as the 'true' custard apple, and is especially popular in the West Indies. The bullock's heart (*A. reticulata*) has buff-coloured flesh. A 100-g portion is a rich *source of vitamin C and supplies 90 kcal (380 kJ).

cutlet *Chop cut from the best end of neck of *lamb, *veal, or *pork.

cutting-and-folding *See* folding-in.

cutting-in Combining the fat with other ingredients in a mixture by cutting with a knife.

CVA Cerebrovascular accident. *See* stroke.

cyamopsis gum *See* guar gum.

cyanocobalamin *See* vitamin B_{12}.

cyanogen(et)ic glycosides Organic compounds of cyanide found in a variety of plants; chemically cyanhydrins linked by glycoside linkage to one or more sugars. Toxic through liberation of the cyanide when the plants are cut or chewed. *See also* almond; amygdalin.

cyclamate A non-nutritive *sweetener, 30 times as sweet as sugar, used as the free acid or the calcium salt; synthesized in 1937. Useful in low-calorie foods. Unlike *saccharin, it is stable to heat and can therefore be used in cooking. Chemically sodium cyclohexyl-sulphamate, also known as Sucaryl (trade name).

cyclitols Cyclic *sugar alcohols such as inositol, quercitol, and tetritol.

cyder *See* cider.

Cymogran Trade name for a protein-rich food which is low in *phenylalanine for feeding patients with *phenylketonuria.

cynar Italian; liqueur made from artichoke hearts.

cystathioninuria A *genetic disease affecting the metabolism of the *amino acid *methionine and its conversion to *cysteine. May result in mental retardation if untreated. Treatment is by feeding a diet low in methionine and supplemented with cysteine, or, in some cases, by administration of high intakes of *vitamin B_6 (about 100–500 times the normal requirement).

cysteine A non-essential *amino acid, but nutritionally important since it spares the essential amino acid *methionine. In addition to its role in protein synthesis, cysteine is important as the precursor of taurine, in formation of coenzyme A from the *vitamin *pantothenic acid and in formation of the tripeptide *glutathione. It is used as a dough 'improver' in baking. See also cystine.

cysticercosis Infection by the larval stage of *tapeworms caused by ingestion of their eggs in food and water contaminated by human faeces. Normally the larval form develops in the animal host, and human beings are infected with the adult form by eating undercooked infected meat.

cystic fibrosis A *genetic disease due to a failure of the normal transport of chloride ions across cell membranes. This results in abnormally viscous mucus, affecting especially the lungs and secretion of pancreatic juice, hence impairing digestion.

cystine The dimer of *cysteine produced when its sulphydryl group (—SH) is oxidized forming a disulphide (—S—S—) bridge. Such disulphide bridges are especially important in maintaining the structure of proteins, and also in the rôle of the tripeptide *glutathione as an *antioxidant. Hair protein (keratin) is especially rich in cystine, which accounts for about 12% of its total amino acid content.

cystinuria A *genetic disease in which there is abnormally high excretion of the amino acids *cysteine and cystine, resulting in the formation of kidney stones. Treatment is by feeding a diet low in the sulphur amino acids methionine, cysteine, and cystine.

cytochrome P_{450} A family of *cytochromes which are involved in the *detoxication system of the body. They act on a wide variety of (potentially toxic) compounds, both endogenous metabolites and foreign compounds (*xenobiotics), rendering them more water-soluble, and more readily conjugated for excretion in the urine.

cytochromes *Haem-containing proteins present in every type of living cell (except the strictly *anaerobic bacteria). Some cytochromes react with oxygen directly; others are intermediates in the oxidation of reduced *coenzymes. Unlike *haemoglobin, the iron in the haem of cytochromes undergoes oxidation and reduction.

cytokinins Substances that stimulate cell division (cytokinesis) and control the development of plants; found in seed embryos, developing fruits, and buds. They are derivatives of the purine *adenine.

cytosine One of the *pyrimidine bases of *nucleic acids.

D-, L-, and DL- Prefixes to chemical names for compounds that have a centre of asymmetry in the molecule, and which can therefore have two forms (*isomers).

Most naturally occurring sugars have the D-conformation; apart from a few microbial proteins and some invertebrate peptides, all the naturally occurring amino acids have the L-configuration. Chemical synthesis yields a mixture of the D- and L-isomers (the racemic mixture), generally shown as DL-. *See also* R-.

d- and l- An obsolete way of indicating dextrorotatory and laevorotatory *optical activity, now replaced by (+) and (−).

D value *See* decimal reduction time.

dabberlocks Edible seaweed, *Alaria esculenta*.

dadhi *See* milk, fermented.

dahlin *See* inulin.

daily value Reference amounts of energy, fat, saturated fat, carbohydrate, fibre, sodium, potassium and cholesterol, as well as protein, vitamins, and minerals, introduced for food labelling in the USA in 1994. The nutrient content of a food must be declared as a percentage of the daily value provided by a standard serving.

daiquiri Correctly a trade name for *rum; commonly used for a mixture of rum and fresh lime juice, or other fruit juice.

dal-chini *See* cassia.

Daltose Trade name for a carbohydrate preparation consisting of maltose, glucose and dextrin for infant feeding.

damascene Original name for *damson.

damson Small dark purple *plum (*Prunus damascena*); very acid and mainly used to make jam. An 80-g portion provides 2.4 g of dietary fibre and supplies 30 kcal (125 kJ).

dandelion The leaves of the weed *Taraxacum officinale* may be eaten as a salad or cooked. In France dandelion greens are known as *pis-en-lit* because of their diuretic action. A 50-g portion of the leaves is a good *source of vitamins C and A (4000 μg carotene); a source of calcium and iron; supplies 25 kcal (105 kJ). The root can be cooked as a vegetable, or may be roasted and used as a substitute for *coffee.

Danish agar *See* furcellaran.

Danish pastry Rich, sweet, yeast pastry confection filled with fruit or nuts. Originally Viennese, not Danish; indeed in Danish it is known as *Wienerbrod*.

dariole Small narrow mould with sloping sides used to make individual sweets and savouries; originally the name of a small cake.

dark adaptation In the eye, the visual pigment rhodopsin is formed by reaction between *vitamin A aldehyde and the protein opsin, and is bleached by exposure to light, stimulating a nerve impulse (this is the basis of *vision). At an early stage of vitamin A deficiency it takes considerably longer than normal to adapt to see in dim light after exposure to normal bright light, because of the limitation of the amount of rhodopsin that can be reformed. Measuring the time taken to adapt to dim light (the dark adaptation time) thus provides a sensitive index of early vitamin A deficiency. More severe vitamin A deficiency results in *night blindness, and eventually complete blindness.

darne French; thick cut from the middle of a fish.

dartois (d'Artois) Small light pastry, filled and flavoured (either sweet or savoury) served as an hors d'œuvre or dessert.

dasheen *See* taro.

date Fruit of date palm, *Phoenix dactylifera*, known as far back as 3000 BC. There are three types: 'soft' (about 80% of the dry matter is *invert sugars); semi-dry (about 40% of the dry matter is invert sugars and 40% sucrose); and dry (20–40% of the dry matter is invert sugars and 40–60% is sucrose). A 100-g portion of fresh dates (five weighed with stones) is a good *source of vitamin C and supplies 230 kcal (960 kJ); 100 g of dried dates (three weighed with stones) provides 3 g of dietary fibre and supplies 270 kcal (1130 kJ).

date, Chinese Fruit of *Ziziphus jujuba* (also called jujube), smaller than the true date; a 50-g portion is a rich *source of vitamin C.

DATEM Diacetyl tartaric esters of mono- and diglycerides used as *emulsifiers to strengthen bread doughs and delay staling of the bread (E-472(e)).

date marking On packaged foods, 'Best before' is the date up until the food will remain in optimum condition, i.e. will not be stale. Foods with a shelf life of up to 12 weeks are marked 'best before day, month, year'; foods with a longer shelf life are marked 'best before end of month, year'.

Perishable foods with a shelf life of less than a month may have a 'sell-by' date instead. 'Use by' date is given for foods that are microbiologically highly perishable and could become a danger to health; it is the date up to and including which the food may be safely used if stored properly.

Frozen foods and ice cream carry star markings which correspond to the star marking on freezers and frozen food compartments of refrigerators. Food in a 1-star rated compartment (−4 °C, 25 °F) will keep for one week; 2-star rated (−11 °C, 12 °F), 1 month; 3-star rated (−18 °C, 0 °F), 3 months. Corresponding times for ice cream are 1 day, 1 week, 1 month (after such times they are still fit to eat but the texture changes).

date plum *See* persimmon.

daube, en Braised or stewed.

dauphinois Dish containing milk and cream or cheese.

DBD process *See* dry-blanch-dry process.

DE *See* dextrose equivalent value.

decaffeinated *See* caffeine; coffee.

decanting Careful pouring of wine from a bottle into a jug or decanter to leave any sediment in the bottle.

deciduous teeth The first set of 20 teeth that appear during infancy and are lost during childhood and early adolescence as the adult (permanent) teeth erupt. Also known as milk teeth, first teeth.

decimal reduction time (D value) Term used in sterilizing canned food, etc.; the duration of heat treatment required to reduce the number of micro-organisms to one-tenth of the initial value, with the temperature shown as a subscript, e.g. D_{121} is time at 121 °C.

deficiency disease Disease associated with characteristic and identifiable symptoms, signs, or pathological findings, due to insufficient intake, defective absorption or utilization, or excessive utilization of one or more nutrients, or of energy. *See also* anaemia; beriberi; pellagra; protein-energy malnutrition; scurvy.

degorger Procedure in which vegetables (e.g. aubergine, cucumber) are lightly salted after slicing, then drained, to remove any strong taste.

degumming agents Compounds used in the refining of fats and oils to remove mucilaginous matter consisting of gum, resin, proteins, and phosphatides. They include hydrochloric and phosphoric acids and phosphates.

dehydration A scientific term for drying, which tends to be used for factory-dried as distinct from wind-dried materials.

dehydroascorbic acid The oxidized form of *vitamin C which is readily reduced back to the active form in the body, and therefore has vitamin activity.

dehydrocanning A process in which 50% of the water is removed from a food before canning. The advantages are that the texture is retained by the partial dehydration and there is a saving in bulk and weight.

dehydrocholesterol The precursor for the synthesis of *vitamin D in the skin.

Delaney Amendment A provision in the US Federal Food, Drug, and Cosmetic Act (1958) which states that no food additive shall be deemed safe after it is found to induce cancer when ingested by man or animals, at any dose level. Such an additive therefore must not be used.

deli North American abbreviation for *delicatessen.

delicatessen Ready-to-eat foods such as cooked meats, salami, pickled and smoked fish, salads, olives, etc. Also used as the name for the shop where such foods are sold. From the German *delikat Essen*, 'fine foods'. Abbreviated to deli in North America.

demerara sugar *See* sugar.

demersal fish Those fish found living on or near the bottom of the sea, including cod, haddock, whiting, and halibut. They contain little oil (1–4%). *See* white fish.

denaturation, protein A change in the structure of protein by heat, acid, alkali, or other agents which results in loss of solubility and *coagulation (as in boiled egg). It is normally irreversible. Denatured proteins lose their biological activity (e.g. as *enzymes), but not their nutritional value. Indeed, their digestibility is improved compared with the original structures, which are relatively resistant to enzymic hydrolysis.

denatured alcohol The addition of dyestuffs and unpleasant flavours (such as pyridine) to prevent the consumption of *alcohol which is intended for domestic or industrial purposes; up to 5% (toxic) methyl alcohol is added.

dendritic salt A form of ordinary table *salt, sodium chloride, with the crystals branched or star-like (dendritic) instead of the normal cubes. This is claimed to have a number of advantages: lower bulk density, more rapid solution, and an unusually high capacity to absorb moisture before becoming wet.

denominacion de origen (DO) *See* wine classification, Spanish.

denominazione di origine controllata (DOC) *See* wine classification, Italian.

dental caries *See* caries.

dental fluorosis *See* fluoride; mottled teeth.

dental plaque *See* plaque, dental.

dent corn *See* maize.

deodorization The removal of an undesirable flavour or odour. Fats are deodorized during refining by bubbling superheated steam through the hot oil under vacuum, when most of the flavoured substances are distilled off.

deoxyribonucleic acid *See* DNA; nucleic acids.

depectinization The removal of *pectins from fruit juice to produce a clear, thin juice instead of a viscous, cloudy liquid, by the use of enzymes which hydrolyse pectins to smaller, soluble compounds.

Derbyshire neck *See* goitre.

dermatitis A lesion or inflammation of the skin; many nutritional deficiency diseases include more or less specific skin lesions (e.g. *ariboflavinosis, *kwashiorkor, *pellagra, *scurvy), but most cases of dermatitis are not associated with nutritional deficiency, and do not respond to nutritional supplements.

desmosine The compound that forms the cross-linkage between chains of the *connective tissue protein *elastin.

detoxication The metabolism of (potentially) toxic compounds to yield less toxic derivatives which are more soluble in water and can be excreted in the urine or *bile. A wide variety of 'foreign compounds' (i.e. compounds that are not normal metabolites in the body), sometimes referred to as xenobiotics, and some hormones and other normal body metabolites, are metabolized in the same way.

devilled Food grilled or fried after coating with condiments or breadcrumbs. *See also* butter, devilled.

devitalized gluten *See* gluten.

dewberry A hybrid fruit, a large variety of *blackberry; rather than climbing, the plant trails on the ground.

dexedrine Anorectic (*appetite suppressing) drug used in the treatment of *obesity.

dexfenfluramine Anorectic (*appetite suppressing) drug used in the treatment of *obesity.

dextran A *polysaccharide composed of linked *fructose units, produced by the action of *Betacoccus arabinosus* on *sugar. It can cause problems in sugar factories, but is clinically useful as a plasma extender for transfusion.

dextrin, limit *See* limit dextrin.

dextrins A mixture of soluble compounds formed by the partial breakdown of *starch by heat, acid or enzymes (*amylases). Formed when bread is toasted. Nutritionally equivalent to starch; industrially used as adhesives, in the sizing of paper and textiles, and as gums.

dextronic acid *See* gluconic acid.

dextrose Alternative name for *glucose. Commercially the term 'glucose' is often used to mean *corn syrup (a mixture of glucose with other sugars and *dextrins) and pure glucose is called dextrose.

dextrose equivalent value (DE) A term used to indicate the degree of hydrolysis of starch into *glucose syrup. It is the percentage of the total solids that have been converted to reducing sugars: the higher the DE, the more sugars and less dextrins are present.

Liquid glucoses are commercially available ranging from 2 DE to 65 DE. A complete acid hydrolysis converts all the starch into glucose but produces bitter degradation products. Glucose syrups above 55 DE are termed 'high conversion' (of starch); of 35–55 DE, regular conversion; below 20 DE the products of hydrolysis are maltins or maltodextrins.

DFD meat Stands for 'dark, firm, dry'; the condition of meat when the *pH remains high through lack of *glycogen (which would form *lactic acid). It poses a microbiological hazard. *See also* meat conditioning; rigor mortis.

DGO Declared geographical origin; *see* wine classification, Bulgaria.

DHA Docosahexaenoic acid, a long-chain polyunsaturated *fatty acid; *see* fish oils.

dhal Indian term for split peas of various kinds, e.g. the pigeon pea (*Cajanus indicus*) and khesari (*Lathyrus sativus*). Red dhal or Massur dhal is the lentil (*Lens esculenta*).

dhanyia *See* coriander.

dhool The name given to leaves of *tea up to the stage of drying.

diabetes There are two distinct conditions: diabetes insipidus and diabetes mellitus. The latter condition is more common, and is generally referred to simply as diabetes or sugar diabetes.

Diabetes insipidus is a metabolic disorder characterized by extreme thirst, excessive consumption of liquids and excessive urination, due to failure of secretion of the antidiuretic hormone.

Diabetes mellitus is a metabolic disorder involving impaired metabolism of *glucose due to either failure of secretion of the *hormone *insulin (insulin-dependent diabetes) or impaired responses of tissues to insulin (non-insulin-dependent diabetes). If untreated, the blood concentration of glucose rises to abnormally high levels (hyperglycaemia) after a meal and glucose is excreted in the urine (glucosuria). Prolonged hyperglycaemia may damage nerves, blood vessels, and kidneys, and lead to development of cataracts, so effective control of blood glucose levels is important.

Type I diabetes mellitus develops in childhood (juvenile-onset diabetes) and is due to failure to secrete *insulin, and hence is called insulin-dependent diabetes. Treatment is by injection of insulin (either purified from beef or pig pancreas or, more commonly now, biosynthetic human insulin), together with restriction of the intake of sugars.

Type II diabetes mellitus generally arises in middle age (maturity-onset diabetes) and is due to resistance of the tissues to insulin action, probably as a result of reduced insulin receptor activity; secretion of insulin by the pancreas may be normal or higher than normal. It is referred to as non-insulin-dependent diabetes and can sometimes be treated by restricting the consumption of sugars and reducing weight, or by the use of oral drugs which stimulate insulin secretion and/or enhance the insulin responsiveness of tissues (sulphonylureas and biguanides). It is also treated by injection of insulin to supplement secretion from the pancreas and overcome the resistance. Impairment of *glucose tolerance similar to that seen in diabetes mellitus sometimes occurs in late pregnancy, when it is known as gestational diabetes. Sometimes pregnancy is the stress that precipitates diabetes, but more commonly the condition resolves when the child is born.

Renal diabetes is the excretion of glucose in the urine without undue elevation of the blood glucose concentration. It is due to a reduction of the renal threshold which allows the blood glucose to be excreted.

See also glucose tolerance.

diabetic foods Loose term for foods that are specially formulated to be suitable for consumption by people with *diabetes mellitus; generally low in carbohydrate (and especially sugar), and frequently containing *sorbitol, xylulose, or sugar derivatives that are slowly or incompletely absorbed.

diable, à la (diablé) Highly spiced, *see* devilled.

diacetyl The main flavour and aroma agent in butter, formed during the ripening stage by the organism *Streptococcus lactis cremoris*. Synthetic

diacetyl is added to margarine as 'butter flavour'. Chemically it is
$CH_3.CO.CO.CH_3$.

diarrhoea Frequent passage of loose watery stools, commonly the result
of intestinal infection; rarely as a result of *adverse reaction to foods
or *disaccharide intolerance. Severe diarrhoea in children can lead to
dehydration and death; it is treated by feeding a solution of salt and
sugar to replace fluid and electrolyte losses.

Osmotic diarrhoea is diarrhoea associated with retention of water in
the bowel as a result of an accumulation of non-absorbable water-
soluble compounds; especially associated with excessive intake of
*sorbitol and *mannitol. Also occurs in *disaccharide intolerance.

diastase See amylase.

diastatic activity of flour A measure of the ability of flour to produce
maltose from its own starch by the action of its own *maltase
(diastase). This sugar is needed for the growth of the yeast during
fermentation. See also amylograph.

dieppoise, à la Sea fish garnished with crayfish tails and mussels,
served with a white wine sauce.

diet Strictly, a diet is simply the pattern of foods eaten; the normal or
habitual intake of food of an individual or population. Commonly used
to mean a modified pattern of food consumption for some special
purpose, e.g. a *slimming, *therapeutic, or low-salt diet (see salt-free
diets) and sometimes named for the person who originated it.

dietary fibre Material mostly derived from plant cell walls which is not
digested by human digestive enzymes but is partially broken down by
intestinal bacteria to volatile *fatty acids that can be used as a source
of energy. A large proportion consists of *non-starch polysaccharides
(NSP); these include soluble fibre that reduces levels of blood
cholesterol and increases the viscosity of the intestinal contents: and
insoluble fibre (cellulose and cell walls) that acts as a laxative. Earlier
known as roughage or bulk.

dietary guidelines Advice to the public on desirable eating behaviour
and patterns of food intake, based on *reference nutrient intakes or
nutrient and food goals to achieve public health objectives.

Dietary Reference Values A UK set of standards of the amounts of
each nutrient needed to maintain good health. People differ in the
daily amounts of nutrients they need; for most nutrients the measured
average need plus 20% (statistically 2 standard deviations) takes care of
the needs of nearly everyone and in the UK this is termed *Reference
Nutrient Intake, elsewhere known as *Recommended Daily Allowances
or Intakes (RDA or RDI), or Population Reference Intake (PRI). This
figure is used to calculate the needs of large groups of people in
institutional or community planning. Obviously some people require
less than the average (up to 20% or 2 standard deviations less). This
lower level is termed the Lower Reference Nutrient Intake, LRNI (also
known as the Minimum Safe Intake, MSI, or Lower Threshold Intake).
This is an intake at or below which it is unlikely that normal health
could be maintained. If the diet of an individual indicates an intake of

any nutrient at or below LRNI then detailed investigation of his/her nutritional status would be recommended.

For energy (total calorie) intake only a single Dietary Reference Value is used, the average (Estimated Average Requirement), because there is potential harm (of *obesity) from ingesting too much. *See also* Energy balance, and Appendices II–VI.

diet, diabetic For the control of *diabetes mellitus, designed not to cause a rapid increase in blood *glucose. Recommendation in the UK is 50–55% carbohydrates, with limits on sucrose, and 35% fat; in the USA, 55–60% carbohydrates.

dietetic foods Foods prepared to meet the particular nutritional needs of people whose assimilation and metabolism of foods are modified, or for whom a particular effect is obtained by a controlled intake of foods or individual nutrients. They may be formulated for people suffering from physiological disorders or for healthy people with additional needs. *See also* PARNUTS.

dietetics The study or prescription of diets under special circumstances (e.g. metabolic or other illness) and for special physiological needs such as pregnancy, growth, weight reduction. *See also* dietitian.

diethylpropion Anorectic (*appetite suppressing) drug used in the treatment of *obesity.

diet-induced thermogenesis The increase in heat production by the body after eating. It is due to both the metabolic energy cost of digestion (the secretion of digestive enzymes, active transport of nutrients from the gut, and gut motility) and the energy cost of forming tissue reserves of fat, glycogen, and protein. It can be up to 10–15% of the energy intake. Also known as the specific dynamic action (SDA) or thermic effect of foods and luxus konsumption.

dietitian, dietician According to the US Department of Labor, *Dictionary of Occupational Titles*, one who applies the principles of nutrition to the feeding of individuals and groups; plans menus and special diets; supervises the preparation and serving of meals; instructs in the principles of nutrition as applied to selection of foods. In the UK the training and state registration of dietitians (i.e. legal permission to practice) is controlled by law. *See also* nutritionist.

differential cell count *See* leucocytes.

digester *See* autoclave.

digestibility The proportion of a foodstuff absorbed from the digestive tract into the bloodstream, normally 90–95%. It is measured as the difference between intake and faecal output, with allowance being made for that part of the faeces that is not derived from undigested food residues (such as shed cells of the intestinal tract, bacteria, residues of digestive juices). Digestibility measured in this way is referred to as 'true digestibility', as distinct from the approximate measure, 'apparent digestibility', which is simply the difference between intake and output.

digestif French term for a *liqueur or *spirit drunk after dinner, supposedly to aid digestion.

digestion The breakdown of a complex compound into its constituent
parts, achieved either chemically or enzymically. Most frequently refers
to the digestion of food, which means breakdown by the digestive
enzymes of *proteins to *amino acids, *starch to *glucose, *fats to
*glycerol and *fatty acids. These breakdown products are then
absorbed into the bloodstream. *See also* gastro-intestinal tract.

digestive juices The secretions of the *gastro-intestinal tract which are
involved in the *digestion of foods: *bile, *gastric secretion, *intestinal
juice, *pancreatic juice, *saliva.

digestive tract *See* gastro-intestinal tract.

Dijon mustard *See* mustard, French.

dill The aromatic herb *Anethum graveolens* (a member of the parsley
family). The dried ripe seeds are used in pickles, sauces, etc. The young
leaves are also used, fresh, dried, or frozen (dill weed) to flavour fish
and other dishes. Dill pepper is a mixture of dill seed, dill weed, and
ground black *pepper, used as a condiment, especially with salmon.

dim-sum (dim-sim) Chinese; steamed dumplings and other delicacies.

dipeptide A *peptide consisting of two amino acids.

diphenyl Also known as biphenyl (E-230), one of two compounds (the
other is orthophenylphenol, OPP, E-231) used for the treatment of fruit
after harvesting to prevent the growth of mould. For making
*marmalade, *citrus fruits that have not been treated with diphenyl
are available.

diphosphopyridine nucleotide (DPN) Obsolete name for
nicotinamide adenine dinucleotide, *NAD.

dipsa Foods that cause thirst.

dipsesis (dipsosis) Extreme thirst, a craving for abnormal kinds of
drinks.

dipsogen A thirst-provoking agent.

dipsomania A morbid craving for alcoholic drinks.

direct extract *See* meat extract.

dirty dick *See* fat hen.

disaccharidases Enzymes that hydrolyse *disaccharides to their
constituent monosaccharides in the intestinal mucosa: sucrase (also
known as invertase) acts on sucrose, lactase on lactose, and maltase on
maltose.

disaccharide Sugars composed of two monosaccharide units; the
nutritionally important disaccharides are *sucrose, *lactose, and
*maltose. *See* carbohydrate.

disaccharide intolerance Impaired ability to digest lactose, maltose, or
sucrose, due to lack of lactase, maltase, or sucrase in the small
intestinal mucosa. The undigested sugars remain in the intestinal
contents, and are fermented by bacteria in the large intestine,
resulting in painful, explosive, watery *diarrhoea. Treatment is by
omitting the offending sugar from the diet.
    Lack of all three enzymes is generally caused by intestinal infections,

and the enzymes gradually recover after the infection has been cured. Lack of just one of the enzymes, and hence intolerance of just one of the disaccharides, is normally an inherited condition.

Lactose intolerance due to loss of lactase is normal in most ethnic groups after puberty; it is only among people of northern ethnic origin that lactase persists into adult life.

disc mill One or more revolving circular plates between which substances are ground; the discs are separated by projecting teeth or pins. Used to grind grain, fruit, sugar, chocolate, pastes, etc.

distillers' dried solubles See spent wash.

DIT See diet-induced thermogenesis.

diuresis Increased formation and excretion of urine; it occurs in diseases such as *diabetes, and also in response to *diuretics.

diuretics Substances that increase the production and excretion of urine. They may be either compounds that occur naturally in foods (including *caffeine and *alcohol), or drugs used medically to reduce the volume of body fluid (e.g. in the treatment of *hypertension and *oedema).

diverticular disease Diverticulosis is the presence of pouch-like hernias (diverticula) through the muscle layer of the colon, associated with a low intake of *dietary fibre and high intestinal pressure due to straining during defecation. Faecal matter can be trapped in these diverticula, causing them to become inflamed, causing pain and diarrhoea, the condition of diverticulitis. See also gastro-intestinal tract.

diverticulitis, diverticulosis See diverticular disease.

djenkolic acid A sulphur-containing amino acid found in the djenkol bean, *Pithecolobium lobatum*, which grows in parts of Sumatra. It is a derivative of *cysteine, and is metabolized but, being relatively insoluble, any djenkolic acid that escapes metabolism can crystallize in the kidney tubules and cause damage.

DNA Deoxyribonucleic acid, the genetic material in the nuclei of all cells. Chemically it is a polymer of deoxyribonucleotides; the purine bases adenine and guanine, and the pyrimidine bases thymidine and cytidine, linked to deoxyribose phosphate. The sugar-phosphates form a double-stranded helix, with the bases paired internally. See also nucleic acids.

DO Denominacion de origen, see wine classification, Spain.

doan choy Chinese; brine-pickled cabbage.

DOC Denominazione di origine controllata, see wine classification, Italy.

doce Portuguese; sweet wines.

DOCG Denominazione di origine controllata e garantita, see wine classification, Italy.

dockage Name given to foreign material in wheat which can be removed readily by a simple cleaning procedure.

docosanoids Long-chain polyunsaturated (essential) *fatty acids with 22 carbon atoms.

docosahexaenoic acid A long-chain polyunsaturated *fatty acid; *see* fish oils.

dogfish A cartilaginous *fish, *Scilliorinus caniculum*, or *Squalis acanthias*, related to the sharks; sometimes called rock salmon or rock eel.

doh peeazah Indian dish; a variant of *korma. The name means 'double onion'.

dolce Italian; sweet wines.

dolma (dolmades, dolmathes) Greek, Turkish; stuffed vegetables, especially vine leaves stuffed with rice and minced meat.

dolomite Calcium magnesium carbonate.

Do-Maker Process For continuous bread making. Ingredients are automatically fed into a continuous dough mixer, the yeast suspension being added in a very active state.

döner kebab Middle-Eastern, Greek, and Turkish (*showarma* in Arabic). Slices of lamb, highly flavoured with herbs and spices, wound around a revolving spit, cooked in front of a vertical charcoal (or sometimes gas) fire. *See also* kebab.

doppelkorn *See* korn.

dosha Indian; pancakes made with rice and lentil flour.

dough Mixture of flour and liquid (water or milk) used to make bread and pastry. May contain yeast or baking powder as leavening agent.

dough cakes A general term to include crumpets, muffins, and pikelets, all made from flour, water and milk. The batter is raised with yeast and baked on a hot plate or griddle (hence sometimes known as griddle cakes). Crumpets have sodium bicarbonate added to the batter; muffins are thick and well aerated, less tough than crumpets; pikelets are made from crumpet batter that has been thinned down.

doughnut Cake made from fried, sweetened dough leavened with yeast or baking powder; may be filled with jam or cream.

Douglas bag An inflatable bag for collecting expired air to measure the consumption of oxygen and production of carbon dioxide, for the measurement of energy expenditure by indirect *calorimetry. *See also* spirometer.

Dowex An *ion exchange resin.

DPN (diphosphopyridine nucleotide) Obsolete name for nicotinamide adenine dinucleotide, *NAD.

dragée French; whole nuts with hard sugar or sugared chocolate coating. Silver dragées are coated with silver leaf.

Drambuie Scottish liqueur based on malt whisky, sweetened with heather honey, and flavoured with herbs.

drawn butter *See* butter, drawn.

dredging Sprinkling food with flour, sugar, etc. Fish and meat are often dredged with flour before frying, while cakes and biscuits are dredged with fine sugar as a decoration.

dressing food To prepare food for cooking or serving in such a way that it looks as attractive as possible. Sometimes denotes a special method of preparation, as in dressed *crab. *See also* salad dressing.

dried solubles, distiller's *See* spent wash.

dripping Unbleached and untreated fat from the fatty tissues or bones of sheep or oxen. Also the rendered fat that drips from meat as it is roasted.

drisheen Irish; blood pudding; *see* black pudding.

drop scones *See* scones, drop.

drug-nutrient interactions Deficiency caused by effects of drugs on the absorption or metabolism of vitamins or minerals. Sometimes this is the mode of action of the drug in treating the disease; in other cases it is an undesirable side-effect.

drumstick The thigh of chicken or other poultry.

drunken foods Chinese; meat or fish is highly seasoned and marinated, then steamed or lightly simmered. After draining it is steeped in wine for several days before serving.

drupe Botanical term for a fleshy fruit with a single stone enclosing the seed that does not split along defined lines to liberate the seed, e.g. apricot, cherry, date, mango, olive, peach, plum.

DRV *See* Dietary Reference Values; Reference Intakes.

dry-blanch-dry process A method of drying fruit so as to retain the colour and flavour; it is faster than drying in the sun and preserves flavour and colour better than hot air drying. The material is dried to 50% water at about 82 °C, blanched for a few minutes, then dried at 68 °C over a period of 6–24 h to 15–20% water content.

dry brining *See* brining.

dry frying Frying without the use of fat by using an anti-stick agent of silicone or a vegetable extract.

dry ice Solid carbon dioxide, which has a temperature of −79 °C; used to refrigerate foodstuffs in transit and for carbonation of liquids. It sublimes from the solid to a gas without liquefying.

drying Method of preserving food by removing most of the water, so as to prevent bacterial and mould growth. Freeze-drying is evaporation of the water from a frozen food, so retaining textural properties and nutrients.

drying oil Any highly unsaturated oil that absorbs oxygen and, when in thin films, polymerizes to form a skin. Linseed and tung oil are examples of drying oils used in paints and in the manufacture of linoleum, etc. Nutritionally they are similar to edible oils, but when polymerized, are toxic. *See also* iodine value.

dubarry, à la A rich cauliflower soup or a cauliflower garnish.

Dublin Bay prawn Scampi or Norway lobster; a shellfish, *Nephrops norvegicus, see* lobster.

du Bois formula A formula for calculating *body surface area.

Dubonnet Trade name; an *aperitif wine.

duchesse potatoes Sieved boiled potato mixed with cream and egg, glazed with beaten egg, and baked until browned.

duck (French: *canard*; German: *Ente*.) Wild duck or wildfowl; mallard (*Anas platyrhynchos*), teal, small dabbling ducks of genus *Anas*. A 150-g portion is a rich *source of protein, vitamins B_1, B_2, B_{12}, niacin, and copper; a good source of iron and zinc; a source of vitamin B_6; contains 15 g of fat of which one-third is saturated; supplies 200 kcal (840 kJ).

ductless glands *See* endocrine glands.

dugléré Method of cooking white fish in white wine and water, adding cream and a velouté sauce.

dulce Spanish; sweet wines.

dulcin A synthetic material (*p*-phenetylurea or *p*-phenetolcarbamide, discovered in 1883) which is 250 times as sweet as sugar but is not permitted in foods. Also called sucrol and valzin.

dulcite *See* dulcitol.

dulcitol A six-carbon *sugar alcohol which occurs in some plants and is formed by the reduction of galactose; also known as melampyrin, dulcite, or galacticol.

dulse Edible purplish-brown seaweeds, *Rhodymenia palmata* and *Dilsea carnosa*, used in soups and jellies.

dumned Indian term for *steamed. *See also* bhoona.

dumpling A ball of *dough, usually boiled, but may be baked. Generally served with soups and stews.

dun Brown discoloration in salted fish caused by mould growth.

Dunaliella bardawil A red marine alga discovered in 1980 in Israel, which is extremely rich in β-*carotene, containing 100 times more than most other natural sources.

Dundee cake Rich fruit cake decorated with split almonds.

dung weed *See* fat hen.

dunst Very fine *semolina (starch from the endosperm of the wheat grain) approaching the fineness of flour. Also called break middlings (not to be confused with middlings, which is branny *offal).

duodenal ulcer *See* ulcer.

duodenum First part of the small intestine, between the stomach and the jejunum; the major site of *digestion. Pancreatic juice and bile are secreted into the duodenum. So called because it is about twelve fingerbreadths in length. *See also* gastro-intestinal tract.

durian Fruit of tree *Durio zibethinum*, grown in Malaysia and Indonesia. Each fruit weighs 2–3 kg and has a soft, cream-coloured pulp, with a smell considered disgusting by the uninitiated. A 100-g portion is a rich *source of vitamin C; a good source of vitamin B_1; a source of vitamin B_2; supplies 125 kcal (500 kJ).

durum wheat A hard type of *wheat of the species *Triticum durum* (most bread wheats are *Triticum vulgare*); largely used for the production of semolina intended for the preparation of *pasta.

Dutching *See* cocoa, Dutch.

Dutch oven A semicircular metal shield which may be placed close to an open fire; fitted with shelves on which food is roasted. It may also be clamped to the fire bars.

duxelles Mince of mushrooms with chopped shallot and herbs, used to flavour stuffing, soups, and sauces.

Dyox Trade name for chlorine dioxide used to treat flour. *See* ageing.

dyspepsia Any pain or discomfort associated with eating. Dyspepsia may be a symptom of gastritis, peptic ulcer, gall-bladder disease, etc., or, if there is no structural change in the intestinal tract, it is called 'functional dyspepsia'. Treatment includes a *bland diet. *See also* indigestion.

dysphagia Difficulty in swallowing, commonly associated with disorders of the *oesophagus. Inability to swallow is aphagia.

E- *See* E-numbers.

e On food labels, before the weight or volume, to indicate that this has been notified to the regulatory authorities of the EU as a standard package size.

EAA index Essential amino acid index, an index of *protein quality.

earth almond *See* tiger nut.

earth-nut The small edible tuber of the umbellifer *Conopodium denudatum*, or *C. majus*, also called pignut or fairy potato. Also another name for the *peanut.

Easter soup (*Mayieritsa*) Greek soup traditionally prepared to celebrate the end of the Lenten fast, made from the pluck (i.e. tripe, intestines, heart, and liver) and feet of a lamb.

eau de vie Spirit distilled from fermented grape juice (sometimes other fruit juices); may be flavoured with fruits, etc. *See also* marc.

eau-de-vie de miel Honey brandy made by distilling mead (which, in turn, is made by fermenting honey).

Eccles cake Pastry filled with dried fruit, melted butter, and sugar. Named originally for the town of Eccles in greater Manchester.

éclair Small finger-shaped cake prepared from *choux pastry, filled with cream or *confectioner's custard, coated with chocolate or coffee-flavoured icing.

E. coli *Escherichia coli*, a group of bacteria including both harmless ones that inhabit human intestines and some types that can cause *food poisoning.

écrévisse *See* crayfish.

ectomorph Description given to a tall, thin person, possibly with underdeveloped muscles. *See also* endomorph; mesomorph.

ecuelle A device for obtaining peel oil from citrus fruit. It consists of a shallow funnel lined with spikes on which the fruit is rolled by hand. As the oil glands are pierced, the oil and cell sap collect in the bottom of the funnel.

Edam Pale yellow, semi-hard Dutch *cheese usually round in shape with red wax coating (black for well-matured Edam). A 30-g portion is a rich *source of vitamin B_{12}, a source of protein and niacin, contains 8 g of fat, 230 mg of calcium and 300 mg of sodium; supplies 100 kcal (415 kJ).

eddo *See* taro.

edema *See* oedema.

edentulous Without teeth.

edetate *See* EDTA.

edgebone Incorrect name for the *aitchbone.

Edifas Trade name for *cellulose derivatives: Edifas A is methyl ethyl cellulose (E-465); Edifas B, sodium carboxymethylcellulose (E-466).

Edosol Trade name for a low-sodium milk substitute, containing 43 mg of sodium/100 g, compared with dried milk at 400 mg.

EDTA Ethylene diamine tetra-acetic acid, a compound that forms stable chemical complexes with metal ions (i.e. a *chelating agent). Also called versene, sequestrol, and sequestrene. It can be used both to remove metal ions from a solution (or at least to remove them from activity) and also to add metal ions, for example in plant fertilizers (E-385).

eel A long thin fish, *Anguilla anguilla*; the conger eel is *Conger myriaster*. Eels live in rivers but go to sea to breed. A 100-g portion is a rich *source of protein, niacin, and vitamins A, D, and B_{12}; a good source of niacin and vitamin B_2; a source of vitamins B_1 and B_6; contains 20 g of fat and supplies 300 kcal (1260 kJ).

EFA Essential fatty acids; *see* fatty acids, essential.

egg Hens' eggs are sold by size (EU); size 0 (weighs 75 g or more); size 1: 70g; size 2: 65 g; size 3: 60 g; size 4: 55 g; size 5: 50–55 g (weighed with shell which is about 10% of the total weight). Useful in food preparation to thicken *sauces and *custard, as an emulsifier, to hold air in meringues and sponges, and as a binder in *croquettes.

Average portion of two eggs is a rich *source of vitamins D and B_{12}; a good source of protein, niacin, and vitamins A and B_2; a source of zinc; contains 170 mg of sodium; 13 g of fat, of which 35% is saturated and 50% mono-unsaturated; supplies 175 kcal (735 kJ). The egg-white is 60% of the whole and the yolk 30%.

Duck eggs weigh about 85 g of which 10% is shell. One egg is a rich *source of vitamins A, D, and B_{12}; a good source of protein and vitamin B_2; contains 90 mg of sodium and 9 g of fat of which 30% is saturated and 20% polyunsaturated; supplies 120 kcal (500 kJ).

egg albumin *See* egg proteins; egg-white.

egg nog Hot, sweetened milk with an egg and brandy or sherry mixed in.

egg-plant *See* aubergine.

egg proteins What is generally referred to as egg protein is a mixture of individual proteins, including ovalbumin, ovomucoid, ovoglobulin, conalbumin, vitellin, and vitellenin. *Egg-white contains 10.9% protein, mostly ovalbumin; yolk contains 16% protein, mainly two phosphoproteins, vitellin and vitellenin. *See also* avidin.

eggs, Chinese (hundred years old) *See* Chinese eggs.

eggs flamenca (Spanish: *huevos a la flamenca*); Andalusian dish of eggs baked on a bed of fried potato, onion, peppers, chorizo, etc.

egg, Scotch *See* Scotch egg.

egg substitute Name formerly used for golden raising powder, a type of *baking powder.

egg-white The white of an egg is in three layers: an outer layer of thin white, a layer of thick white, richer in ovomucin, and an inner layer of thin white surrounding the yolk. The ratio of thick to thin white varies, depending on the individual hen. A higher proportion of thick white is desirable for frying and poaching, since it helps the egg to coagulate into a small firm mass instead of spreading; thin white produces a larger volume of froth when beaten than does thick. *See also* egg proteins.

egg-white injury *See* biotin.

EGRAC test *See* enzyme activation tests; glutathione reductase.

EH *See* equilibrium humidity.

eicosanoids Compounds formed in the body from long-chain polyunsaturated *fatty acids (*eicosenoic acids), including the prostaglandins, prostacyclins, thromboxanes, and leukotrienes, all of which act as local hormones and are involved in wound healing, inflammation, *platelet aggregation, and a variety of other functions.

eicosapentaenoic acid (EPA) A long-chain polyunsaturated *fatty acid; *see* fish oils.

eicosenoic acids Long-chain polyunsaturated *fatty acids; with 20 carbon atoms.

einkorn A type of *wheat, the wild form of which, *Triticum boeoticum*, was probably one of the ancestors of all cultivated wheats. Still grown in some parts of southern Europe and the Middle East, usually for animal feed. The name means 'one seed', from the single seed found in each spikelet.

eiswein *Wine made from grapes that have frozen on the vine, picked and processed while still frozen, so that the juice is highly concentrated and very sweet. Similar Canadian wines are known as ice wine. *See* wine classification, Germany.

eiweiss milch *See* protein milk.

elaichi *See* cardamom.

elastin Insoluble protein in *connective tissue, which is not changed by cooking, and hence is the cause of tough meat.

elder A common hedgerow bush (*Sambucus nigra*); the flowers are used to flavour cordials, syrups, fruit jellies, and elderflower wine. The fruit is used for making jelly and wine (elderberry wine).

electrolytes Chemically salts that dissociate in solution and will carry an electric current; generally used to mean the mineral salts of blood plasma and other body fluids, especially sodium and potassium.

electronic heating *See* microwave cooking.

electropure process A method of *pasteurizing milk by passing through it low-frequency, alternating current.

elemental diet *See* formula diet.

elements, minor *See* trace elements.

elixir Alcoholic extract (tincture) of a naturally occurring substance; originally devised by medieval alchemists (the elixir of life), now used for a variety of medicines, liqueurs, and *bitters.

elute To wash off or remove. Rather specifically applied to removal of adsorbed chemicals from the substance that adsorbed them, as in chromatography. *See also* ion exchange resins.

elver Young *eel, about 5 cm in length.

emaciation Extreme thinness and wasting, caused by disease or undernutrition. *See also* cachexia; protein-energy malnutrition.

Embden groats *See* groats.

emblic Berry of the South-East Asian malacca tree, *Emblica officinalis*, similar in appearance to the gooseberry. Also known as the Indian gooseberry. An exceptionally rich source of vitamin C: 600 mg per 100 g.

embolism Blockage of a blood vessel caused by a foreign object (embolus) such as a quantity of air or gas, a piece of tissue or tumour, a blood clot (thrombus), or fatty tissue derived from *atheroma, in the circulation.

emetic Substance that causes vomiting.

emincé French; a dish of meat cut into thin slices, covered with sauce, and baked in an earthenware dish.

emmental Semi-hard cow's milk cheese originally from Switzerland; has large round holes formed by gases from bacterial fermentation during ripening.

emmer A type of *wheat known to have been used more than 8000 years ago. Wild emmer is *Triticum dicoccoides* and true emmer is *T. dicoccum*. Nowadays grown mainly for animal feed.

empanadas Spanish (Galician); pies and pasties with a variety of savoury fillings.

Emprote Trade name for a dried milk and cereal preparation consumed as a beverage, containing 33% protein.

emulsifying agents Substances that are soluble in both fat and water and enable fat to be uniformly dispersed in water as an *emulsion. Foods that consist of such emulsions include *butter, *margarine, *salad dressings, mayonnaise, and *ice cream. *Stabilizers maintain emulsions in a stable form. Emulsifying agents are also used in baking to aid the smooth incorporation of fat into the dough and to keep the crumb soft.

   Emulsifying agents used in foods include *agar, *albumin, *alginates, *casein, egg yolk, *glycerol monostearate, *gums, *Irish moss, *lecithin, soaps.

emulsifying salts Sodium citrate, sodium phosphates, and sodium tartrate, used in the manufacture of milk powder, evaporated milk, sterilized cream, and processed cheese.

emulsin A mixture of *enzymes (glycosidases) in bitter *almond which hydrolyse the glucoside *amygdalin to benzaldehyde, glucose, and cyanide.

emulsion An intimate mixture of two immiscible liquids (for example oil and water), one being dispersed in the other in the form of fine droplets. They will stay mixed only as long as they are stirred together, unless an *emulsifying agent is added.

enchilada Mexican; *tortilla fried in oil, filled with meat, cheese, or vegetables and served with chilli sauce. *See also* tacos; tamales.

endive Curly serrated green leaves of *Cichorium endivia*. Called chicory in the USA and *chicorée frisée* in France. A 50-g portion is a *source of vitamin A (1000 μg carotene); it supplies 5 kcal (20 kJ), but little vitamin C. There is also broad-leaved Batavian endive which resembles lettuce. *See also* chicory.

endocrine glands Those (ductless) glands that produce and secrete *hormones, including the *thyroid gland (secreting thyroxine and tri-iodothyronine), *pancreas (*insulin and *glucagon), *adrenal glands (*adrenaline, *noradrenaline, *glucocorticoids, *mineralocorticoids), ovary and testes (sex steroids).

Some endocrine glands respond directly to chemical changes in the bloodstream; others are controlled by hormones secreted by the pituitary gland, under the control of the hypothalamus.

endomorph In relation to body build, means short and stocky. *See* ectomorph; mesomorph.

endomysium *See* muscle.

endopeptidases *Enzymes that hydrolyse proteins (i.e. proteinases or peptidases), by cleaving *peptide bonds inside protein molecules, as opposed to *exopeptidases, which remove amino acids from the end of the protein chain. The main endopeptidases in *digestion are chymotrypsin, elastase, pepsin, and trypsin.

endosperm The inner part of cereal grains; in wheat it comprises about 83% of the grain. Mainly starch, it is the source of *semolina. Contains only about 10% of the vitamin B_1, 35% of the vitamin B_2, 40% of the niacin, and 50% of the vitamin B_6 and pantothenic acid of the whole grain. *See also* flour, extraction rate.

endotoxins Toxins produced by bacteria as an integral part of the cell, so they cannot be separated by filtration; unlike *exotoxins, they do not usually stimulate antitoxin formation but the antibodies that they induce act directly on the bacteria. They are relatively stable to heat compared with exotoxins.

enema *See* nutrient enemata.

Energen rolls Trade name for a light *bread roll of wheat flour plus added wheat *gluten.

energy The ability to do work. The SI unit of energy is the joule, and nutritionally relevant amounts of energy are kilojoules (kJ, 1000 J) and megajoules (MJ, 1,000,000 J). The *calorie is still widely used in nutrition; 1 cal = 4.186 J (approximated to 4.2). While it is usual to speak of the calorie or joule content of a food it is more correct to refer to the energy content or yield.

The total chemical energy in a food, as released by complete combustion (in the bomb *calorimeter) is gross energy. Allowing for the losses of unabsorbed food in the faeces gives digestible energy. Allowing for loss in the urine due to incomplete combustion in the body (e.g. urea from the incomplete combustion of proteins) gives metabolizable energy. Allowing for the loss due to *diet-induced thermogenesis gives net energy, i.e. the actual amount available for use in the body. *See also* energy conversion factors.

energy balance The difference between intake of energy from foods and *expenditure on *basal metabolism and physical activity. Positive energy balance leads to increased body tissue, the normal process of growth. In adults positive energy balance leads to creation of body reserves of fat, resulting in overweight and *obesity. Negative energy balance leads to utilization of body reserves of fat and protein, resulting in wasting and undernutrition.

energy conversion factors Various factors are used to calculate the energy yields of foodstuffs.

The complete *heats of combustion (gross energy) as determined by *calorimetry are: protein, 5.7 kcal (23.9 kJ); fat, 9.4 kcal (39.5 kJ); carbohydrate, 4.1 kcal (17.2 kJ)/gram.

The Rubner conversion factors for metabolic energy yield are: protein, 4.1 kcal (17 kJ); fat, 9.3 kcal (39 kJ); carbohydrate, 4.1 kcal (17 kJ)/gram.

The Atwater factors also allow for losses in digestion and incomplete oxidation of the nitrogen of proteins: protein, 4 kcal (16.8 kJ); fat, 9 kcal (37.8 kJ); carbohydrate, 4 kcal (16.8 kJ)/gram.

The following factors are used in general practice: carbohydrate 4 kcal (17 kJ); fat, 9 kcal (38 kJ); carbohydrate (as monosaccharides), 4 kcal (17 kJ); *alcohol, 7 kcal (29 kJ); *sugar alcohols, 2.4 kcal (10 kJ); *organic acids, 3 kcal (13 kJ).

energy expenditure The total energy cost of maintaining constant conditions in the body, i.e. homeostasis (*basal metabolism, BMR) plus the energy cost of physical activities. The average total energy expenditure in Western countries is about 1.4 times BMR; a desirable level of physical activity should be about 1.7 times BMR.

energy metabolism The various reactions involved in the oxidation of metabolic fuels (mainly carbohydrates, fats, and proteins), to provide energy (linked to the formation of *ATP (adenosine triphosphate) from ADP (adenosine diphosphate) and phosphate ions).

energy requirements Energy requirements are calculated from estimated *basal metabolic rate and physical activity. Average energy requirements for adults are 1900 kcal (8 MJ)/day for women and 2400 kcal (10 MJ)/day for men.

energy-rich bonds An outdated and chemically incorrect concept in *energy metabolism, which suggested that the bond between ADP and phosphate in *ATP, and between *creatine and phosphate in creatine phosphate, which have a high chemical free energy of hydrolysis, somehow differs from 'ordinary' chemical bonds.

enfleurage A method of extracting essential oils from flowers by placing them on glass trays covered with purified *lard or other fat, which eventually becomes saturated with the oil.

English wine *See* wine.

enocianina Desugared grape extract used to colour fruit flavours. Prepared by acid extraction of the skins of black grapes; it is blue in neutral conditions and turns red in acid.

en papillote French method of cooking in a closed container, a parchment paper or aluminium foil case. *See also* sous vide.

enrichment The addition of nutrients to foods. Although often used interchangeably, the term *fortification is used of legally imposed additions, and enrichment means the addition of nutrients beyond the levels originally present. *See also* nutrification; restoration.

ensete *See* banana, false.

enteral nutrition Tube feeding with a liquid diet directly into the stomach or small intestine. *See also* gastrostomy feeding; nasogastric tube; nutrient enemata; parenteral nutrition.

enteritis Inflammation of the mucosal lining of the small intestine, usually resulting from infection. Regional enteritis is *Crohn's disease.

enterocolitis Inflammation of the mucosal lining of the small and large intestine, usually resulting from infection.

enterogastrone Hormone secreted by the small intestine which inhibits the activity of the stomach. Its secretion is stimulated by fat; hence, fat in the diet inhibits gastric activity.

enterokinase Obsolete name for the intestinal *enzyme *enteropeptidase.

enteropathy Any disease or disorder of the intestinal tract.

enteropeptidase An enzyme secreted by the small intestinal mucosa which activates trypsinogen (from the pancreatic juice) to the active proteolytic enzyme *trypsin. *See also* protein digestion.

enterotoxin Substances more or less specifically toxic to the cells of the intestinal mucosa, normally produced by bacteria.

enteroviruses Viruses that multiply mainly in the intestinal tract.

entoleter A machine used to disinfest cereals and other foods. The material is fed to the centre of a high-speed rotating disc carrying studs so that it is thrown against the studs; the impact kills any insects and destroys their eggs.

entrecôte Steak cut from the middle part of the sirloin of *beef; in France a steak taken from between two ribs.

entrée A dressed savoury dish, served hot or cold, complete in its dish with the sauce. The term is used both for the main part of a meal (especially in France) and also to describe courses intermediate between hors d'œuvre and main course.

entremeses Spanish; mixed hors d'œuvre dishes served as a prelude to a meal.

entremets French; originally a dish served between courses, now the dessert course.

E-numbers Within the EU food *additives may be listed on labels either by name or by their number in the EU list of permitted additives. *See* Appendix VIII.

enzyme A *protein that speeds up (catalyses) a metabolic reaction. Enzymes are specific for both the compounds acted on (the substrates) and the reactions carried out. Because of this, enzymes extracted from plant or animal sources or from micro-organisms, or those produced by *genetic manipulation are widely used in the chemical, pharmaceutical, and food industries (e.g. *chymosin in cheese making, *maltase in beer production, synthesis of *vitamin C and *citric acid), as well as in washing powders.

Because they are proteins, enzymes are permanently inactivated by heat, strong acid or alkali, and other conditions which cause *denaturation of proteins.

Many enzymes contain non-protein components which are essential for their function. These are known as prosthetic groups, *coenzymes, or cofactors, and may be metal ions, metal ions in organic combination (e.g. haem in *haemoglobin and *cytochromes) or a variety of organic compounds, many of which are derived from *vitamins. The (inactive) protein without its prosthetic group is known as the apo-enzyme, and the active assembly of protein plus prosthetic group is the holo-enzyme. *See also* enzyme activation assays; tenderizers.

enzyme activation A number of compounds increase the activity of enzymes; sometimes this is a part of normal metabolic regulation and integration (e.g. the responses to *hormones), and sometimes it is the action of drugs.

enzyme activation assays Used to assess the nutritional status of an individual with respect to *vitamins B_1, B_2, and B_6. A sample of red blood cells in a test-tube is tested for activity of the relevant *enzyme before and after adding extra vitamin; enhancement of the enzyme activity beyond a standard level serves as a biochemical index of a shortage of the vitamin in question. The enzymes involved are transketolase for vitamin B_1, glutathione reductase for vitamin B_2 and either aspartate or alanine aminotransferase for vitamin B_6.

enzyme induction Synthesis of new enzyme protein in response to some stimulus, normally a hormone, but sometimes a metabolic intermediate or other compound (e.g. a drug or food additive).

enzyme inhibition A number of compounds reduce the activity of enzymes; sometimes this is a part of normal metabolic regulation and integration (e.g. the responses to *hormones), and sometimes it is the action of drugs. Some inhibitors are reversible, others act irreversibly on the enzymes, and therefore have a longer duration of action (the activity of the enzyme remains low until more has been synthesized).

enzyme precursors *See* zymogens.

enzyme repression Reduction in synthesis of enzyme protein in response to some stimulus such as a hormone or the presence of large amounts of the end-product of its activity.

EPA Eicosapentaenoic acid; *see* fish oils.

epicarp *See* flavedo.

epigramme French; small pieces of neck or breast of lamb, cooked, then dipped in egg and breadcrumbs and grilled or fried.

epinephrine *See* adrenaline.

Epsom salts Magnesium sulphate, originally found in a mineral spring in Epsom, Surrey, England; acts as a purgative because the *osmotic pressure of the solution causes it to retain water in the intestine and so increase the bulk and moisture content of the faeces.

Equal Trade name for *aspartame.

equilibrium humidity The relative humidity of the atmosphere with which the substance under consideration is in equilibrium.

equilibrium, nitrogen *See* nitrogen balance.

ercalciol *See* vitamin D.

erdbeergeist German spirit distilled from strawberries with added alcohol.

erepsin Name given to a mixture of enzymes contained in *intestinal juice, including aminopeptidases and dipeptidases.

ergocalciferol *See* vitamin D.

ergosterol A sterol isolated from yeast; when treated with ultra-violet light, it is converted to ercalciol (ergocalciferol, vitamin D_2). This is the main source of manufactured *vitamin D.

ergot A fungus that grows on grasses and cereal grains; the ergot of medical importance is *Claviceps purpurea*, which grows on rye. The consumption of infected rye is harmful, causing the disease known as St Anthony's fire (*ergotism), and can be fatal.

    The active principles in ergot are alkaloids (ergotinine, ergotoxine, ergotamine, ergometrine, etc.), which yield lysergic acid on hydrolysis. This is believed to be the active component. Its effect is to increase the tone and contraction of smooth muscle, particularly of the pregnant uterus. For this reason ergot has been used in obstetrics, but pure ergonovine maleate and ergotonine tartrate are preferable.

ergotism Poisoning due to an *ergot infection of rye which occurs from time to time among people eating rye bread. The last outbreak in the UK was in Manchester in 1925, when there were 200 cases. Symptoms appear when as little as 1% of ergot-infected rye is included in the flour.

eriodictin A *flavonoid (flavonone) found in citrus pith, a constituent of what is sometimes called vitamin P.

erucic acid A mono-unsaturated *fatty acid, *cis*-13-docosenoic acid found in *rape seed (*Brassica napus*) and mustard seed (*B. junca* and *B. nigra*) oils; it may constitute 30–50% of the oil in some varieties. It causes fatty infiltration of heart muscle in experimental animals, and the amount of ordinary rape seed oil used in margarines is consequently limited. Low erucic acid varieties of rape seed have been developed for food use.

eructation The act of bringing up air from the stomach, with a characteristic sound. Also known as belching.

erythorbic acid The D-isomer of *ascorbic acid, also called D-araboascorbic acid and iso-ascorbic acid, with only slight *vitamin C activity. It is as powerful an antioxidant as vitamin C and is used in foods for that purpose.

erythroamylose An old name for *amylopectin.

erythrocytes See blood cells, red.

erythropoiesis The formation and development of the red *blood cells in the bone marrow.

erythrosine BS Red colour permitted in foods in most countries (E-127, known as Red number 3 in USA). Used in preserved cherries, sausages, and meat and fish pastes; it is unstable to light and heat. Chemically the disodium or potassium salt of 2,4,5,7-tetraiodofluorescein.

escabeche Caribbean; fish, poultry, or game cooked in oil and vinegar or cooked and then pickled in oil and vinegar marinade. From the Spanish for pickled. Fish prepared in this way is also known as escovitch or caveached fish.

escalope Thin slice of meat (generally veal or pork), round or oval shaped, cut from the top of the leg or fillet. Also a thin slice of fish.

escargot See snail.

escarole See endive.

escovitch See escabeche.

esculin See aesculin.

espagnole sauce Spanish *sauce; basically a thick, brown *roux, diluted with stock made from meat or bones, with onion, carrot, garlic, herbs, tomato pulp, and sherry.

ESPEN European Society for Parenteral and Enteral Nutrition.

espresso Italian; strong black coffee made by forcing steam through finely ground coffee.

espumante Portuguese; sparkling wines.

espumoso Spanish; sparkling wines.

essential amino acid index An index of *protein quality.

essential amino acid pattern, provisional The quantities of essential *amino acids considered desirable in the diet.

essential amino acids See amino acids, essential.

essential fatty acids See fatty acids, essential.

essential nutrient Those nutrients that are required by the body and cannot be synthesized in the body in adequate amounts to meet requirements, so must be provided by the diet: includes the essential *amino acids and *fatty acids, *vitamins, and *minerals. Really a tautology, since by definition nutrients are essential dietary constituents.

essential oils Volatile, aromatic, or odoriferous oils found in plants and used for flavouring foods. Chemically they are quite distinct from the edible oils, since they are not glycerol esters. See also terpenes.

esterases *Enzymes that hydrolyse *esters, i.e. cleave the ester linkage to form free acid and alcohol. Those that hydrolyse the ester linkages of fats are generally known as *lipases, and those that hydrolyse *phospholipids as phospholipases.

esters The chemical name for the compounds formed by condensation between an acid and an alcohol, e.g. ethyl alcohol and acetic acid yield the ester ethyl acetate. *Fats are esters of the alcohol glycerol, and long-chain *fatty acids. Many esters are used as synthetic *flavours.

ester value *See* saponification value.

estouffade Meat cooked very slowly in very little liquid; braised or casseroled.

ethanoic acid *See* acetic acid.

ethanol Systematic chemical name for ethyl *alcohol.

ethanolamine One of the water-soluble bases of *phospholipids, chemically it is 2-aminoethanol. Used as softening agent for hides, as dispersing agent for agricultural chemicals, and to peel fruits and vegetables.

ethene *See* ethylene.

ethyl alcohol *See* alcohol.

ethyl carbamate *See* urethane.

ethylene Ethene; a gas of the formula $CH_2{=}CH_2$, produced by fruit as a hormone to speed ripening. This explains why some fruits ripen faster if they are stored in a plastic bag. It is used commercially in very small amounts to speed fruit ripening after harvesting.

ethylene diamine tetra-acetic acid *See* EDTA.

ethyl formate Used as a fumigant against raisin moth, dried fruit beetle, fig moth, etc., and as a flavour; an ingredient of lemon, strawberry, and artificial rum flavours.

ethylmethylcellulose *See* cellulose derivatives.

ethyl vanillin A synthetic compound, chemically the ethyl analogue of vanillin, the major flavouring principle of *vanilla.

eukeratins *See* keratin.

eutectic ice The solid formed when a mixture of 76.7% water and 23.3% salt (by weight) is frozen. It melts at −21 °C. It has about three times the refrigerant effect of solid carbon dioxide (*dry ice), and is especially useful for icing fish on board trawlers.

eutrophia Normal nutrition.

evaporation, flash A short, rapid application of heat so that a small volume (about 1% of the total) is quickly distilled off, carrying with it the greater part of the volatile components. The flash distillate is collected separately from the later distillate and is added back to the concentrate to restore the flavour; applied to the concentration of products such as fruit juices.

evening primrose *Oenothera biennis*, the oil from the seeds is a rich source of *γ-linolenic acid, which may account for 8% of total *fatty acids. It is used as a dietary supplement and may have beneficial effects in a number of conditions, although there is little firm scientific evidence of its efficacy.

Evian water A still mineral water from a source in Evian in southern France.

exchange list List of portions of foods in which energy yield, fat, carbohydrate, and/or protein content are equivalent, so simplifying meal and diet planning for people with special needs.

exclusion diet A limited diet excluding foods known possibly to cause food intolerance, to which foods are added in turn to test for intolerance (allergy). *See* adverse reactions to foods.

exergonic Chemical reactions that proceed with the output of energy, usually as heat (then sometimes known as exothermic reactions) or light. The reactions involved in the oxidation of food-stuffs are generally exergonic.

exopeptidases Proteolytic enzymes that hydrolyse the peptide bonds of the terminal amino acids of proteins or peptides, as opposed to *endopeptidases, which cleave at sites in the middle of a peptide chain. There are two groups: aminopeptidases which remove the amino acid at the amino terminal of the protein, and carboxypeptidases, which remove the amino acid at the carboxyl terminal.

exothermic *See* exergonic.

exotic foods Foods introduced from a foreign country.

exotoxins Toxic substances produced by bacteria which diffuse out of the cells and stimulate the production of antibodies which specifically neutralize them (antitoxins). They are generally heat-labile and inactivated in about 1 hour at 60 °C. Exotoxins include those produced by the organisms responsible for *botulism, tetanus, and diphtheria. *See also* endotoxins.

expansion rings In relation to cans, the concentric rings stamped into the ends of the can to allow bulging during heat processing without straining the seams unduly.

expeller cake The residue from oilseeds after most of the oil has been removed by pressing; it is a valuable source of protein, especially for animal feeding.

extensograph (extensometer) An instrument for measuring the stretching strength of dough as an index of its baking quality.

extraction rate *See* flour, extraction rate.

extract of malt *See* malt.

extract of meat *See* meat extract.

extract of yeast *See* yeast extract.

extremophiles Micro-organisms that can grow under extreme conditions of heat (*thermophiles and extreme thermophiles, some of which live in hot-springs at 100 °C), or cold (*psychrophyles), in high concentrations of salt (*halophiles), high pressure, or extremes of acid or alkali.

extrinsic factor *See* anaemia, pernicious; vitamin B_{12}.

FAD Flavin adenine dinucleotide, one of the *coenzymes formed from *vitamin B₂ (riboflavin).

faeces Body waste, composed of undigested food residues, remains of digestive secretions that have not been reabsorbed, bacteria from the intestinal tract, cells, cell debris and mucus from the intestinal lining, and substances excreted into the intestinal tract (mainly in the *bile). The average amount is about 100 g/day, but varies widely depending on the intake of *dietary fibre.

faggot 1 Traditional British meatball made from pig *offals and meat. A 150-g portion is an exceptionally rich *source of iron and a rich source of vitamins B₁, B₂, and niacin; contains 28 g of fat; supplies 400 kcal (1680 kJ).
   2 Bundle of herbs, *bouquet garni.

fair maids Cornish name for *pilchards (thought to be a corruption of the Spanish *fumade*, 'smoked').

fairy cakes *See* cup cake.

fairy potato *See* earth-nut.

fakasoupa Greek *lentil soup.

falafel Israeli, Middle Eastern; small deep-fried balls of spiced *chick pea flour, normally served in *pita bread with salad and a piquant sauce.

familial hypercholesterolaemia *See* hypercholesterolaemia.

fansi *See* beans, French.

FAO Food and Agriculture Organization of the United Nations, founded in 1943; headquarters in Rome. Its goal is to achieve freedom from hunger worldwide. According to its constitution the specific objectives are 'raising the levels of nutrition and standards of living ... and securing improvements in the efficiency of production and distribution of all food and agricultural products'.

farce Stuffing, hence forcemeat as a name for meats used as stuffing.

Farex Trade name for an infant cereal food.

farfals *See* pasta.

farina General term for starch. More specifically in the UK refers to *potato starch; in the USA is defined as the starch obtained from wheat other than *durum wheat; starch from the latter is *semolina.

farinaceous Starchy.

farina dolce Italian; flour made from dried chestnuts.

farinograph An instrument for measuring the physical properties of a dough.

farl Scottish; triangular oatmeal cake.

fasolada Greek; bean soup.

fassolia Greek; a variety of dishes prepared with dried beans.

fast foods (fast service foods) General term used for a limited menu of foods that lend themselves to production-line techniques; suppliers tend to specialize in products such as *hamburgers, *pizzas, chicken, or *sandwiches.

fasting Going without food. The metabolic fasting state begins some 4 hours after a meal, when the digestion and absorption of food are complete and body reserves of fat and *glycogen begin to be mobilized. In more prolonged fasting the blood concentration of *ketone bodies rises, as they are exported from the liver for use by muscle and other tissues as a metabolic fuel.

fat 1 Chemically fats (or lipids) are substances that are insoluble in water but soluble in organic solvents such as ether, chloroform, and benzene, and are actual or potential esters of *fatty acids. The term includes triacylglycerols (triglycerides), phospholipids, waxes, and sterols.

   2 In more general use the term 'fats' refers to the neutral fats which are mixtures of esters of *fatty acids with *glycerol, triacylglycerols (or triglycerides).

fat, blood Total blood fat in the fasting state is about 590 mg per 100 mL plasma: 150 mg neutral fats (*triacylglycerols), 160 mg (4 mmol) cholesterol, 200 mg phospholipids. This is mainly in the plasma *lipoproteins. After a meal the total fat increases, as a result of the *chylomicrons containing the recently absorbed dietary fat. *See also* lipids, plasma.

fat, brown See brown adipose tissue.

fat-extenders See superglycinerated fats.

fat-free EU regulations restrict use of the term 'fat-free' to foods that contain less than 0.15 g of fat/100 g; in the USA low-fat foods must state the percentage of fat; thus a product described as 95% fat-free contains only 5 g of fat/100 g.

fat hen A common wild plant (*Chenopodium album*); The leaves have a strong scent when crushed, akin to that of chrysanthemum leaves, and can be used in soup or fried as a vegetable. The name comes from the fact that it was formerly used to feed hens. The seeds can be ground into a flour for preparation of bread, cakes, and gruel; they have a flavour similar to that of *buckwheat. Also known as bacon weed, dirty dick, muck hill, or dung weed (because it commonly grows around dung heaps), goose foot (because of the shape of the leaves), and pig weed.

fat, neutral *Fats that are chemically *triacylglycerols (triglycerides).

fat-replacers Substances that provide a creamy, fat-like texture used to replace or partly replace the fat in a recipe food. Made from a variety of substances, e.g. Slendid is the trade name for such a product derived from pectin, Olestra is *sucrose polyester which is not absorbed by the body, Simplesse is a protein product, N-oil is made from tapioca.

fat, saturated *Fats containing only or mainly saturated *fatty acids.

fats, high-ratio *See* superglycinerated fats.

fats, hydrogenated *See* hydrogenated oils.

fats, non-saponifiable, saponifiable *See* saponification.

fat-soluble vitamins *Vitamins A, D, E, and K; they occur in food dissolved in the fats and are stored in the body to a greater extent than the water-soluble vitamins.

fat spread A general term for fatty bread spreads (yellow fats), including *butter, *margarine, and low-fat spreads. Reduced fat spreads contain not more than 60% fat, and low-fat spreads not more than 40%, compared with 80% fat in butter and margarine. Very low-fat spreads contain less than 20% fat.

fats, yellow *See* fat spread.

fatty acids Organic *acids consisting of carbon chains with a carboxyl group at the end. The nutritionally important fatty acids have an even number of carbon atoms, commonly between twelve and twenty-two.

Saturated fatty acids are those in which every carbon atom carries its full 'quota' of hydrogen atoms, and therefore there are only single bonds between adjacent carbon atoms. It is recommended that intake should not exceed about 11% of food energy intake, since they increase levels of blood *cholesterol (a major risk factor in *heart disease).

Unsaturated fatty acids have one or more carbon-carbon double bonds in the molecule. Chemically these double bonds can take up hydrogen, which is the process of hydrogenation, forming saturated fatty acids. Fatty acids with only one double bond are termed mono-unsaturated, *oleic acid is the main one found in fats and oils. Fatty acids with two or more double bonds are termed polyunsaturated fatty acids, often abbreviated to pufa.

Unsaturated fatty acids not only do not raise the levels of cholesterol in the blood but may be beneficial; their dietary value depends to a great extent on replacing saturated fatty acids. Vegetable and fish oils are generally rich sources of unsaturated fatty acids.

In general fats from animal sources are high in saturated and relatively low in unsaturated fatty acids; vegetable and fish oils are generally higher in unsaturated and lower in saturated fatty acids.

In addition to their accepted names, fatty acids can be named by a shorthand giving the number of carbon atoms in the molecule (e.g. C18), then a colon and the number of double bonds (e.g. C18 : 2), followed by the position of the first double bond from the methyl end of the molecule as n- or ω (e.g. C18 : 2 n-6, or C18 : 2 ω6). *See* Appendix X.

fatty acids, essential (EFA) Fatty acids that cannot be made in the body and are therefore dietary essentials; two polyunsaturated fatty acids: linoleic (C18 : 2 ω6) and α-linolenic (C18 : 3 ω3). Several other fatty acids have some EFA activity in that they cure some, but not all, of the signs of (experimental) EFA deficiency. *Arachidonic, *eicosapentaenoic (EPA), and *docosahexaenoic (DHA) acids are physiologically important, although they are not dietary essentials since they can be formed from linoleic and α-linolenic acids. *See* Appendix X.

The requirement to prevent deficiency is about 1% of total energy intake, equivalent to 260 mg/MJ; a desirable intake, and the basis of *Reference Intakes is 8–10% of energy intake, about 2–2.6 g/MJ. Although all fatty foods contain some essential fatty acids, the richest sources are vegetable and fish oils.

fatty acids, free (FFA) Fatty acids may be liberated from triacylglycerols (triglycerides) either by enzymic hydrolysis (when they are generally known as non-esterified fatty acids, nefa, or unesterified fatty acids, ufa) or as a result of hydrolytic rancidity of the fat. Determination of FFA is therefore an index of the quality of fats.

Free fatty acids circulate in the bloodstream, bound to albumin. They are released from *adipose tissue, especially in the fasting state, as a fuel for muscle and other tissues. The normal concentration in plasma is between 0.5 and 2 μmol/L, increasing with fasting and exercise.

fatty acids, unesterified, non-esterified (NEFA) *See* fatty acids, free.

fatty acids, volatile Refers to acetic, propionic, and butyric acids which, apart from their presence in some foods, are produced by bacteria in the human intestine and rumen of cattle from undigested starch and dietary fibre. To some extent they can be absorbed and used as a source of energy. Butyric acid formed in the colon may have some anti-carcinogenic action.

fat, unsaturated *Fats containing a high proportion of unsaturated *fatty acids.

fat, white *See* adipose tissue.

favism Acute haemolytic *anaemia induced in genetically sensitive people by eating broad beans, *Vicia faba*. The disease is due to deficiency of the *enzyme glucose-6-phosphate dehydrogenase in the red *blood cells, which are then vulnerable to the toxins, vicine and convicine, in the beans. The condition affects some 100 million people world-wide, and is commonest in people of Mediterranean and Middle-Eastern descent.

FDA Food and Drug Administration; US government regulatory agency.

fecula (fécule) Foods that are almost solely starch; prepared from roots and stems by grating, e.g. *tapioca, *sago, and *arrowroot; starchy powder from rice, potatoes, etc.

feijoa beans *See* beans, adzuki.

Feingold diet Exclusion of foods containing synthetic colours, flavours, and preservatives and limitation of intake of fruits and vegetables such as oranges, apricots, peaches, tomatoes, and cucumbers; intended to treat hyperactive children. There is little evidence either that these foods are a cause of hyperactivity or that the exclusion diet is beneficial.

fenfluramine Anorectic (*appetite suppressing) drug used in the treatment of *obesity.

feng kuo Chinese (Cantonese); savoury filling of chopped roast meat or seafood with mushrooms and bamboo shoots, flavoured with oyster sauce and wrapped in dough made from flour, cornflour, and lotus root flour, then fried.

fennel 1 Aromatic seeds and feathery green leaves of the perennial plant, *Foeniculum vulgare*, used to flavour a variety of dishes.
  2 *Foeniculum dulce* (or *F. vulgare* var. *azoricum*). Annual plant, also called Florence fennel or finnochio; the swollen bases of the leaves are eaten as a vegetable, raw or cooked (aniseed flavour). Seeds used as flavouring; a 60-g portion supplies 10 kcal (40 kJ).

fenugreek *Trigonella feonumgraecum*, a leguminous plant eaten as a vegetable; the seeds are used for flavouring. It is traditionally eaten by women in the Orient to help gain weight.

ferment As a noun, the old name for *enzyme. As a verb, to carry out the process of *fermentation.

fermentation Anaerobic *metabolism. Used generally of alcohol fermentation of sugars, also production of lactic acid, citric acid, etc., by micro-organisms.

fermented milk *See* milk, fermented.

fermentograph An instrument for measuring the gas-producing power of a dough.

Fernet Branca Italian; bitter *digestif; herbs and spices steeped in white wine and brandy.

ferric ammonium citrate The chemical form in which *iron is sometimes added to foods. Occurs as brown-red scales (16.5–18.5% iron) and as green scales (14.5–16% iron).

ferritin *See* iron storage.

ferrum redactum See iron, reduced.

feta Greek, general Balkan; semi-hard white cheese from ewe's or goat's milk; preserved in salt water. A 30-g portion is a rich *source of vitamin B_{12}, a source of protein, contains 6 g of fat of which three-quarters is saturated, 450 mg of sodium, and 100 mg of calcium; supplies 75 kcal (310 kJ).

fettucini Ribbon-shaped *pasta.

FFA Free fatty acids. *See* fatty acids, free.

fibre, crude The term given to the indigestible part of foods, defined in the UK Fertilizer and Feedingstuffs Act of 1932 as the residue left after successive extraction under closely specified conditions with petroleum ether, 1.25% sulphuric acid, and 1.25% sodium hydroxide, minus ash. No real relation to *dietary fibre.

fibre, dietary *See* dietary fibre.

fibre, insoluble The part of *dietary fibre (or *non-starch polysaccharide) that is not soluble in water, i.e. *cellulose, hemicelluloses, and lignin. These increase the bulk of the intestinal contents.

fibre, soluble The part of the *dietary fibre (or *non-starch polysaccharide) that forms a gel in water and hence is soluble, i.e.

*pectins and plant *gums. These increase the viscosity of the intestinal contents.

fibrin The blood protein formed from *fibrinogen which is responsible for the clotting of *blood.

fibrinogen One of the proteins of the blood plasma which is responsible for the clotting of *blood. When *prothrombin is activated to thrombin in response to injury, it converts fibrinogen to fibrin, which is deposited as strands that trap the red cells and form the clot.

fibrous proteins See albuminoids.

ficin Proteolytic *enzyme from the *fig.

fiddleheads Canadian name for *bracken fronds.

field egg See aubergine.

field mushroom Agaricus campestris, A. vaporarius; see mushrooms.

fig The fruit of Ficus carica; eaten fresh or dried. Figs have mild laxative properties, e.g. syrup of figs is a medicinal preparation. A 40-g portion of dried figs (two figs) is a *source of calcium, iron, and copper; provides 3 g of dietary fibre; supplies 80 kcal (335 kJ) and contains 50% sugars. A 100-g portion of fresh figs (two figs) supplies 60 kcal (245 kJ).

fig, Adam's See plantain.

fig, berberry or Indian See prickly pear.

figgy pudding Pudding made with raisins; originally dried figs stewed in wine. Figgy duff or figgie hobbin is the Cornish name for a pastry containing raisins.

FIGLU test A test for *folic acid nutritional status, based on excretion of formiminoglutamic acid (FIGLU), a metabolite of the *amino acid *histidine, which is normally metabolized by a folic acid-dependent enzyme.

figueredas Spanish (Valenciana); a spiced seafood dish similar to *paella, but served on a bed of pasta rather than rice.

filbert See hazel nut.

filé powder Dried powdered young leaves of the sassafras tree (Sassafras albidum); very aromatic, an essential ingredient of *gumbo.

filled milk See milk, filled.

fillet 1 The lean, tender strip of meat beneath an animal's ribs, especially beef. Now also used to mean a lean cut of veal, lamb, or pork from the top of the hind leg.
   2 To remove the bones from fish. Filet mignon (French 'dainty fillet') is a small, round cut of beef from the centre of the fillet, similar to *tournedo.

film yeasts See yeasts.

filo pastry See phyllo pastry.

filter To strain a liquid through a porous paper, fine cloth, etc., to remove small particles, as in making coffee or clarifying fruit juice to make jelly. Water may be filtered through charcoal to remove unpleasant flavours and colours; bacterial filters for water have pores fine enough to remove bacteria.

filth test Name given to a test originated in the USA for determining the contamination of a food with rodent hairs and insect fragments as an index of the hygienic handling of the food.

financière, à la Meat or poultry in a rich Madeira sauce containing mushrooms and truffles, or with a garnish of cocks' combs, cocks' kidneys, truffles, olives, and mushrooms.

fines herbes Mixture of chopped parsley, tarragon, chives, chervil, marjoram, and sometimes watercress.

fingerware Edible seaweed, *Laminaria digitata*.

fining agents Substances used to clarify liquids by precipitation, e.g. *egg albumin, casein, bentonite, *isinglass, *gelatine, etc.

finnan haddock Smoke-cured haddock (named after Findon in Scotland). *See also* Arbroath smokie.

fino Very dry *sherry.

finocchio Variety of *fennel with swollen leaf base; *Foeniculum vulgare* var. *azoricum*.

fior d'Alpi Italian; liqueur flavoured with alpine herbs and flowers; there is a sugar-encrusted twig in each bottle.

fireless cooker *See* haybox cooking.

fire point The temperature at which a frying oil will sustain combustion. It ranges between 340 and 360 °C for different fats. *See also* flash point; smoke point.

firkin A quarter of a barrel of beer, 9 imperial gallons (40 L); also 56 lb (25.5 kg) of butter.

firmi Indian; rice dessert with almonds and pistachio nuts.

firming agents Fresh fruits contain insoluble *pectins as a firm gel around the fibrous tissues which keeps the fruit firm. Breakdown of cell structure allows conversion of pectin to pectic acid, with loss of firmness. The addition of calcium salts (chloride or carbonate) forms a calcium pectate gel which protects the fruit against softening; these are known as firming agents. Alum is sometimes used to firm pickles.

first teeth *See* teeth, deciduous.

fish cakes Chopped or minced fish, bound with egg and flour (or *matzo meal) and seasoned with onion, pepper, and sometimes herbs, then deep fried. *See also* gefillte fish.

fish, fatty or oily Anchovies, herring, mackerel, pilchard, salmon, sardine, trout, tuna, whitebait, containing about 15% fat (varying from 5 to 20% through the year) and containing 10–40 µg vitamin D per 100 g, as distinct from white fish, which contain 1–2% fat and only a trace of vitamin D. *See also* herring.

fish fingers Shaped fish fillets covered with breadcrumbs; approximately 50% fish. Two fish fingers, grilled (55 g) are a rich *source of iodine; a source of protein and niacin; contain 5 g of fat, of which one-third is saturated and one-third polyunsaturated; and supply 120 kcal (500 kJ).

fish flour *See* fish protein concentrate.

fish ham Japanese product made from a red fish such as tuna or marlin, pickled with salt and nitrite, mixed with whale meat and pork fat and stuffed into a large sausage-type casing.

fish meal Surplus fish, waste from filleting (fish-house waste), and fish unsuitable for human consumption are dried and powdered. The resultant meal is a valuable source of protein for animal feed, or, after deodorization, as human food since it contains about 70% protein of biological value up to 0.7. That made from white fish is termed white fish meal, distinct from the oily type which is sometimes of very poor quality and is consequently used as fertilizer.

fish oils These contain long-chain polyunsaturated *fatty acids which appear to offer some protection against problems associated with heart disease. The two main ones are EPA (eicosapentaenoic acid; twenty carbon atoms and five double bonds) and DHA (docosahexaenoic acid; twenty-two carbon atoms and six double bonds). Fish oil concentrates containing these fatty acids are sold as pharmaceutical preparations. *See also* cod liver oil; halibut liver oil; menhaden; Appendix X.

fish, oily *See* fish, fatty.

fish paste A spread made from ground fish and cereal. In the UK it legally contains not less than 70% fish.

fish protein concentrate Deodorized, decolorized, defatted *fish meal, also known as fish flour. A cheap source of protein for enrichment of foods. Approximately 70% protein; *biological value 0.7.

fish sausage Japanese product made from chopped fish fillet, spiced and flavoured, with added fat and starch, and packed into sausage casing.

fish stick *See* seafood stick; also American name for *fish fingers.

fish tapeworm *See* tapeworm.

fish, white Non-oily fish, i.e. 1–2% fat, e.g. cod, dogfish, haddock, halibut, plaice, saithe, skate, sole, and whiting. All are similar in nutrient composition; a 150-g portion, steamed (200 g with skin and bones) is an exceptionally rich *source of iodine; a rich source of protein, niacin, and selenium; supplies 120 kcal (500 kJ). When fried (coated in breadcrumbs) the fat content increases to about 10 g and the energy increases to 240 kcal (1000 kJ). These figures are higher for fish fried in batter.

five-spice powder Chinese; a mixture of star *anise, anise pepper, fennel, cloves, and cinnamon, and sometimes also powdered dried orange peel.

flageolet Small green variety of haricot bean. *See* bean, haricot.

flaky pastry *See* pastry.

flamande, à la Dish served with a garnish of braised vegetables and bacon or small pork sausages.

flambé (flamber) Brandy or other spirit is poured over the food (particularly crêpes and Christmas pudding) and set alight before serving. Also the process of singeing poultry before cooking.

flan Open fruit tart, on a base of pastry or sponge.

flán Spanish; *see* caramel cream.

flapjack 1 Biscuit made from fat, sugar, rolled oats and syrup. **2** A thick pancake.

flash evaporation *See* evaporation, flash.

flash-pasteurization *See* pasteurization.

flash point With reference to frying oils, the temperature at which the decomposition products can be ignited, but will not support combustion; range between 290 and 330 ˚C. *See also* fire point; smoke point.

flatfish *Fish with a flattened shape, including dab, flounder, halibut, plaice, sole and turbot.

flatogens Substances that cause gas production, *flatulence, in the intestine, by providing fermentable substrate for intestinal bacteria. Those identified include small *oligosaccharides such as raffinose, stachyose, and verbascose in a variety of beans. *See also* non-starch polysaccharides.

flat sours Bacteria such as *Bacillus stearothermophilus* render canned food sour by fermenting carbohydrates to lactic, formic, and acetic acids, without gas production. This means that the ends of the can are not swelled out but remain flat. Economically they are the most important of the *thermophilic spoilage agents; some species can grow slowly at 25 ˚C and thus spoil products after long storage periods.

flatulence (flatus) Production of gas in the intestine; hydrogen, carbon dioxide, and methane. May be caused by a variety of foods including beans, Brussels sprouts, cabbage, cauliflower, onion, radishes, melon, and avocado, which contain *flatogens.

flavanols, flavanones *See* flavonoids.

flavedo The coloured outer peel layer of citrus fruits, also called the epicarp or zest. It contains the oil sacs, and hence the aromatic oils, and numerous plastids which are green and contain chlorophyll in the unripe fruit, turning yellow or orange in the ripe fruit, when they contain carotene and xanthophyll.

flavin The group of compounds containing the iso-alloxazine ring structure, as in riboflavin (*vitamin B_2), and hence a general term for riboflavin derivatives.

flavin adenine dinucleotide (FAD) A *coenzyme in oxidation reactions, derived from *vitamin B_2, phosphate, ribose, and adenine.

flavin mononucleotide (FMN) A *coenzyme in oxidation reactions, chemically the phosphate of *vitamin B_2 (riboflavin).

flavone *See* flavonoids.

flavonoids Compounds widely distributed in nature as pigments in flowers, fruit, vegetables, and tree barks. Chemically they are glycosides of flavones; the sugar moiety may be either rhamnose or rhamnoglucose, and depending on the different reactive groups in the flavone may be flavonols, flavanones, flavonals, or isoflavones.

Some of the flavonoids have pharmacological actions, but they are not known to be dietary essentials, although claims have been made (they were at one time classified as *vitamin P), and are sometimes called bioflavonoids. They may make a useful contribution to the total *antioxidant activity of foods.

flavonols *See* flavonoids.

flavoproteins Enzymes that contain the vitamin *riboflavin, or a derivative such as flavin adenine dinucleotide or riboflavin phosphate, as the *prosthetic group. Mainly involved in oxidation reactions in *metabolism.

flavour *See* taste; organoleptic.

flavour enhancer *See* flavour potentiator.

flavour potentiator A substance that enhances the flavours of other substances without itself imparting any characteristic flavour of its own, e.g. *monosodium glutamate and ribotide as well as sugar, salt, and vinegar in small quantities.

flavour profile A method of judging the flavour of foods by examination of a list of the separate factors into which the flavour can be analysed, the so-called character notes.

flavours, synthetic Mostly mixtures of *esters, e.g. banana oil is ethyl butyrate and amyl acetate; apple oil, ethyl butyrate, ethyl valerianate, ethyl salicylate, amyl butyrate, glycerol, chloroform, and alcohol; pineapple oil is ethyl and amyl butyrates, acetaldehyde, chloroform, glycerol, and alcohol.

flea seed *See* psyllium.

fleishig Jewish term for dishes containing meat, which cannot be served with or before milk dishes. *See also* milchig, pareve.

fleuron Small crescent-shaped piece of puff pastry used as a garnish.

flint corn *See* maize.

flip Drink made with beaten egg and milk, with added wine or spirit, and sweetened.

flippers *See* swells.

flitch Side of bacon; half a pig, slit down the back, with the legs and shoulders removed.

floats Caribbean (Trinidad); fried biscuits made with yeast dough. *See also* bakes.

flor de Jamaica *See* rosella.

Florence oil Name given to a high grade of *olive oil.

florentine 1 Thin biscuits with nuts and dried fruit coated with chocolate.
    2 Garnished with spinach.

floridean starch A polysaccharide (chemically a glucosan) resembling *glycogen, obtained from red algae (*Florideae* spp.).

flounder Small flatfish, *Platichthys* spp., also called fluke.

flour Most commonly refers to the ground wheat berry, although also used for other cereals and applied to powdered dried matter such as *fish flour, potato flour, etc. The ground wheat berry yields wholemeal flour (100% extraction); whiter flours are obtained by separation of the bran and the germ from the starchy endosperm. See also bread; flour, extraction rate.

flour, ageing and bleaching See ageing.

flour, agglomerated A dispersible form, easily wetted, produced by agglomerating the fine particles in steam; particles are greater than 100 μm in diameter, so the flour is dust-free.

flour enrichment The addition of certain vitamins and minerals to flour, to contain not less than: in the UK, vitamin B_1, 0.24 mg; niacin, 1.6 mg; iron, 1.65 mg; calcium, 120 mg/100 g; in the USA, vitamin B_1, 0.44–0.56 mg; vitamin B_2, 0.2–0.33 mg; niacin, 3.6–4.4 mg; iron, 2.9–3.7 mg/100 g; calcium not specified.

flour, enzyme inactivated Flour in which the *enzyme α-amylase has been inactivated by heat to prevent degradation when the flour is used as a thickening agent in gravies, soups, etc.

flour, extraction rate The yield of flour obtained from wheat in the milling process. A 100% extraction (or straight-run flour) is wholemeal flour containing all of the grain; lower extraction rates are the whiter flours from which progressively more of the *bran and *germ (and thus B vitamins and iron) are excluded, down to a figure of 72% extraction, which is normal white flour. 'Patent' flours are of lower extraction rate, 30–50%, and so comprise mostly the *endosperm of the grain. See also bread; Fig. 2 on page 150.

flour, high-ratio Flour of very fine, uniform particle size, treated with chlorine to reduce the *gluten strength. Used for making cakes, since it is possible to add up to 140 parts sugar to 100 parts of this flour, whereas only half this quantity of sugar can be incorporated into ordinary flour. See flour strength.

flour improvers See ageing.

flour, national See wheatmeal.

flour, patent See flour, extraction rate.

flour, self-raising Wheat flour to which *baking powder has been added to produce carbon dioxide in the presence of water and heat; the dough is thus aerated without prolonged fermentation. Usually 'weaker' flours are used (see flour strength). Legally, self-raising flour must contain not less than 0.4% available carbon dioxide.

flour strength A property of the flour proteins enabling the dough to retain gas during fermentation to give a 'bold' loaf. 'Strong' flour is higher in protein content, has greater elasticity and resistance to extension, and greater ability to absorb water. A 'weak' flour gives a loaf that lacks volume. See also extensometer, farinograph.

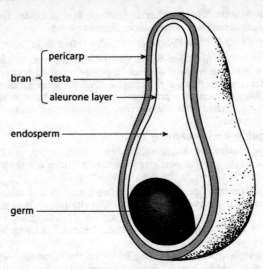

bran { pericarp
testa
aleurone layer

endosperm

germ

FIGURE 2.

flour, wholemeal Flour made from the entire grain of wheat, i.e. a 100% extraction rate.

fluid balance *See* water balance.

fluid bed dryer A bed of solid particles is supported on a cushion of hot air jets (fluidized) and the material may be conveyed this way, while being dried. The method achieves intimate mixing without mechanical damage; applied to cereals, tabletting granules, salt, coffee, and dried vegetables.

fluke Small flatfish, *Platichthys* spp., also called flounder.

flummery Old English pudding made by boiling down the water from soaked oatmeal until it becomes thick and gelatinous. Similar to *frumenty. Dutch flummery is made with gelatine or isinglass and egg yolk; Spanish flummery with cream, rice flour, and cinnamon.

fluoridation The addition of *fluoride to drinking water.

fluoride The *ion of the element fluorine, one of the halogens (the other members of this group of elements are chlorine, bromine, and iodine). Although it occurs in small amounts in plants and animals, and has effects on the formation of dental enamel and bones, it is not considered to be a dietary essential and no deficiency signs are known.

Drinking water containing about 1 part per million of fluoride protects teeth from decay (the mechanism of this effect is not known), and in some areas fluoride is added to drinking water to achieve this level. Naturally, the fluoride content of water ranges between 0.05 and 14 ppm.

Water containing more than about 12 ppm fluoride can lead to chalky white patches on the surface of the teeth, known as mottled enamel. At higher levels there is strong brown mottling of the teeth and inappropriate deposition of fluoride in bones known as fluorosis.

fluorosis Damage to teeth (brown mottling of the enamel) and bones caused by an excessive intake of *fluoride.

FMN Flavin mononucleotide (chemically riboflavin phosphate), one of the *coenzymes derived from vitamin B_2.

foam-mat drying A method of drying food. The liquid concentrate is whipped to a foam with the aid of a foaming agent, spread on a tray and dried in a stream of warm air. It reconstitutes very rapidly with water because of the fine structure of the foam.

foccacia *See* bread.

foie gras (French for 'fat liver'). The liver of goose or duck that has been specially fed and fattened; may be cooked whole or used as the basis of *pâté de foie gras, the most highly prized of the pâtés.

folacin, folate *See* folic acid.

folding-in A method of combining a mixture of flour and other ingredients so that it retains its lightness; it is used for mixing meringues, soufflés, and some cakes. Sometimes called cutting and folding.

folic acid A *vitamin that functions as a carrier of one-carbon units in a variety of metabolic reactions. Essential for the synthesis of purines and pyrimidines (and so for *nucleic acid synthesis and hence cell division); the principal deficiency disease is megaloblastic *anaemia, due to failure of the normal maturation of red *blood cells, with release into the circulation of immature precursors of red blood cells. Occurs in foods in several complex combinations, of which probably about half are nutritionally useful.

The *reference intake is 200 µg/day, increasing to 300 µg/day in pregnancy. However, giving supplements of 400 µg free folic acid per day to a mother, beginning before conception, reduces the incidence of spina bifida and other neural tube defects in babies; it is unlikely that ordinary foods could provide this much folate, so supplements are advised; rich sources include liver, kidney, green leafy vegetables, and yeast, and average UK intakes of mixed folates are around 200–300 µg/day.

folinic acid The 5-formyl derivative of the vitamin *folic acid; more stable to oxidation than folic acid itself, and commonly used in pharmaceutical preparations. The synthetic (racemic) compound is known as leucovorin.

fondant Minute sugar crystals in a saturated sugar syrup; used as the creamy filling in chocolates and biscuits and for decorating cakes. Prepared by boiling sugar solution with the addition of *glucose syrup or an inverting agent (*see* invert sugar) and cooling rapidly while stirring.

fondue Swiss; cheese melted with wine and herbs, eaten by dipping small squares of bread into the hot mixture. Fondue bourguignonne is small cubes of marinated meat, cooked on a long fork in a vessel of hot oil at the table.

fonduta Italian (Piedmontese); dish made from Fontina cheese and truffles.

food Any solid or liquid material consumed by a living organism to supply *energy, build and replace tissue, or participate in such reactions. Defined by the FAO/WHO *Codex Alimentarius Commission as a substance, whether processed, semi-processed, or raw, which is intended for human consumption and includes drink, chewing gum, and any substance that has been used in the manufacture, preparation, or treatment of food but does not include cosmetics, tobacco, or substances used only as drugs.

food-borne disease Infectious or toxic disease caused by agents that enter the body through the consumption of food. The causative agents may be present in food as a result of infection of animals from which food is prepared or contamination at source or during manufacture, storage, and preparation.

There are three main categories: (1) diseases caused by micro-organisms (including parasites) that invade and multiply in the body; (2) diseases caused by toxins produced by micro-organisms growing in the gastro-intestinal tract; (3) diseases caused by the ingestion of food contaminated with poisonous chemicals or containing natural toxins or the toxins produced by micro-organisms in the food.

food chain The chain between green plants (the primary producers of food energy) through a sequence of organisms in which each eats the one below it in the chain, and is eaten in turn by the one above. Also used for the chain of events from the original source of a foodstuff (from the sea, the soil, or the wild) through all the stages of handling until it reaches the table.

food combining *See* Hay diet.

food composition tables Tables of the chemical composition, energy, and nutrient yield of foods, based on chemical analysis. Although the analyses are performed with great precision, they are, of necessity, only performed on a few samples of each type of food. There is, however, considerable variation, especially in the content of vitamins and minerals, between different samples of the same food. Therefore, calculation of energy and nutrient intakes based on use of food composition tables, even when intake has been weighed, can only be considered to be accurate to within about ±10%, at best.

food exchange *See* exchange list.

food poisoning May be due to (1) contamination with harmful bacteria or other micro-organisms; (2) toxic chemicals; (3) *adverse reactions to certain proteins or other natural constituents of foods; (4) chemical contamination.

The commonest bacterial contamination is due to species of *Salmonella*, *Staphylococcus*, *Campylobacter*, *Listeria*, *Bacillus cereus*, and *Clostridium welchii*. Very rarely, food poisoning is due to *Clostridium botulinum*, or *botulism.

Staphylococcal poisoning causes rapid symptoms (within 2–4 hours): abdominal cramp, nausea, vomiting, and diarrhoea; recovery is normally rapid. Salmonellae produce an endotoxin which is not destroyed by cooking and causes acute gastro-enteritis after 12–24 hours: nausea, vomiting, and diarrhoea may persist for several weeks.

food science The study of the basic chemical, physical, biochemical, and biophysical properties of foods and their constituents, and of changes that these may undergo during handling, preservation, processing, storage, distribution, and preparation for consumption. Hence, the term food scientist.

food standard A set of criteria that a food must meet if it is to be suitable for human consumption, such as source, composition, appearance, freshness, permissible additives, and maximum bacterial content.

Food Standards Committee Permanent advisory body to the Ministry of Agriculture, Fisheries, and Food in the UK.

foodstuffs Defined in EU Directives as products intended for human consumption in an unprocessed, processed, or mixed state, with the exception of tobacco products, cosmetics, and pharmaceuticals.

food tables See food composition tables.

food technology The application of science and technology to the treatment, processing, preservation, and distribution of foods. Hence the term food technologist.

food yeast See yeast.

foo-foo Caribbean, West African; small dumplings made by pounding boiled green *plantain.

fool A purée of fruit with cream or custard.

forbidden fruit See grapefruit.

forcemeat A highly seasoned *stuffing made from chopped or minced veal, pork, or sausage meat mixed with onion and a range of herbs (French: *farce*, stuffing).

forestière, à la Meat or poultry with a garnish of mushrooms, ham or bacon, and fried potatoes.

formiminoglutamic acid test See FIGLU test.

formula diet Composed of simple substances that do not require digestion, are readily absorbed, and leave a minimum residue in the intestine: glucose, amino acids or peptides, mono- and diglycerides rather than starch, proteins, and fats.

fortification The deliberate addition of specific nutrients to foods in order to increase their content, sometimes to a higher level than normal, as a means of providing the population with an increased level of intake. Generally synonymous with enrichment, supplementation, and restoration; in the USA enrichment is used to mean the addition to foods of nutrients that they do not normally contain, while fortification is the restoration of nutrients lost in processing. See also wine, fortified.

four ale Originally sold at four pence per quart. The four ale bar is the public bar.

four, au Cooked in the oven.

fovantini *See* pasta.

FPC *See* fish protein concentrate.

fractional test meal A method of examining the secretion of gastric juices; the stomach contents are sampled at intervals via a stomach tube after a test meal of gruel. It is usual to test for total and free acidity, and in addition peptic activity may be measured.

frail A rush basket for raisins, figs, etc.; also a quantity of raisins, usually about 75 lb (34 kg).

frangipane (frangipani) Originally a jasmine perfume which gave its name to an almond cream flavoured with the perfume. The term is used for cake-filling made from eggs, milk, and flour with flavouring, and also for a pastry filled with an almond-flavoured mixture.

frankfurter A seasoned, smoked beef and pork *sausage (hot dog). A 100-g portion (two large sausages) is a good *source of protein and niacin; a source of vitamin B_1 and iron; contains 25 g of fat and 1000 mg of sodium; supplies 270 kcal (1140 kJ).

frappé 1 Iced, frozen, or chilled.
    2 Egg-white and sugar syrup whipped until so aerated that the density reaches 5 lb per gallon (100 g in 200 mL).

free fatty acids (FFA) *See* fatty acids.

free from For a food label or advertising to bear a claim that it is free from fat, saturates, cholesterol, sodium, or alcohol it must contain no more than a specified (low) amount. The precise levels at which such claims are permitted differ from one country to another. In the USA the food so described must contain only a trivial or physiologically insignificant amount of the specified nutrient.

free radicals Highly reactive molecules with an unpaired electron. *See* antioxidant nutrients.

freeze concentration Concentration of a liquid by freezing out pure ice, leaving a more concentrated solution; it requires less input of energy, and causes less loss of flavour, than concentration by evaporation. Used especially in the concentration of fruit juices, *vinegar, and *beer.

freeze drying Also known as lyophilization. A method of drying in which the material is frozen and subjected to high vacuum. The ice sublimes off as water vapour without melting. Materials dried in this way are damaged little, if at all.
    Freeze-dried food is very porous, since it occupies the same volume as the original and so rehydrates rapidly. There is less loss of flavour and texture than with most other methods of drying. Controlled heat may be applied to the process without melting the frozen material; this is accelerated freeze drying.

freezerburn A change in the texture of frozen meat, fish, and poultry during storage due to sublimation of the ice.

freezer temperatures For long-term storage of frozen foods (up to 2–3 months), domestic freezers run at −18 ˚C (0 ˚F); in the UK this is a 3-star rated deep freeze. A freezing compartment of a refrigerator (for short-term storage of frozen foods) is between −11 ˚C (12 ˚F), 2-star rated, for storage up to 4 weeks; and −4 ˚C (25 ˚F), 1-star rated, for storage up to a week. *See also* date marking.

A 3-star rated deep freeze with a snowflake symbol is one that is suitable for freezing foods, as opposed to storing ready-frozen food; it has a higher cooling capacity than a simple deep freeze storage cabinet.

French dressing *See* salad dressing.

French fried onions American name for onion rings, fried in batter.

French fries *See* chips.

frenching Breaking up the fibres of meat by cutting, usually diagonally or in a criss-cross pattern.

French mustard *See* mustard.

French toast North American breakfast dish; slices of bread dipped in beaten egg, fried, and served with cinnamon and sugar. Known in France as *pain perdu* ('bread lost' in egg).

Freons *See* refrigerants.

fresh For food labelling and advertising purposes, the US Food and Drug Administration has defined fresh to mean a food that is raw, has never been frozen or heated, and contains no preservatives. (*Irradiation at low levels is permitted.) 'Fresh frozen' and 'frozen fresh' may be used for foods that are quickly frozen while still fresh, and *blanching before freezing is permitted.

friandises A variety of small sweets, preserved fruits, etc., served as *petits fours or desserts.

fricadelle Minced meat balls.

fricandeau Dish made from the long fillet of *veal, braised or roasted.

fricassée A combination of sautéing and stewing; food is fried briefly with a small amount of fat, then stewed.

frijole bean *Phaseolus acutifolius*, also known as Mexican haricot bean, tepary, or pinto. Able to withstand drought.

frijoles A Mexican dish based on boiled fava or lima (butter) beans which have been left to cool, then fried. Also known as refried beans.

frisée Alternative name for *endive.

frites *See* chips.

fritter A portion of sweet or savoury food, coated in batter and fried.

fritto misto Italian; small thin pieces of a variety of types of meat, fish, or vegetables, coated with egg and breadcrumbs or batter, and deep fried.

frizzante Italian; lightly sparkling wines, equivalent to French pétillant. *See also* spumante.

frogs' legs The back and legs of the edible frog, *Rana esculenta*. A 100-g portion is a rich *source of protein; a source of vitamins B_1, B_2, and iron; has a trace of fat; supplies 75 kcal (315 kJ).

fromage à la crème (cœur à la crème) French; sour milk cheese. The curd is drained, mixed with cream, and pressed in heart-shaped moulds.

fromage frais (fromage blanc) French equivalent of *quark ('fresh cheese'). A soft, unripened cheese, 80% water, made from skim milk or semi-skim milk, and may include added cream; 1–8% fat; a 100-g portion of 8% fat variety is a rich *source of vitamin B_{12}, and a good source of vitamin B_2; a source of protein and vitamin A; contains 8 g of fat, 30 mg of sodium, 90 mg of calcium; supplies 115 kcal (470 kJ).

frosting 1 American name for icing on cakes; in the UK icing made from sugar and egg white (known as American icing).
   2 A way of decorating the rim of a glass in which a cold drink is to be served; the edge is coated with whipped egg white, dipped into caster sugar, and allowed to dry.
   3 For a *margarita cocktail the edge of the glass is frosted by dipping it into lemon juice, then salt.

frothing *Dredging the surface of roast joints and poultry with flour before *basting, in order to give an attractive brown finish.

fructosan A general name for polysaccharides of *fructose, such as *inulin. Not digested, and hence a part of *dietary fibre or *non-starch polysaccharides.

fructose Also known as fruit sugar or laevulose. A six-carbon monosaccharide *sugar (hexose) differing from *glucose in containing a ketone group (on carbon-2) instead of an aldehyde group (on carbon-1). Found as the free sugar in fruits and honey, and as a constituent of the *disaccharide *sucrose (together with glucose). It is 1.7 times as sweet as sucrose. Commercially it is prepared by the hydrolysis of the polysaccharide *inulin from the Jerusalem artichoke. *See also* invert sugar.

fructose syrups Glucose *syrups made by hydrolysis of starch and half the glucose then being converted into fructose, similar to invert syrup produced from sucrose but cheaper. Also known as iso-syrups, high fructose syrups, and high fructose corn syrups (HFS, HFCS).

fruit The fleshy seed-bearing part of plants (including tomato and cucumber, which are usually called *vegetables). They contain negligible protein and fat, with carbohydrate varying from 3% in melon to 25% in banana, and supply varying amounts of vitamin C. Yellow- and orange-coloured fruits (e.g. apricot, peach, papaya) are sources of vitamin A (as carotene).

fruit acids *See* acids, fruit.

fruitarian A person who eats only fruits, nuts, and seeds; an extreme form of *vegetarianism.

fruit cordials, drinks, squash *See* soft drinks.

fruit, dried Dried currants, dates, figs, prunes, raisins, and sultanas all have similar analyses; a 100-g portion is a *source of iron and supplies 250 kcal (1050 kJ).

fruit gums *See* gumdrops.

fruit mince *See* mincemeat.

frumenty An old English pudding made from whole wheat stewed in water for 24 hours until the grains have burst and set in a thick jelly, then boiled with milk. Similar to *flummery.

frying Cooking foods with oil at temperatures well above the boiling point of water. Deep frying, in which a food is completely immersed in oil, reaches a temperature around 185 °C. Nutrient losses are less than in roasting, about 10–20% thiamin, 10–15% riboflavin and nicotinic acid from meat; about 20% thiamin from fish.

fu-yung Chinese dishes prepared with egg-white and cornflour mixed with minced chicken; commonly applied to a variety of dishes with egg scrambled into the mixture.

fudge *Caramel in which crystallization of the sugar (graining) is deliberately induced by the addition of *fondant (saturated *syrup containing sugar crystals).

fuga The Japanese puffer fish, *Fuga* spp., responsible for *tetrodontin poisoning.

fuller's earth An adsorbent clay, calcium montmorillonite, or bentonite; adsorbs both by physical means and by ion extraction. Used to bleach oils, clarify liquids, and absorb grease.

fumeol Refined smoke with the bitter principles removed; used for preparing 'liquid' smokes for dipping foods such as fish to give them a smoked flavour. *See also* smoking.

fumet French; concentrated stock from meat, fish, or vegetables prepared by boiling down to a syrupy consistency, used to give flavour and body to sauces.

funchi Caribbean; corn meal pudding.

functional foods Foods eaten for specified health purposes, because of their (rich) content of one or more nutrients or non-nutrient substances which may confer health benefits.

fungal protein *See* mycoprotein.

fungi Subdivision of Thallophyta, plants without differentiation into root, stem, and leaf; they cannot photosynthesize, and all are parasites or saprophytes. Microfungi are *moulds, as opposed to larger fungi, which are mushrooms and toadstools. *Yeasts are sometimes classed with fungi.

 Species of moulds such as *Penicillium*, *Aspergillus*, etc., are important causes of food spoilage in the presence of oxygen and relatively high humidity. Those that produce toxins (*mycotoxins) are especially problematical. On the other hand species of *Penicillium* such as *P. cambertii* and *P. roquefortii* are desirable and essential in the ripening of certain *cheeses.

A number of larger fungi (*mushrooms) are cultivated, and other wild species are harvested for their delicate flavour. The mycelium of smaller fungi (including *Graphium*, *Fusarium*, and *Rhizopus* species) are grown commercially on waste carbohydrate as a rich source of protein for food manufacture. *See* mycoprotein.

furcellaran Danish agar; an anionic, sulphated polysaccharide extracted from the red alga, *Furcellaria fastigiata*, structurally similar to *carrageenan; used as a gelling agent.

fusel oil Alcoholic fermentation produces about 95% alcohol and 5% fusel oil: a mixture of organic acids, higher alcohols (propyl, butyl, and amyl), aldehydes, and esters, known collectively as congeners.

It is present in low concentration in wines and beer, and in high concentration in pot-still spirit. On maturation of the liquor fusel oil changes and imparts the special flavour to the spirit. Many of the symptoms of *hangover can be attributed to fusel oil in alcoholic beverages.

fussol Monofluoroacetamide, a systemic insecticide for treating fruit.

F value A unit of measurement used to compare relative sterilizing effects of different procedures; equal to 1 minute at 121.1 °C.

G

gaffelbitar 'Semi-preserved' *herring in which microbial growth is checked by the addition of salt at a concentration of 10–12%, and sometimes by the addition of *benzoic acid as a preservative.

gage *See* greengage.

gajjar *See* carrot.

galacticol *See* dulcitol.

Galactomin Trade name for preparation free from lactose and galactose, used for patients suffering from lactose intolerance.

galactosaemia *Genetic disease, inability to metabolize the sugar *galactose. Unless galactose is excluded from the diet, the subjects suffer mental retardation, growth failure, vomiting, and jaundice, with enlargement of liver and spleen and development of cataracts. Special baby foods are therefore prepared entirely free from *lactose, which is the only important source of galactose in the diet.

galactose A six-carbon sugar (a monosaccharide) differing from *glucose only in position of the hydroxyl group on carbon-4. It is about one-third as sweet as sucrose. The main dietary source is as part of the disaccharide *lactose in milk, and it is important in formation of the galactolipids (*cerebrosides) of nerve tissue. *See also* galactosaemia.

galantine A dish of white meat or poultry, boned, rolled, cooked with herbs, glazed with *aspic jelly, and served cold.

galenicals Crude drugs, infusions, decoctions, and tinctures prepared from medicinal plants.

galette Round, flat cake of flaky pastry, or thin fried potato cakes or pancakes.

gallates Salts and esters of gallic acid, found in many plants. Used in making dyes and inks, and medicinally as an astringent. Propyl, octyl, and dodecyl gallates are legally permitted antioxidants in foods (E-310–312).

gall-bladder The organ situated in the liver which stores the *bile formed in the liver before its secretion into the small intestine. *See* gastro-intestinal tract.

Galliano Italian; liqueur flavoured with herbs, roots, berries, and flowers; the basis of the Harvey Wallbanger cocktail.

gallimaufry Medieval; chicken stew with bacon, mustard, and wine.

gallon A unit of volume. The imperial gallon is 4.546 litres, and the US gallon is 3.7853 litres; therefore 1 imperial gallon = 1.2 US gallons.

gallstones (cholelithiasis) Concretions composed of cholesterol, bile pigments, and calcium salts, formed in the bile duct of the *gall-bladder when the bile becomes supersaturated.

gamay A *grape variety widely used for *wine making, although not one of the classic varieties. The grape of the Beaujolais and Mâcon districts of France, making light, fragrant, red wines that are best drunk young.

game Non-domesticated (i.e. wild) animals and birds shot for sport and eaten. *Rabbit and *pigeon may be shot at any time, but other game species, such as *grouse, *hare, *partridge, *pheasant, *quail, deer (*venison), and wild *duck may not be shot during the close season, to protect breeding stocks. Game birds are generally raised on farms to provide sport, rather than being hunted in the wild, and increasingly game species are farmed and killed in conventional humane ways to provide food. Traditionally, game is hung for several days to soften the meat, whereupon it develops a strong flavour.

game chips Thin slices of fried potato chips, called crisps in the UK and chips in the USA. *See* potato chips.

gammon Hind legs of bacon pig, cured while still part of the carcass. Ham is the same part of the pig but is cured after removal from the carcass. *See also* bacon; pork.

garam masala A mixture of aromatic spices widely used in Indian cooking; contains powdered black pepper, cumin, cinnamon, cloves, mace, cardamom seeds, and sometimes also coriander and/or bay leaf.

garbanzo *See* chickpea.

garbure Southern France, Spain; thick soup or vegetable purée.

garhi yakhni *See* yakhni.

Garibaldi biscuit Square or rectangular biscuit with a layer of currants inside (popularly known as squashed-fly biscuits).

garlic The bulb of *Allium sativum* with a pungent odour when crushed, widely used to flavour foods. There is some evidence that garlic has a beneficial effect in lowering blood *cholesterol.

garlic mustard A common wild plant of hedgerows and woodland (*Alliaria petiolata*); the leaves have a garlic-like flavour and can be used in salads or cooked as a vegetable.

garnish Small pieces of vegetables, herbs, croûtons, pastry, etc., used to decorate a dish before serving.

garrafeira Portuguese; aged, strong table wines.

gas storage, controlled (modified) Storage of fruits, vegetables, and prepacked red meat in a controlled atmosphere in which a proportion of the oxygen is replaced by carbon dioxide, sometimes with the addition of other gases. In modified atmosphere (MA) storage the control is less precise.

gastric acidity A number of digestive disorders are popularly called 'gastric acidity', but the principal nutritional problem in this area is the reduction in gastric acid secretion that occurs with advancing age; this limits the absorption of *iron and *vitamin B_{12}. *See also* achlorhydria; anaemia, pernicious; gastric secretion.

gastric inhibitory peptide A hormone secreted by the mucosa of the duodenum and jejunum in response to absorbed fat and carbohydrate which stimulates the pancreas to secrete *insulin. Also known as glucose-dependent insulinotropic polypeptide.

gastric secretion Gastric juice contains the *enzymes *chymosin and lipase, the inactive precursor of pepsin (pepsinogen), *intrinsic factor, mucin, and hydrochloric acid. The acid is secreted by the parietal cells at a strength of 0.16 mol/L (0.5–0.6% acid); the same cells also secrete intrinsic factor, and failure of acid secretion (*achlorhydria) is associated with a failure to absorb *vitamin B_{12} because of lack of intrinsic factor. See anaemia, pernicious.

Pepsinogen is secreted by the 'chief' cells of the gastric mucosa, and is activated to pepsin by either gastric acid or the action of existing pepsin; it is a proteolytic enzyme. The only function of chymosin is to coagulate milk; the lipase hydrolyses a small proportion of dietary fat.

gastric ulcer See ulcer.

gastrin Polypeptide *hormone secreted by the stomach in response to foods (especially meat) which stimulate *gastric and *pancreatic secretion.

gastritis Inflammation of the mucosal lining of the stomach; may result from infection or excessive alcohol consumption.

gastro-enteritis Inflammation of the mucosal lining of the stomach and/or small or large intestine, normally resulting from infection. See also gastro-intestinal tract.

gastroenterology The study and treatment of diseases of the *gastro-intestinal tract.

gastro-intestinal tract The whole of the digestive tract, from the mouth to the anus. Average length 4.5 m (15 feet). See Fig. 3 on page 162.

gastrostomy feeding Feeding a liquid diet directly into the stomach through a tube that has been surgically introduced through the abdominal wall. See also enteral nutrition; nasogastric tube.

gâteau Elaborate cake with sponge, biscuit, or pastry base and topped with fruit, jelly, and cream.

gaufre See waffle.

gaufrette French; wafer.

gavage The process of feeding liquids by stomach tube. Also feeding an excessive amount (hyperalimentation).

gazpacho Spanish; vegetable soup made by blending green pepper, cucumber, onions, and tomatoes, uncooked, with bread crumbs, olive oil, vinegar, and garlic; served ice-cold with a garnish of chopped onion, cucumber, red and green peppers, etc.

gean Scottish name for the fruit of *Prunus avium avium*; also known as wild cherry, sweet cherry, and mazzard.

gefillte fish (Also gefilte, gefültte). Literally, German for stuffed fish. The dish is of Russian or Polish origin where it is commonly referred to as Jewish fish. The whole fish is served and the filleted portion

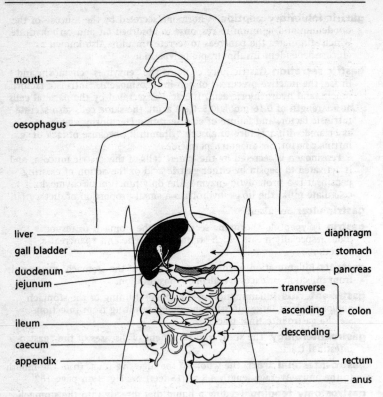

mouth

oesophagus

liver

gall bladder

duodenum

jejunum

ileum

caecum

appendix

diaphragm

stomach

pancreas

transverse

ascending

descending
} colon

rectum

anus

FIGURE 3.

chopped and stuffed back between the skin and the backbone. More frequently today, the fish is simply chopped and made into balls, which are either fried or boiled. In the UK it has been legally referred to as 'fish cutlets in fish sauce' rather than fish cake.

geist German name for liqueur made by macerating soft fruit in alcohol, then distilling.

gel A sol or colloidal suspension that has set to a jelly.

gelatine A soluble protein prepared from *collagen or bones by boiling with water: used for sugar confectionery, in canned meats, for table jellies, and in pharmaceutical capsules. Gelatine from fish (especially the swim bladder) is *isinglass. As a protein it is of poor nutritive value, since it lacks *tryptophan.

gelatine, Chinese *See* agar.

gelatine sugar *See* glycine.

gellan gum A *polysaccharide produced by fermentation of the bacterium, *Pseudomonas elodea*, used in some foods.

gelometer *See* Bloom gelometer.

generic descriptor The name used to cover the different chemical forms of a *vitamin; compounds that have the same *vitamin activity.

generoso Portuguese, Spanish; fortified wines.

genetic diseases Also known as inborn errors of metabolism. Diseases due to a single defective gene, with a characteristic pattern of inheritance in families. Many affect the ability to metabolize individual *amino acids or *carbohydrates and can be treated by dietary restriction. *See also* amino acid disorders; disaccharide intolerance.

genetic modification A change in the genes in a living organism, as occurs in nature, and which has been used for many years in selective breeding, or, more quickly and specifically, in the laboratory (genetic engineering).

geneva *See* gin.

genoa cake A rich, dark, fruit cake containing glacé cherries and decorated with almonds or brazil nuts.

genoese Whisked sponge mixture of eggs, sugar, flour, and soft creamed butter. Victoria sponge is a type of genoese.

gentiobiose A disaccharide consisting of two molecules of glucose joined 1,6-β.

Gentleman's relish Trade name for a paste of anchovies, butter, cereal, salt, and spices developed in the UK in the nineteenth century; also called patum peperium.

Gerber test An analytical test for the fat (*cream) in milk.

German pound cake Similar to *genoa cake, but containing less fruit and no almonds.

germ, wheat The embryo or sprouting portion of the wheat berry, comprising about 2.5% of the seed. Contains 64% of the vitamin B_1, 26% of the vitamin B_2, 21% of the vitamin B_6, and most of the fat of the wheat grain. It is discarded, with the bran, when the grain is milled to white *flour. See flour, extraction rate.

gewürztraminer A *grape variety widely used for *wine making, although not one of the classic varieties; the wines have a characteristic spicy flavour and aroma.

ghee Clarified butter fat, *see* butter.

gherkin Young green *cucumber of a small variety (*Cucumis anguira*), used mainly for pickling.

ghrt Alternative name for *ghee.

giardiasis Intestinal inflammation and *diarrhoea caused by infection with the protozoan parasite *Giardia lamblia*.

giberellins Plant growth substances derived from giberellic acid, originally found in the fungus *Gibberella fujikori* growing on rice. About thirty giberellins are known; they cause stem extension and allow mutant dwarf forms of plants to revert to normal size, induce flower formation, and break bud dormancy. They are used to accelerate the germination of barley for *malting.

gibier French; wild animals that are hunted for food, *game.

giblets The edible part of the entrails of a bird; gizzard, liver, heart, and neck.

gigot French; leg of lamb or mutton. In Ireland gigot chops are neck chops used for stewing.

gill Obsolete British measure of liquid, 5 or 10 fl oz ($^1/_4$ or $^1/_2$ pint), varying regionally. Still used as the basis for measure of *spirits in the UK, a standard measure is $^1/_5$ or $^1/_6$ of a 5 fl oz gill.

gin Alcoholic drink made by distilling fermented starch or other carbohydrate, flavoured mainly with juniper berries together with coriander seeds, angelica, cinnamon, and orange and lemon peel. Distillate is diluted to 40% *alcohol by volume, 220 kcal (925 kJ) per 100 mL. The name is derived from the French *genièvre* (juniper); originally known as geneva, schiedam, or hollands, since it is Dutch in origin.

There are two types of English gin: Plymouth gin, with a fuller flavour, and London gin. Dutch and German gins are more strongly flavoured than English or American; steinhäger and schinkenhäger are distilled from a mash of wheat, barley, and juniper berries; wacholder is made from neutral spirit flavoured with juniper. Dutch gin may be *jonge* (young) or *oude* (aged, matured).

gingelly (gingili) *See* sesame.

ginger The rhizome of *Zingiber officinale*, used as a spice. Preserved ginger is made from young fleshy rhizomes boiled with sugar and either packed in syrup or crystallized.

gingerbread Cake flavoured with ginger and treacle, often baked in the shape of an animal or person, and glazed.

ginger paralysis *See* Jamaica ginger paralysis.

gingivitis Inflammation, swelling, and bleeding of the gums; may be due to *scurvy, but most commonly the result of poor dental hygiene.

gin, pink Gin flavoured with *angostura bitters.

GIP *See* gastric inhibitory peptide.

gipping (of fish) Partial evisceration to remove intestines but not pyloric caeca which contains enzymes responsible for the characteristic flavour of *herring when it is subsequently salted.

girdle Griddle.

girolle French name for the chanterelle, an edible wild *mushroom, *Cantharellus cibarius*.

GI tract *See* gastro-intestinal tract.

glacé 1 Iced or frozen.
2 Having a smooth glossy surface or glaze.

glacé cherry *Cherry preserved in a heavy syrup of sugar and glucose, generally also with added colour. Used in confectionery and fruit cakes. Little or none of the original vitamin C content of the cherry will remain.

Glamorgan sausage A dish based on Caerphilly cheese, breadcrumbs, and egg, fried in sausage shape (traditional Welsh dish).

Glasgow magistrate *See* red herring.

Glayva Scottish whisky-based liqueur, flavoured with herbs and sweetened with heather honey.

glaze Glossy surface on sweet or savoury food.

glessie *See* toffee.

gliadin One of the proteins that make up wheat *gluten. Allergy to, or intolerance of, gliadin is *coeliac disease.

globins *Proteins that are rich in the *amino acid *histidine (and hence basic), relatively deficient in *isoleucine, and contain average amounts of *arginine and *tryptophan. Often found as the protein part of conjugated proteins such as haemoglobin.

globulins Class of *proteins that are heat-coagulated and soluble in dilute solutions of salts; they differ from *albumins in being relatively insoluble in water. They occur in blood (serum globulins), milk (lactoglobulins), and some plants, e.g. edestin from hemp seed and amandin from almonds.

glossitis Inflammation of the tongue; may be one of the signs of *riboflavin deficiency.

Gloucester cheese Originally there were single and double Gloucester versions with minor differences; by far the commonest now is double Gloucester, similar in chemical and nutrient composition to *Cheddar cheese.

glucagon A *hormone secreted by the α-cells of the *pancreas which causes an increase in blood sugar by increasing the breakdown of liver *glycogen and stimulating the synthesis of *glucose from *amino acids.

glucans Soluble but undigested complex made of glucose units; found particularly in oats, barley, and rye. *See also* fibre, soluble; non-starch polysaccharides.

glucaric acid Alternative name for saccharic acid, the dicarboxylic acid derived from glucose.

glucide (gluside) Name occasionally used for *saccharin.

glucitol Obsolete name for sorbitol, one of the *sugar alcohols or *glycitols.

glucocorticoids The *steroid *hormones secreted by the *adrenal cortex which regulate carbohydrate metabolism.

glucomannan A polysaccharide consisting of glucose and mannose.

gluconeogenesis The metabolic processes involved in the formation of *glucose from non-carbohydrate precursors, such as glycerol, lactate, and a variety of amino acids.

gluconic acid The acid formed by oxidation of the hydroxyl group on carbon-1 of glucose to a carboxylic acid group. Also termed dextronic acid, maltonic acid, and glycogenic acid.

glucono-δ-lactone (glucono-delta-lactone) A derivative (chemically the lactone) of *gluconic acid; slowly liberates acid at a controlled rate; used in chemically leavened (aerated) *bread to liberate carbon dioxide from bicarbonate.

glucosaccharic acid *See* saccharic acid.

glucosamine The amino derivative of *glucose, a constituent of a variety of complex *polysaccharides.

glucosan A general term for polysaccharides of *glucose, such as *starch, *cellulose, and *glycogen.

glucose A six-carbon monosaccharide sugar (hexose), with the chemical formula $C_6H_{12}O_6$, occurring free in plant and animal tissues and formed by the hydrolysis of *starch and *glycogen. Also known as dextrose, grape sugar, and blood sugar.

The major dietary carbohydrates are starches, which are polymers of glucose and disaccharides: sucrose (glucose-fructose); lactose (glucose-galactose); maltose and isomaltose, which are dimers of glucose.

The circulating carbohydrate in the bloodstream (blood sugar) is glucose; the normal concentration is between 4.5 and 5.5 mmol/L (80–100 mg/100 mL). In the fed state excess glucose is used for the synthesis of glycogen in liver and muscle, as well as for synthesis of fats; in the fasting state glycogen is hydrolysed as a source of glucose to maintain the blood concentration.

It is used in the manufacture of confectionery, since its mixture with *fructose prevents sucrose from crystallizing (*see* boiled sweets); it is 74% as sweet as sucrose.

glucose, confectioners' Glucose *syrups are known as glucose in confectionery making (*glucose is referred to as dextrose).

glucose metabolism Process through which glucose is oxidized to carbon dioxide and water as a metabolic fuel (i.e. to provide energy). The overall reaction is: $C_6H_{12}O_6 + 6O_2 \rightarrow 6CO_2 + 6H_2O$ + 3.9 kcal per gram, occurring in a series of stages. The oxidation of glucose to carbon dioxide and water yields 3.9 kcal (16.4 kJ)/g, or 686 kcal (2.88 MJ)/mol.

The first series of reactions does not require oxygen and is referred to as (anaerobic) glycolysis or glucose fermentation, yielding two molecules of the three-carbon compound pyruvic acid. Under anaerobic conditions this can be reduced to *lactic acid.

Pyruvic acid is normally oxidized to acetyl CoA, which is then oxidized to carbon dioxide and water in a series of reactions known as the citric acid or Krebs cycle. Both glycolysis and the citric acid cycle are linked to the formation of *ATP from ADP and phosphate, as a metabolically usable energy source.

glucose oxidase *Enzyme that oxidizes glucose to gluconic acid, with the formation of hydrogen peroxide. Used for specific quantitative determination of glucose, including urinary glucose excreted in *diabetes, and also to remove traces of glucose from foodstuffs (e.g. from dried egg to prevent the *Maillard reaction during storage). Originally isolated from the mould *Penicillium notatum* and called notatin.

glucose-6-phosphate dehydrogenase deficiency *See* favism.

glucose syrups *See* syrup; dextrose equivalent value.

glucose tolerance The ability of the body to deal with a relatively large dose of glucose is used as a test for *diabetes mellitus. The fasting subject ingests 50 or 75 g of glucose and the concentration of blood sugar is measured at intervals. In normal subjects the fasting sugar concentration is between 4.5 and 5.5 mmol/L, and rises to about 7.5 mmol/L, returning to the starting level within $1-1^1/2$ hours. In diabetics, the blood sugar concentration rises considerably higher and takes longer to return to the baseline value. The graph of the results forms a glucose-tolerance curve.

glucose tolerance factor *See* chromium.

glucosides Complexes of substances with glucose. The general name for such complexes with other sugars is glycosides.

glucosinolates Substances occurring widely in plants of the family Crucifera, genus *Brassica* (e.g. Brussels sprouts, cabbage, watercress, radishes); broken down by the *enzyme myrosinase to yield, among other products, the mustard oils which are responsible for the pungent flavour (especially in mustard and horseradish). Several of the glucosinolates interfere with the metabolism of *iodine by the *thyroid gland, and hence are *goitrogens; chemically they are thio-esters. There is evidence that the various glucosinolates in vegetables may have useful anti-cancer activity, since they increase the rate at which a variety of potentially toxic and carcinogenic compounds are conjugated and excreted.

glucostatic mechanism A theory that appetite depends on the difference between arterial and venous concentrations of glucose; when the difference falls low enough, the hunger centres in the hypothalamus are stimulated.

glucosuria (Also glycosuria); appearance of *glucose in the urine, as in *diabetes and after the administration of drugs that lower the renal threshold.

glucuronic acid The acid derived from glucose by the oxidation of the hydroxyl group on carbon-6. Many substances, including hormones and potentially toxic ingested substances, are excreted as conjugates with glucuronic acid, known as glucuronides. It is present in various complex polysaccharides.

glucuronides A variety of compounds are metabolized by conjugation with *glucuronic acid to yield water-soluble derivatives for excretion from the body.

glühwein Austrian, German; spiced hot wine punch, generally fortified by the addition of rum.

glutamate Salts of *glutamic acid.

glutamic acid A non-essential *amino acid; it is acidic since it has two carboxylic acid groups; its amide is glutamine. *See also* monosodium glutamate.

glutamine A non-essential amino acid, chemically the amide of *glutamic acid.

glutathione A tripeptide of *glycine, *glutamic acid, and *cysteine (γ-glutamyl-cysteinyl-glycine) which is involved in oxidation-reduction reactions, the conjugation of foreign substances for excretion and possibly the transport of amino acids into cells.

glutathione peroxidase *Selenium-containing *enzyme that protects tissues from oxidative damage by removing peroxides resulting from free radical action, linked to oxidation of *glutathione; part of the body's *antioxidant protection.

glutathione reductase *Enzyme in red *blood cells for which flavin adenine dinucleotide (derived from *vitamin B_2) is the cofactor. Activation of this enzyme *in vitro* by added cofactor provides a means of assessing vitamin B_2 nutritional status, sometimes known as the erythrocyte glutathione reductase activation coefficient (EGRAC) test. *See also* enzyme activation assays.

glutelins Proteins insoluble in water and neutral salt solutions but soluble in dilute acids and alkalis, e.g. wheat glutenin.

gluten The protein complex in wheat, and to a lesser extent rye, which gives dough the viscid property that holds gas when it rises. There is none in oats, barley, or maize. It is a mixture of two proteins, gliadin and glutelin. Allergy to, or intolerance of, the gliadin fraction of gluten is *coeliac disease (gluten sensitive enteropathy).

In the undamaged state with extensible properties it is termed vital gluten; when overheated, these properties are lost and the product is termed devitalized gluten, used for protein enrichment of foods.

gluten-free foods Formulated without any wheat or rye protein (although the starch may be used) for people suffering from *coeliac disease.

gluten-sensitive enteropathy *See* coeliac disease.

glutose A six-carbon sugar (hexose) with a keto group on carbon-3; it is not metabolized and non-fermentable.

glycaemic index The ability of a carbohydrate to increase blood glucose, compared with the same amount of glucose: the increase in blood glucose over 2 hours after ingesting 50 g of available carbohydrate, expressed as a percentage of that after 50 g of glucose.

glycerides Esters of *glycerol with *fatty acids. Since glycerol has three hydroxyl groups, it can be esterified with three molecules of fatty acid to form a triglyceride (correctly known as a *triacylglycerol), the main type of *fat in the diet and body, sometimes known as simple fats or neutral fats. If all three molecules of fatty acid are the same, the product is a simple triglyceride, e.g. tristearin, triolein; mixed glycerides may also be formed such as distearo-olein and stearo-oleo-palmitin.

glycerides, partial *See* superglycerinated fats.

glycerine *See* glycerol.

glycerol A trihydric alcohol, chemically 1,2,3-propane triol
($CH_2OH-CHOH-CH_2OH$), also known as glycerine. Simple or neutral
*fats are esters of glycerol with three molecules of *fatty acid, i.e.
triacylglycerols, sometimes known as triglycerides. *See also* glycerides.
　　Glycerol is a clear, colourless, odourless, viscous liquid, sweet to
taste; it is made from fats by alkaline hydrolysis (saponification). Used
as a solvent for flavours, as a humectant to keep foods moist, and in
cake batters to improve texture and slow down staling.

glycerose A three-carbon sugar, derived from the *glycerol. Formula
$CHO-CHOH-CH_2OH$.

glyceryl lactostearate Also known as lactostearin. Formed by
glycerolysis of hydrogenated soya bean oil followed by esterification
with lactic acid, which results in a mixture of mono- and diglycerides
and their lactic mono-esters. Used as an emulsifier in shortenings
(E-472(b)).

glyceryl monostearate *See* superglycerinated fats.

glycine A non-essential *amino acid, chemically the simplest of the
amino acids, it is amino-acetic acid, CH_2NH_2COOH. It has a sweet taste
(70% of the sweetness of sucrose) and is sometimes mixed with
*saccharin as a sweetening agent. Known at one time as collagen sugar.

glycinin Globulin protein in soya bean.

glycitols *See* sugar alcohols. Glycitol was used at one time as an
alternative name for *sorbitol.

glycocholic acid One of the *bile acids.

glycogen The storage carbohydrate in the liver and muscles, a branched
polymer of *glucose units. It has the same structure as the
amylopectin form of *starch, and is sometimes referred to as animal
starch. In an adult there are about 250 g of glycogen in the muscles
and 100 g in the liver in the fed state.
　　Since glycogen is rapidly broken down to glucose after an animal is
killed, meat and animal liver do not contain glycogen; the only dietary
sources are oysters, cockles, mussels, scallops, clams, whelks, and
winkles that are eaten virtually alive and contain about 5% glycogen.

glycogenesis The synthesis of glycogen from glucose in liver and
muscle after a meal, stimulated by the hormone *insulin.

glycogenic acid *See* gluconic acid.

glycogenolysis The breakdown of *glycogen to *glucose for use as a
metabolic fuel and to maintain the normal blood concentration of
glucose in the fasting state. Stimulated by the hormone *glucagon.

glycogen storage diseases A group of rare *genetic diseases
characterized by excessive accumulation of *glycogen in liver and/or
muscles and, in some forms, profound *hypoglycaemia in the fasting
state. Treatment is by feeding small frequent meals, rich in
carbohydrate.

glycolysis The first sequence of reactions in *glucose metabolism, leading to the formation of two molecules of pyruvic acid from each glucose molecule.

glycoproteins Proteins conjugated with carbohydrates such as uronic acids, polymerized glucosamine-mannose, etc., including mucins and mucoids; found in the vitreous humour of the eye, cornea, cartilage, and gastric mucosa. *See also* mucoproteins.

glycosides Compounds of a sugar attached to another molecule. When glucose is the sugar, they are called glucosides. A wide variety occur in plants and some, such as digitalis and rutin, are useful medicinally.

glycosuria (Also glucosuria); appearance of *glucose in the urine, as in *diabetes and after the administration of drugs that lower the renal threshold.

glycyrrhizin Triterpenoid glycoside extracted from *liquorice root *Glycyrrhiza glabra*; 50–100 times as sweet as sucrose but with liquorice flavour. Used to flavour tobacco and pharmaceutical preparations, and as a foaming agent in some non-alcoholic beverages.

GMP *See* Good Manufacturing Practice.

GMS Glyceryl monostearate, *see* superglycerinated fats.

gnocchi Italian; square, round, or other shaped *pasta used to garnish soups or served as a savoury dish with cheese sauce. May also be made from potato flour (potato gnocchi).

gob stopper Large, spherical, hard sugar sweet (2–4 cm in diameter), usually flavoured with mint and containing a caraway seed in the centre. So called because it fills the mouth for a long time while it is slowly dissolving.

gobhi bund *See* cabbage.

gobhi chote bund *See* Brussels sprouts.

gobhi phool *See* cauliflower.

gofio Spanish (Canary Islands); flour milled from toasted wheat grains.

goflo Spanish (Canary Islands); bread made from powdered bracken roots and barley meal.

goitre Enlargement of the *thyroid gland, seen as a swelling in the neck, most commonly due to deficiency of *iodine in the diet or to the presence of *goitrogens in foods. In such cases there is commonly underproduction of the *thyroid hormones, i.e. hypothyroid goitre. Euthyroid goitre is a condition in which the enlargement of the thyroid gland is sufficient to compensate for a limited dietary deficiency of iodine and permit normal production of thyroid hormones.

In infancy, iodine deficiency can also lead to severe mental retardation, goitrous cretinism. Supplementation with iodide often prevents the condition, hence the use of iodized *salt. Rarely, goitre may be due to other causes, including excessive stimulation of the thyroid gland. In this case there is overproduction of the *thyroid hormones, i.e. hyperthyroid goitre.

goitrogens Substances found in foods (especially *Brassica* spp. but including also groundnuts, cassava, and soya bean) which interfere with the synthesis of thyroid hormones (*glucosinolates) or the uptake of iodide into the *thyroid gland (thiocyanates), and hence can cause *goitre, especially when the dietary intake of iodide is marginal. Although goitrogens are associated with underactivity of the thyroid in animals, it is not established that they are a cause of goitre in human beings.

golden berry See Cape gooseberry.

golden syrup Light-coloured *syrup made by evaporation of cane sugar juice; *see also* treacle; sugar.

Goldwasser Literally 'gold water'; an aniseed- and caraway- or cumin-flavoured liqueur containing minute specks of gold leaf.

Gomez classification One of the earliest systems for classifying *protein-energy malnutrition in children, based on percentage of expected weight for age: over 90% is normal, 76–90% is mild (first degree) malnutrition, 61–75% is moderate (second degree) malnutrition and less than 60% is severe (third degree) malnutrition.

Good Manufacturing Practice (GMP) Part of a food and drink control operation aimed at ensuring that products are consistently manufactured to a quality appropriate to their intended use (detailed in *Good Manufacturing Practice: A Guide to Responsible Management*, Institute of Food Science and Technology, 1987).

goose (French: *oie*; German: *Gans*.) Domesticated water-fowl, *Anser anser*. A 150-g portion is a rich *source of protein, iron, vitamins B_2, B_6, B_{12}, and niacin; a good source of vitamin B_1, copper, and zinc; contains more than 30 g of fat of which one-third is saturated; supplies 470 kcal (1970 kJ).

gooseberry Berry of the shrub, *Ribes grossularia*. The British National Fruit Collection contains 155 varieties. An 80-g portion is a rich *source of vitamin C; provides 2.4 g of dietary fibre; supplies 12 kcal (50 kJ).

gooseberry, Indian See emblic.

goose foot See fat hen.

gorny dubnya Russian; bitter liqueur flavoured with ginger, angelica, and cloves.

gossypol Yellow toxic pigment found in some varieties of cottonseed. When included in chicken feed, it causes discoloration of the yolk, but has not been found to be toxic to human beings, and has been investigated as a possible male contraceptive agent.

Gouda Dutch semi-hard *cheese with random holes formed by gases during the ripening period (2–4 months or longer for well-matured cheese). A 30-g portion is a rich *source of vitamin B_{12}, a source of protein, niacin, and vitamin A; contains 9 g of fat; supplies 110 kcal (460 kJ).

gougère French; savoury *choux pastry containing cheese.

goujon Small, deep-fried pieces of *fish. The name is derived from gudgeon, a small fresh-water fish. The term is now also used for small pieces of chicken breast.

goulash (gulyas) Hungarian; literally 'cowherd'; beef (or other meat) stewed with potatoes, tomatoes, onions, peppers, and paprika. Distinct from Austrian *gulasch.

gourds Vegetables of the family Cucurbitaceae, including calabash or bottle gourd (*Lagenaria vulgaris*), ash gourd (*Benincasa hispida*), snake gourd (*Trichosanthes anguina*), cucumber (*Cucumis sativus*), vegetable marrow (*Cucurbita pepo*), pumpkin (*Cucurbita moschata*), squash (*Cucurbita maxima*), coocha or chayote (*Sechium edule*), cantaloup melon (*Cucumis melo*), water melon (*Citrullus vulgaris*). All contain more than 90% water and have little food value apart from vitamin C at 10 mg per 100 g. In addition, yellow pumpkin contains 900 µg carotene per 100 g. Melons are sometimes grown for their seeds, which contain 20–40% oil and 20% protein.

gout Painful disease caused by accumulation of crystals of *uric acid in the synovial fluid of joints; may be due to excessive synthesis and metabolism of *purines, which are metabolized to uric acid, or to impaired excretion of uric acid. Traditionally associated with a rich diet, although there is little evidence for dietary factors in causing the condition. May be exacerbated by alcohol.

Graham bread Wholewheat bread in which the bran is very finely ground. Graham cakes are made from wholemeal flour and milk. The name is that of a miller of wholemeal flour who advocated its use in the USA (*Treatise on Bread and Bread Making*, 1837). *See also* Allinson bread.

graining Crystallization of refined sugar when boiled. Prevented by adding glucose or cream of tartar as *sugar doctors.

grains of paradise *See* pepper, melegueta.

Gram-negative, Gram-positive A method of classifying bacteria depending on whether or not they retain crystal-violet dye after staining and decolorizing with alcohol. Named after the Danish botanist H. C. J. Gram.

grams, Indian Various small dried peas (*legumes), e.g. green gram (*Phaseolus aureus*), black gram (*Phaseolus mungo*), red gram (*Cajanus indicus*), Bengal gram or *chick pea (*Cicer aretinum*).

granadilla *See* passion fruit.

grand marnier Orange-flavoured liqueur.

grand premier cru *See* wine classification, Luxembourg.

granita Italian; water-ice or *sorbet; *see also* sherbet.

granvas Spanish; sparkling wines made by the tank method.

grape Fresh fruit of a large number of varieties of *Vitis vinifera*. One of the oldest cultivated plants (recorded in ancient Egypt in 4000 BC). Can be grouped as dessert grapes, *wine grapes, and varieties that are used for drying to produce raisins, currants, and sultanas (*see* fruit, dried).

Of the many varieties of grape that are grown for *wine making, nine
are considered 'classic varieties': cabernet sauvignon, chardonnay,
chenin blanc, merlot, pinot noir, riesling, sauvignon blanc, sémillon,
syrah. A 100-g portion is a *source of copper; provides 0.5 g of dietary
fibre; supplies 60 kcal (245 kJ).

grapefruit Fruit of *Citrus paradisi*; thought to have arisen as a sport of
the *pomelo or shaddock (*Citrus grandis*), a coarser *citrus fruit, or as a
hybrid between pomelo and sweet orange. It contains 35–40 mg
vitamin C per 100 g. The pith contains *naringin, which is very bitter.
The name is said to have arisen because the fruit is borne on the tree
in clusters (like grapes!).

grape sugar *See* glucose.

grappa *See* marc.

GRAS (Generally regarded as safe) Designation given to food
additives when further evidence is required before the substance can
be classified more precisely (US usage).

gras, au Cooked and dressed with rich gravy or sauce.

grass tetany *Magnesium deficiency in cattle.

gratin 1 A fireproof dish.
    2 Also known as gratiné, the French term for the thin brown crust
formed on top of foods that have been covered with butter and
breadcrumbs, then heated under the grill or in the oven. Au gratin
means that cheese is also used.

grattons (gratterons) French; crispy remains of melted fatty tissues of
poultry or pork. German equivalent is gribbens.

gravadlax (gravlaks, gravlax) Scandinavian; pickled or marinated
raw salmon.

gravy Sauce made from the juices and extractives which run out from
meat during cooking, normally thickened.

gravy browning Caramelized sugar and starch used to thicken and
colour gravy and sauces; may be powder or liquid.

gravy granules Seasoned and coloured granules of modified *starch
with a savoury flavour, used to make gravy; they form a gel on
addition of boiling water.

Gray (Gy) The SI unit for ionizing radiation (= 100 rad). The Gray is
equivalent to 1 J/kg.

great millet *See* sorghum.

green butter *See* vegetable butters.

greengage (French: *Reine-Claude*; German: *Reinclaude*, named after the
French Queen Claude.) Green variety of *plum introduced into England
in the early eighteenth century by Sir William Gage. A 200-g portion
(four raw gages weighed without stones) is a *source of iron and
vitamin C; contains 500 mg of potassium and 4–5 g of dietary fibre;
supplies 100 kcal (420 kJ).

greens *See* collard; spring greens.

green S Food *colour, also known as Wool green S and Brilliant acid green BS, E-142.

grenache A *grape variety widely used for *wine making, although not one of the classic varieties.

grenadin French; small slice of fillet of veal, *larded and braised.

grenadine French; syrup made from pomegranate juice, used as a beverage and to flavour beer.

gribbens (also greben, gribbenes) German; *see* grattons.

gribbenschmaltz German; dripping containing the crispy remnant of the fatty tissue of the animal (gribbens).

griddle Also girdle; iron plate used for baking scones, etc., on top of stove.

grill To cook by radiant heat; some of the fat is lost. Barbecues cook by grilling.

grillade à l'ardoise Andorran method of cooking on a red-hot roof slate heated over a wood fire (French: *ardoise*, slate).

grilse Young *salmon that has returned to fresh water after one year in the sea.

grind To reduce hard foods such as nuts and coffee beans to small particles using a food mill, grinder, or sometimes a liquidizer.

griskin *Chine of pork, also used for a thin, poor, piece of loin.

grissini Italian 'finger rolls' or stick bread, 15–45 cm (6–18 in) long, and normally crisp and dry.

grist Cereal for grinding.

gristle The *connective tissue of the meat, consisting mainly of the insoluble proteins *collagen and elastin. Usually inedible and accounts for the toughness of some cuts of meat. Prolonged slow cooking converts collagen to *gelatine, but has no effect on elastin.

grits, corn *See* hominy.

groats Oats from which the husk has been entirely removed; when crushed, Embden groats result. Used to make gruel and porridge.

grog British naval drink; sugared rum mixed with hot water. Named after Admiral Vernon (early eighteenth century) whose nickname 'Old Grog' came from his grosgrain (heavy corded silk) coat.

ground meat American term for minced meat.

groundnut *See* peanut.

ground tomato *See* Cape gooseberry.

grouse *Game bird, *Lagopus lagopus*. Shooting period in the UK is 12 August to 10 December; eaten fresh or after being hung for 2–4 days to develop flavour. The whole bird weighs about 700 g; a 150-g portion is an extremely rich *source of iron and vitamin B_2; rich source of protein, niacin, and vitamin B_1; contains about 8 g of fat of which one-fifth is saturated; supplies 250 kcal (1050 kJ).

gruel Thin porridge made from oatmeal, barley, or other cereal.

GTF Glucose tolerance factor, *see* chromium.

guacamole Mexican; sauce made from very ripe *avocado, mashed with garlic, lemon juice, and chilli.

guanine One of the *purines.

guarana A substance from the seeds of a climbing shrub, *Paullina cupana*, native to the Amazon region. It contains caffeine and related compounds; used in the UK as an ingredient of drinks, chewing gum, a powder to be sprinkled on food, and capsules and tablets.

guar gum Cyamopsis gum; from the cluster bean, *Cyamopsis tetragonoloba*. Member of Leguminosae, used in India as livestock feed. The *gum is a water-soluble galactomannan; used in 'slimming' preparations, since it is not digested by digestive enzymes, and experimentally in the treatment of *diabetes, since it slows the absorption of nutrients, and so prevents a rapid rise in blood sugar after a meal.

guava Fruit of the Central and South American tropical shrub *Psidium guajava*, eaten raw or preserved as guava jelly.

guinea corn *See* sorghum.

guinea fowl Game bird, *Numida meleagris*, not seasonal. Nutritionally similar to *chicken.

guinea pepper *See* pepper, melegueta.

gulab jaman Indian dessert; deep-fried balls of ground almond and flour dough, served in syrup.

gulasch Austrian; cubes of meat or poultry fried with onions, then simmered with paprika, tomato, and caraway seed. Distinct from Hungarian *goulash or gulyas.

gullar *See* fig.

gulyas *See* goulash.

gum Substances that can disperse in water to form a viscous mucilaginous mass. Used in food processing to stabilize emulsions (such as salad dressings and processed cheese), as a thickening agent, and in sugar confectionery.
  The substances may be extracted from seeds (*guar gum, locust (*carob), quince, *psyllium), plant sap or exudates (gum arabic, karaya or sterculia, tragacanth, ghatti, bassora or hog gum, shiraz, mesquite, anguo), and seaweeds (*agar, *kelp, *alginate, *Irish moss), or they may be made from starch or *cellulose, or they may be synthetic, such as vinyl polymer. Most of these (apart from dextrins) are not digested and have no food value, although they contribute to the intake of *non-starch polysaccharides. *See also* fibre, soluble.

gum arabic (gum acacia) Exudate from the stems of several species of acacia; the best product comes from *Acacia senegal*. Used as thickening agent, as stabilizer, often in combination with other gums, in gum drops and soft jelly gums, and to prevent crystallization in sugar confectionery. Also used as the adhesive on postage stamps.

gumbo American (*Creole); soup or stew made from okra, onions, celery, and pepper, flavoured with filé powder (powdered dried *sassafras leaves), and containing chicken, meat, fish, or shellfish. Also a name for *okra.

gum, British Partly hydrolysed starch, *dextrin.

gum, chewing *See* chewing gum.

gum dragon *See* gum tragacanth.

gum drops (fruit gums) *Sugar confectionery based on *sucrose and *glucose with *gum arabic (hard gums) or a mixture of *gelatine and gum arabic (soft gums).

gum tragacanth Obtained from the trees of *Astralagus* spp., used as a stabilizer.

gur Mixture of sugar crystals and syrup, brown and toffee-like, made by evaporation of juice of sugar cane; also called jaggery.

gury Russian (Georgian); whole raw white cabbage soaked in brine with beetroot and red peppers.

gut *See* gastro-intestinal tract.

Guthrie test Test for a number of *genetic diseases (especially *phenylketonuria) based on measuring the concentrations of *amino acids in a small sample of blood taken by pricking the heel of the child a few days after birth, by biological assay using mutated bacteria.

gut sweetbread *See* pancreas.

GYE Guinness Yeast Extract, *see* yeast extract.

gyle *Alcohol solution formed in the first stage of *vinegar production, 6–9% alcohol. Subsequent fermentation with *Acetobacter* spp. converts the alcohol to *acetic acid.

haché Minced or chopped.

hachis Minced or chopped mixture of meat and herbs, generally used as *forcemeat.

haddock White *fish, *Melanogrammus aeglefinus*.

haem (heme) The iron-containing pigment which, in combination with the protein globin, forms *haemoglobin and *myoglobin. It is also part of a wide variety of other proteins, collectively known as haem proteins, including the *cytochromes.

haemagglutinins (hemagglutinins) *See* lectins.

haematemesis (hematemesis) Vomiting bright red blood, due to bleeding in the upper *gastro-intestinal tract.

haematin (hematin) Formed by the oxidation of *haem; the iron is oxidized from the ferrous (Fe^{2+}) to the ferric (Fe^{3+}) state.

haematinic (hematin) General term for those nutrients, including iron, folic acid, and vitamin B_{12}, required for the formation and development of blood cells in bone marrow (the process of haematopoiesis), deficiency of which may result in *anaemia.

haemin (hemin) The hydrochloride of *haematin, derived from *haemoglobin. The crystals are readily recognizable under the microscope and are used as a test for blood.

haemoglobin (hemoglobin) The red *haem-containing protein in red blood cells which is responsible for the transport of oxygen and carbon dioxide in the bloodstream. Because haem contains *iron, there is a deficiency of haemoglobin and impaired oxygen transport to tissues in iron deficiency *anaemia.

haemoglobin, glycosylated (glycated) Haemoglobin linked via lysine to *glucose. The reaction occurs non-enzymically, and is increased when blood concentrations of glucose are persistently higher than normal. Measurement of glycosylated haemoglobin is used as an index of the control of *diabetes over the preceding 2–3 months. Normally 3–6% of haemoglobin is glycosylated; as much as 20% may be glycosylated in uncontrolled diabetes.

haemoglobinometer (hemoglobinometer) Instrument to measure the amount of haemoglobin in blood by direct colorimetry or after conversion to another coloured compound.

haemolytic (hemolytic) anaemia *See* anaemia, haemolytic.

haemorrhagic (hemorrhagic) disease of the newborn Excessive bleeding due to *vitamin K deficiency; in most countries infants are given vitamin K by injection shortly after birth to prevent this rare but serious (potentially fatal) condition.

haemorrhoids (hemorrhoids) Or piles, varicosity in the lower rectum or anus due to congestion of the veins; caused or exacerbated by a low-fibre diet and consequent straining to defecate. *See also* dietary fibre.

haemosiderin (hemosiderin) *See* iron storage.

Haff disease Acute paroxysmal myoglobinuria suffered by fishermen around the Koenigsberg Haff in eastern Germany; attributed either to a toxin in the seawater which entered the fish or to *thiaminase in raw or incompletely cooked fish.

Hagberg test Measure of α-amylase activity of flour based on the change in viscosity of flour paste.

haggis Traditional Scottish dish made from sheep's heart, liver, and lungs cooked and chopped with suet, onions, oatmeal, and seasoning, and stuffed into the stomach of a sheep. Said to have originated with the Romans when they were campaigning in Scotland; when they broke camp in an emergency, the food was wrapped in the sheep's stomach. A similar Norman-French dish was afronchemoyle. A 150-g portion is an exceptionally rich *source of iron; a rich source of protein; a good source of vitamins B_1, B_2, niacin, calcium, and copper; a source of zinc; contains about 33 g of fat of which half is saturated; supplies 450 kcal (1900 kJ).

hake A white *fish, *Merluccius bilinearis*.

halal Food conforming to the Islamic (Muslim) dietary laws. Meat from permitted animals (in general grazing animals with cloven hooves, and thus excluding pig meat) and birds (excluding birds of prey). The animals are killed under religious supervision by cutting the throat to allow removal of all blood from the carcass, without prior stunning.

halawa *See* halvah.

halbsüss, halbtrocken *See* wine sweetness.

haldi *See* turmeric.

half-life 1 The time taken for half the *protein or tissue in question to be replaced. Proteins are continuously being degraded and replaced even in the mature adult, and the half-life is used as a quantitative measure of this 'dynamic equilibrium'. The values of half-life of different proteins range from a few minutes or hours for *enzymes which control the rate of metabolic pathways, to almost a year for structural proteins such as collagen. The average half-life of human liver and serum proteins is 10 days, and of the total body protein, 80 days.

2 Of radioactive isotopes, the time in which half the original material undergoes radioactive decay.

halibut A white *fish, *Hippoglossus* spp.

halibut liver oil The oil from the liver of the *halibut, one of the richest natural sources of vitamins A and D; contains 50 mg of vitamin A and 80 µg of vitamin D per gram.

halophiles (halophilic bacteria) Bacteria able to grow in high concentrations of salt (up to 25%). The growth of colonic bacteria is inhibited at 8–9% salt, *Clostridia* at 7–10%, food-poisoning staphylococci at 15–20%, and *Penicillium* at 20%. Film-forming *yeasts can grow in 24% brine.

halvah (halva, halwa, halawa, chalva) 1 A sweetmeat composed of an aerated mixture of glucose, sugar, and crushed sesame seeds; because of the seeds, the sweet contains 25% fat.

    2 Indian desserts of various types, made from carrot, pumpkin, or banana, sweetened and flavoured.

halverine Name sometimes given to low-fat spreads with less than the statutory amount of fat in a *margarine.

ham (French: *jambon*; German: *Schweineschinken*.) The whole hind leg of the pig, removed from the carcass and cured individually; sometimes the process is secret. Hams cured or smoked in different ways have different flavours, e.g. York, Bradenham, Suffolk, and Westphalian hams. A 100-g portion is a rich *source of protein, niacin, and vitamin B_1; a good source of copper; a source of vitamin B_2, iron, zinc, and selenium; contains 5 g of fat of which 40% is saturated; supplies 120 kcal (500 kJ). *See also* bacon; gammon.

Haman's ears Biscuits; very thin pieces of egg dough, deep fried.

Haman taschen Traditional Jewish cakes for the festival of Purim; pastry made from *kuchen dough filled with poppy seed and honey, chopped stewed prunes, or cream cheese.

hamburger Or Hamburg steak, also known as beefburger. A flat cake made from ground (minced) *beef, seasoned with salt, pepper, and herbs, and bound with egg and flour. Commercial beefburgers are usually 80–100% meat, but must by law (in the UK) contain 52% lean meat, of which 80% must be beef. Cereal, cereal fibre, or bean fibre may be added as filler or 'meat extender'. A 100-g portion (4 oz raw weight) is a rich *source of protein, vitamin B_{12}, niacin, copper, and iron; a good source of zinc; a source of vitamins B_2 and B_6; contains 900 mg of sodium and 17 g of fat, of which half is saturated and half mono-unsaturated; supplies 260 kcal (1100 kJ).

ham, green Ham that has been cured but not smoked.

hand of pork The foreleg of *pork; usually salted and boiled.

hangover Headache and feeling of malaise resulting from excessive consumption of *alcoholic beverages. The severity differs with different beverages and is not due to the toxic effects of alcohol alone, but to the presence of higher alcohols and esters (collectively known as *congeners or *fusel oil), the substances that give different beverages their distinctive flavours.

Hansa can An all-aluminium can (developed in Germany) with easily opened ends.

haram Food forbidden by Islamic law (opposite of *halal).

hardening of oils *See* hydrogenated oils.

hardness of water *See* water, hardness.

hard sauce Butter and sugar, flavoured with brandy or rum, served with rich puddings.

hare (French: *lièvre*; German: *Hase*.) Game animal, similar to *rabbit but larger; caught wild but not farmed commercially. *Lepus europaeus* is the common hare, but some twenty *Lepus* species occur in Europe. A 150-g portion is an extremely rich *source of iron (15 mg); a rich source of protein; contains 12 g of fat; supplies 300 kcal (1260 kJ).

hare's lettuce *See* sow thistle.

haricot French for beans; also stewed chopped meat, as haricot mutton.

Hartnup disease A *genetic disease affecting the absorption and tissue uptake of the *amino acid tryptophan, with considerable loss in the urine. Characterized by development of *pellagra, and treated by administration of supplements of *niacin.

Harvard standard Tables of height and weight for age used as reference values for the assessment of growth and nutritional status in children, based on data collected in the USA. Now largely replaced by the NCHS (US National Center for Health Statistics) standards.

Harvey Wallbanger A cocktail based on half a measure of *Galliano floating on four measures of orange juice and half a measure of vodka.

hash Dish of cooked meat reheated in highly flavoured sauce. In the USA canned *corned beef is known as corned beef hash.

hash browns American; cooked potatoes, chopped, formed into small cakes, and fried.

haslet (harslet) Old English country dish made from pig's offal (heart, liver, lungs, and sweetbreads) cooked in small pieces with seasoning and flour. Also known as pig's fry.

hasty pudding English, sixteenth century; made from flour, milk, butter, and spices, which, since they were usually readily available, could be quickly made into a pudding for unexpected visitors. Made in the USA with maize (corn) flour instead of wheat flour.

hâtelet *See* attelette.

haunch Hindquarters of deer, *see* venison.

Hausa groundnut *Legume grown in West Africa, *Kerslingiella geocarpa*; 20% protein, 60% fat.

haybox cooking The food is cooked for only a short time, then placed in a well-lagged container, the haybox, where it remains hot for many hours, so cooking continues without further use of fuel. Also known as the fireless cooker.

Hay diet A system of eating based on the concept that carbohydrates and proteins should not be eaten at the same meal, for which there is no scientific basis. It ignores the fact that almost all carbohydrate-rich foods also contain significant amounts of protein. In any case, in the absence of adequate carbohydrate, protein is oxidized as a metabolic fuel (i.e. to provide energy) and therefore not available for tissue building. Also called combining diet or food combining.

haze Term in general use in brewing to indicate cloudiness of the *beer. Chill haze appears at 0 °C and disappears at 20 °C; permanent haze remains at 20 °C but there is no fundamental difference. It is caused by *gums derived from the barley, leucoanthocyanins from the malt and hops, and glucose, pentoses, and amino acids. *See also* chill-proofing.

hazel nut Fruit of the tree *Corylus avellana*; cultivated varieties include Barcelona nut, cob nut, and filbert (*C. maxima*). A 50-g portion (fifty nuts) is a rich *source of copper and vitamin E; a source of protein, niacin, vitamins B_1 and B_2, calcium, zinc, and iron; contains 32 g of fat (most of which is mono-unsaturated); provides 5 g of dietary fibre; supplies 325 kcal (1300 kJ).

HDL High-density lipoproteins, one of the classes of plasma *lipids.

headcheese Mock *brawn.

health foods Substances whose consumption is advocated by various reform movements, including vegetable foods, whole grain cereals, food processed without chemical additives, food grown on organic compost, 'magic' foods (bees' royal jelly, *lecithin, seaweed, etc.), and pills and potions. Numerous health claims are made but rarely is there any evidence to support these claims.

healthy US legislation permits a claim of 'healthy' for a food that is *low in fat and saturated fat, and contains no more than 480 mg of sodium and 60 mg of cholesterol per serving.

heart (French: *cœur*; German: *Herz*.) Usually from ox, lamb, pig, or sheep; a 150-g portion is a rich *source of protein, niacin, iron, and vitamins B_1 and B_2, also, unusually for a meat product, a good source of vitamin C; contains about 9 g of fat, of which half is saturated; supplies 270 kcal (1130 kJ).

heartburn A burning sensation in the chest usually caused by reflux (regurgitation) of acid digestive juices from the stomach into the oesophagus. A common form of *indigestion, treated by *antacids.

heat of combustion *Energy released by complete combustion, as for example, in the *bomb calorimeter. Values can be used to predict energy physiologically available from foods only if an allowance is made for material not completely oxidized in the body. For example, the end products of protein oxidation in the body are carbon dioxide, water, and urea; the latter contains non-available energy. *See* energy conversion factors.

hedonic scale Term used in tasting panels where the judges indicate the extent of their like or dislike for the food.

heel-prick test Test for *genetic diseases based on measuring the concentrations of amino acids in a small sample of blood taken by pricking the heel of the child a few days after birth.

Helicobacter pyloris Bacterium commonly infecting the gastric mucosa in patients with *ulcers. Believed to be the underlying cause of ulcers, and also implicated in the development of gastric cancer. *See also* Campylobacter.

hemicelluloses Complex *carbohydrates included as *dietary fibre, composed of polyuronic acids combined with xylose, glucose, mannose, and arabinose. Found together with cellulose and lignin in plant cell walls; most *gums and mucilages are hemicelluloses.

hemoglobin American spelling of *haemoglobin; similarly, hematin = haematin, heme = haem, hemosiderin = haemosiderin.

hepatitis Inflammatory liver disease, characterized by jaundice, abdominal pain, and anorexia. May be due to bacterial or viral infection, alcohol abuse, or various toxins. Treatment is usually conservative, with a very low fat diet (secretion of *bile is impaired) and complete abstinence from alcohol.

Even after recovery, people may continue to be carriers of the virus, especially for hepatitis B and C, which are transmitted through blood and other body fluids. Liver cancer and cirrhosis are more common among people who have suffered from hepatitis B or C.

herb butter A mixture of butter and mayonnaise blended with parsley, tarragon, dill, watercress, thyme, green pepper, garlic, and other herbs, used as a savoury spread on biscuits or bread.

herb liqueurs *See* liqueurs.

herbs Soft-stemmed, aromatic plants used fresh or dried to flavour and garnish dishes, and sometimes for medicinal effects. Not clearly distinguished from *spices, except that herbs are usually the leaves or the whole of the plant while spices are only part of the plant, commonly the seeds, or sometimes the roots or rhizomes.

herb tea Or tisane, an infusion made from any kind of herb, fruit, or flower. Camomile, lime blossom, and fennel seeds are commonly used. Medicinal or health claims are sometimes made, largely on traditional rather than scientific grounds.

Hermesetas Trade name for *saccharin tablets.

herring (French: *hareng*; German: *Hering*.) Oily *fish, *Clupea harengus*; young herrings are sild. Sprat is *Clupea sprattus*; young are brislings. Pilchard is *Clupea pilchardus*; young are sardines. Kippers, bloaters, and red herrings are salted and smoked herrings; bucklings are hot-smoked herrings. *Gaffelbitar are preserved herring. A 150-g portion (weighed with bones), grilled, is an exceptionally rich *source of vitamins D, B_{12}, and selenium; a rich source of protein, niacin, and vitamin B_6; a source of vitamins B_1, B_2, iodine, and iron; contains 200 mg of sodium, about 13–28 g of fat, varying with the season, of which one-third is *saturated and half is mono-unsaturated; supplies 200–360 kcal (800–1500 kJ).

hesperidin A *flavonoid found in the pith of unripe citrus fruits; chemically a complex of glucose and rhamnose with the flavonone hesperin. At one time called *vitamin P, since it affects the fragility of the capillary walls, although there is no evidence that it is a dietary essential.

Hess test A test for capillary fragility in *scurvy. A slight pressure is applied to the arm for 5 minutes and a shower of petechiae (small blood spots) appear on the skin below the area of application.

heterosides *See* holosides.

heterotrophes *See* autotrophes.

hexamethylene tetramine Preservative (fungicide), E-239. Also known as hexamine.

hexamic acid Trade name for cyclohexyl sulphamic acid, the free acid of *cyclamate, a synthetic sweetener about 27 times as sweet as sugar.

hexamine *See* hexamethylene tetramine.

hexoses Six-carbon (monosaccharide) *sugars such as *glucose or *fructose.

hexuronic acid The acid derived from a hexose *sugar by oxidation of the hydroxyl group on carbon-6. The hexuronic acid derived from glucose is glucuronic acid.

HFCS High-fructose corn syrup. *See* fructose syrups.

HF heating High-frequency heating. *See* microwave heating.

hiatus hernia Protrusion of a part of the stomach upwards through the diaphragm. The condition occurs in about 40% of the population, most people suffering no ill-effects; in a small number of people there is reflux of stomach contents into the oesophagus, causing *heartburn. *See also* gastro-intestinal tract.

hickory nut North American walnut, *Carya* spp.; the best known is the *pecan nut.

high-density lipoproteins One of the classes of plasma *lipids.

higher in EU legislation (in preparation in 1995) states that for a food label or advertising to bear a claim that it is higher in a nutrient it must contain at least 25% more of the claimed nutrient than a similar food for which no claim is made. *See also* high in.

high-frequency heating *See* microwave heating.

high-fructose corn syrup *See* fructose syrups.

high in EU legislation (in preparation in 1995) states that for a food label or advertising to bear a claim that it is high in a nutrient it must contain 50% more of the claimed nutrient than a similar product for which no claim is made. Claims may also be made for foods containing more than 12 g of protein, 6 g of dietary fibre or more than 30% of the labelling Reference Amount of a vitamin or mineral /100 g (*see* Appendix VI). US legislation permits a claim of 'high in' for foods containing more than 20% of the Daily Value for a particular nutrient in a serving.

high-performance liquid chromatography Also known as high-pressure liquid chromatography, and generally abbreviated to hplc. An extremely sensitive analytical technique, typically able to separate and measure nanograms or smaller amounts of compounds in samples of 10–100 μl.

high-ratio fats *See* superglycerinated fats.

high-ratio flour *See* flour, high-ratio.

high-ratio shortenings *See* superglycerinated fats.

high-temperature short-time treatment (HTST) Sterilization by heat from times ranging from a few seconds to minutes; usually applied to flow sterilization, in which the process time is less than about 1 minute; based on the fact that at higher temperatures bacteria are destroyed more rapidly than damage can occur to nutrients and texture.

Himbeergeist German spirit distilled from raspberries with added alcohol.

hindle wakes Very old English method of cooking chicken, stuffed with fruit and spices, including prunes. Possibly a corruption of *hen de la wake*, a feast of fourteenth-century Flemish introduction.

Hi-soy Trade name for full-fat *soya flour.

histamine The amine formed by decarboxylation of the amino acid *histidine in the body, also found in small amounts in cheeses, beer, chocolate, sauerkraut, and wines. Excessive release of histamine from mast cells is responsible for many of the symptoms of allergic reactions. It also stimulates secretion of *gastric acid, and administration of histamine is used as a test for *achlorhydria.

histidinaemia *Genetic disease due to a defect in the metabolism of the *amino acid histidine. If untreated it leads to mental retardation and nervous system abnormalities. Treatment is by feeding a diet very low in histidine.

histidine A basic *amino acid which can be synthesized in the body, but not in adequate amounts to meet requirements; hence an essential amino acid.

histones Proteins rich in arginine and lysine, soluble in water but not dilute ammonia. They occur mainly in the cell nucleus and are concerned with the regulation of *DNA.

hiyu Japanese name for Chinese spinach (*Amaranthus gangeticus*), also known as bhaji and *callaloo.

HMG CoA reductase inhibitors Drugs which inhibit the enzyme hydroxymethylglutaryl CoA (HMG CoA) reductase, the controlling enzyme of *cholesterol synthesis, used in the treatment of *hypercholesterolaemia.

hock 1 Generic term for white wines from the Rhine region of Germany, known in the USA as Rhine wines; bottled in brown glass, to distinguish from Moselle wines (in green glass).
   2 The knuckle of *pork; also used in the USA for foreleg pork shank.

hogget One-year-old sheep. *See* lamb.

hogshead A traditional UK measure of volume or size of barrel: for beer or cider contains 54 gallons (243 L); for wine contains $52\frac{1}{2}$ gallons (236 L).

hoisin sauce Chinese; spicy vegetable-based brownish-red sauce.

holishkes Middle-European, Jewish; cabbage leaves stuffed with rice, minced meat, and sultanas.

hollandaise sauce Rich *sauce made from egg yolks, butter, and lemon.

hollands *See* gin.

holocellulose Mixture of *cellulose and hemicellulose in wood, the fibrous residue that remains after the extractives, the lignin, and the ash-forming elements have been removed.

holoenzyme An *enzyme protein together with its *coenzyme or *prosthetic group. *See also* enzyme activation tests.

holosides Complexes of sugars that yield only sugars on hydrolysis. As distinct from heterosides which yield other substances as well as sugars on hydrolysis, e.g. tannins, anthocyanins, nucleosides.

homard *See* lobster.

hominy Prepared *maize kernels. Lye hominy has the pericarp and germ removed by soaking in caustic soda. Pearled hominy is degermed hulled maize. Corn grits are ground hominy.

homocysteine An amino acid formed as an intermediate in the metabolism of *methionine, and in the formation of *cysteine from methionine; it is demethylated methionine. Does not occur in foods to any significant extent, and is not generally considered to be of nutritional importance. High blood concentrations of homocysteine (occurring as a result of poor *folic acid, *vitamin B_6, and B_{12} status) have been implicated in the development of *atherosclerosis and heart disease.

homocystinuria A *genetic disease affecting the metabolism of the *amino acid methionine and its conversion to cysteine, characterized by excretion of *homocysteine and its derivatives. May result in mental retardation and early death from *atherosclerosis and coronary thrombosis if untreated, as well as fractures of bones and dislocation of the lens of the eye. Treatment (which must be continued throughout life) is either by feeding a diet low in methionine and supplemented with cysteine or, in some cases by administration of high intakes of *vitamin B_6 (about 100–500 times the normal requirement).

homogenization Emulsions usually consist of a suspension of globules of varying size. Homogenization reduces these globules to a smaller and more uniform size. In homogenized milk the smaller globules adsorb more of the protein, which acts as a stabilizer, and the cream does not rise to the top.

homogenizer, ultrasonic *See* ultrasonic homogenizer.

honey Syrupy liquid made by bees (the honey bee is *Apis mellifera*) from the nectar of flowers (which is essentially sucrose). The flavour and colour depend upon the flowers from which the nectar was obtained and the composition also varies with the source. Average composition: water 18% (12–26%), invert sugar, i.e. glucose and fructose, 74% (69–75%), sucrose 1.9% (0–4%), ash 0.18% (0.1–0.8%), organic acids 0.1–0.4%. If the ratio of fructose to glucose is high, there is a tendency for the honey to crystallize.

Comb honey is honey stored by bees in cells of freshly built, broodless combs and sold in the comb; drained honey is drained from decapped combs.

honeydew honey During periods of prolonged drought, bees may supplement their nectar supplies with honeydew, the sweet fluid excreted on leaves by leaf-sucking insects. The resultant *honey is dark, with an unpleasant taste.

honeyware *See* badderlocks.

Hongroise, à la Dish cooked in a cream sauce seasoned with paprika; the term is synonymous with à l'Autrichienne.

hops Perennial climbing plant, *Humulus lupulus*; the dried female flowers contain bitter resins and *essential oils and are added to beer both to preserve it and to enhance the flavour. The tender shoots are eaten as a vegetable in some countries.

horchata de chufa Spanish; aqueous extract of *tiger nut (*Cyperus esculentus*) used as a drink.

hordein A protein in barley; one of the prolamines.

hordenin Alkaloid found in germinated barley, sorghum, and millet which can cause *hypertension and respiratory inhibition.

Horlick's Trade name for a preparation of malted milk, for consumption as a beverage when added to milk.

hormones Compounds produced in the body in *endocrine glands, and released into the bloodstream, where they act as chemical messengers to affect other tissues and organs.

hormones, sex Male hormones, or androgens, include testosterone, dihydrotestosterone and androsterone; female hormones, or *oestrogens, include oestradiol, oestrone, and progesterone. Chemically, all are *steroids, derived from *cholesterol.
   The synthetic female hormones stilboestrol and hexoestrol have similar biological activities to the oestrogens, but are quite different chemically. Apart from clinical use the oestrogens have been used for chemical *caponization of cockerels and to enhance the growth rate of cattle.

horned melon *See* kiwano.

hors d'œuvre Small savoury dishes served as an appetizer either as the first course of a meal or before the meal with cocktails or an aperitif. It is French for 'outside the main work of the meal'. The Spanish equivalent is *tapas.

horse *Equus caballus* (French: *cheval*; German: *Pferdefleisch*); a 150-g portion is an exceptionally rich *source of iron; a rich source of protein and niacin, and a source of vitamins B_1 and B_2; contains about 5 g of fat of which one-third is *saturated; supplies 175 kcal (735 kJ).

horse mushroom *Agaricus arvensis*, *see* mushrooms.

horseradish The root of *Armoracia lapathifolia*. Its pungency is caused by volatile oils. Used as a condiment, usually as a creamed sauce, or grated and mixed with beetroot (*chrane), it is also an important ingredient in *wasabe powder.

horse's neck A long drink based on ginger ale with ice, *bitters, and a spirit.

Hortvet freezing test Test for the adulteration of milk with water by measuring the freezing point; milk normally freezes between −0.53 to −0.55 °C; if diluted with water it will freeze above −0.53 °C.

horzata Italian; *see* horchata de chufas.

hot breads American term for *waffles and *pancakes.

hotch-potch Thick soup or stew of meat and vegetables.

hot cross bun Spiced yeast bun traditionally eaten in the UK at Easter; the top is decorated with a cross of dough.

hot dog *Frankfurter sausage in a long bread roll.

hotpot Baked stew or casserole of meat or fish, topped with sliced potatoes.

hot sauce A tomato sauce with pungent flavour due to *cayenne.

Hot Springs Conference International Conference held in 1943 at which the Food and Agriculture Organization (FAO) of the United Nations originated.

hot-water crust Pastry made by melting lard into boiling water and pouring the mixture onto the flour, then kneading it into a dough.

Hovis Trade name for a mixture of brown flour and wheatgerm; from Latin *hominis vis*, 'strength of man'; originally, in the 1880s, called Smith's Old Patent Germ Bread. It is not baked centrally but franchised to local bakers. Four large slices (140 g) are a rich *source of vitamin B_1, iron, and niacin; a good source of protein, calcium, and zinc; supply 4.5 g of dietary fibre and 300 kcal (1260 kJ).

Howard mould count Standardized microscopical technique for measuring mould contamination.

howtowdie Scottish; boiled chicken with poached egg and spinach.

hplc *See* high-performance liquid chromatography.

hsiao mai Chinese; fish-filled wraplings or *wuntun.

5HT *See* 5-hydroxytryptamine.

HTST *See* high-temperature short-time treatment.

huckleberry Wild North American berry, the fruit of *Gaylussacia baccata* and other species (named after the French chemist Gay-Lussac). Similar to *blueberry but has larger seeds; used in tarts, pies, and preserves.

huevos a la flamenca *See* eggs flamenca.

huff paste Northern British name for pastry made from suet, flour, and water, used to enclose meat, fish, or poultry while baking.

hull *See* husk.

humble pie *See* umbles.

humbug Hard boiled sweet, normally peppermint-flavoured, cushion-shaped.

humectants Substances such as *glycerol, *sorbitol, *invert sugars, *honey which prevent loss of moisture from foods, especially flour confectionery, which would make them unappetizing; they also prevent sugar crystallizing and the growth of ice crystals in frozen foods. They are used in other products too, such as tobacco, inks, glues, etc.

humidity The moistness of air. Weight of water per unit weight of air is absolute or specific humidity. Saturation humidity is the absolute humidity of air that is saturated with water vapour at a given temperature. Relative humidity is the degree of saturation: the ratio of water vapour pressure in the atmosphere to water vapour pressure that would be exerted by pure water at the same temperature.

hummus Middle Eastern; hors d'œuvre, a purée of *chickpeas and *tahini with garlic, oil, and lemon juice. A 100-g portion is a *source of protein, niacin, vitamin B_1, iron, and zinc; provides 2.5 g of dietary fibre; contains 13 g of fat; supplies 190 kcal (760 kJ).

hurricane A New Orleans cocktail based on rum, passion fruit juice, and lime juice, in equal measures.

hush puppies Southern USA; fried, seasoned, batter cakes, served especially with fish.

husk (or hull) The outer woody cellulose covering of seeds and grains. In wheat it is loosely attached and removed during threshing; in rice it is firmly attached. High in fibre content and of limited use as animal feed.

hydrogenated oils Liquid oils hardened by *hydrogenation.

hydrogenation Conversion of liquid oils to semi-hard fats by the addition of hydrogen to the unsaturated double bonds; used for margarines and shortenings intended for bakery products. *See* fatty acids, unsaturated.

hydrogen-ion concentration A measure of the acidity or alkalinity of a solution by the concentration of hydrogen (H^+) ions present, usually expressed as *pH.

hydrogen peroxide Anti-microbial agent; can be used at 0.1% to preserve milk (Buddeized milk), but destroys vitamin C, methionine, and tryptophan. Not permitted in the UK. Formula H_2O_2, readily loses active oxygen, the effective sterilizing agent, forming water.

hydrogen swells *See* swells.

hydrolyse (hydrolysis) To split a complex compound into its constituent parts by the action of water, either enzymically or catalysed by the addition of acid or alkali. For example, sucrose is hydrolysed to glucose and fructose; proteins to amino acids; triacylglycerols to fatty acids and glycerol.

hydromel Reputedly the most popular beverage of the ancient world, prepared by mixing honey with water, sometimes flavoured with herbs and spices, and leaving it in the sun to ferment.

hydroponics The practice of growing plants without soil in a solution of inorganic salts.

hydrostatic sterilizer Continuous sterilizer in which the process is carried out under sufficient depth of water to maintain the required pressure. Used for continuous sterilization of canned foods on a large scale.

hydroxyapatite The calcium phosphate complex which is the main mineral of bones.

hydroxybenzoic acid esters *See* parabens.

hydroxycholecalciferol *See* vitamin D.

hydroxylysine Amino acid found only in *connective tissue proteins (collagen and elastin); incorporated into the protein as *lysine and then hydroxylated in a vitamin-C-dependent reaction.

hydroxyproline Amino acid mainly in *connective tissue proteins (collagen and elastin); incorporated into the protein as *proline and then hydroxylated in a vitamin-C-dependent reaction. Peptides of hydroxyproline are excreted in the urine and the output is increased when collagen turnover is high, as in rapid growth or resorption of tissue.

hydroxyproline index Urinary excretion of *hydroxyproline is reduced in children suffering *protein-energy malnutrition. The index is the ratio of urinary hydroxyproline to creatinine per kg of body weight, and is low in malnourished children.

5-hydroxytryptamine (5HT) Also called serotonin. A neurotransmitter amine synthesized from the *amino acid *tryptophan, also formed in blood platelets; it acts as a vasoconstrictor. Found in *plantains and some other foods, but metabolized in the intestinal mucosa.

hygroscopic Readily absorbing water, as when table salt becomes damp. Materials such as calcium chloride and silica gel absorb water so readily that they are used as drying agents.

hyper- Prefix meaning above the normal range, or abnormally high.

hyperalimentation Provision of unusually large amounts of energy, either intravenously (*parenteral nutrition) or by *nasogastric or *gastrostomy tube (*enteral nutrition).

hyperammonaemia High blood ammonia concentrations, especially after protein intake, leading to coma, convulsions, and possibly death. May be due to a variety of *genetic diseases affecting amino acid metabolism. Treatment is normally by severe restriction of protein intake. *See also* amino acid disorders.

hypercalcaemia, idiopathic Elevated plasma concentrations of calcium believed to be due to hypersensitivity of some children to *vitamin D toxicity. There is excessive absorption of calcium, with loss of appetite, vomiting, constipation, flabby muscles, and deposition of calcium in the soft tissues and kidneys. It can be fatal in infants.

hyperchlorhydria Excess secretion of hydrochloric acid in the stomach due to secretion of a greater volume of *gastric juice rather than to a higher concentration.

hypercholesterolaemia Abnormally high concentrations of *cholesterol in the blood. Generally considered to be a sign of high risk for *atherosclerosis and *ischaemic heart disease. Treatment is by

restriction of fat (especially *saturated fat) and cholesterol intake and a
high intake of non-starch polysaccharides, which increase the excretion
of cholesterol and its metabolites (the *bile salts) in the faeces. In
severe cases, *ion-exchange resins may be fed, to increase further the
excretion of bile salts, and drugs (*HMG CoA reductase inhibitors) may
be given to inhibit the synthesis of cholesterol in the body.

Familial hypercholesterolaemia is a *genetic disease in which
affected individuals have extremely high blood concentrations of
cholesterol, frequently dying from ischaemic heart disease in early
adulthood; treatment is as for other forms of hypercholesterolaemia,
but more rigorous. *See also* lipids, plasma.

hyperglycaemia High blood sugar; elevated plasma concentration of
*glucose concentration, caused by a failure of the normal hormonal
mechanisms of blood glucose control. *See also* diabetes mellitus; glucose
tolerance.

hyperlipidaemia (hyperlipoproteinaemia) A variety of conditions in
which there are increased concentrations of *lipids in plasma:
*phospholipids, *triglycerides, free and esterified *cholesterol, or
*unesterified fatty acids. Familial hyperlipidaemias are due to genetic
diseases; less severe hyperlipidaemia is commonly seen in people in
affluent developed countries, associated with increased risk of
*atherosclerosis and *ischaemic heart disease. *See also* lipids, plasma.

hyperlipoproteinaemia *See* hyperlipidaemia.

hyperoxaluria *Genetic disease leading to excessive formation of
*oxalic acid, which causes the formation of kidney stones. Treatment
includes a diet low in those fruits and vegetables that are sources of
oxalic acid and in some cases supplements of *vitamin B_6 some 50–100
times greater than reference intakes.

hypersalivation Excessive flow of *saliva.

hypertension High blood pressure; a risk factor for ischaemic disease,
stroke, and kidney disease. May be due to increased sensitivity to *salt
(correctly sensitivity to *sodium), and treated by restriction of salt
intake, together with drugs; increased intake of fruits and vegetables
(as a safe source of potassium) is recommended.

When the heart contracts (systolic pressure) the normal blood
pressure of females is 120 mm mercury at the age of 12 rising to 175
at 70. In males it is 120 rising to 160. When the heart relaxes (diastolic
pressure) the normal range for females is 70 rising to 95; males 70 to
85. Diastolic blood pressure above 105 is moderate, and above 115
severe, hypertension. *See also* 'salt-free' diet.

hyperthyroidism *See* thyrotoxicosis.

hypertonic A solution more concentrated than the body fluids;
see isotonic.

hypervitaminosis Overdosage with vitamins, leading to toxic effects. A
problem with high levels of intake of *vitamins A, D, B_6, and *niacin,
normally at levels of intake from supplements considerably higher
than might be obtained from foods, although hypervitaminosis A and
D may result from (enriched) foods. *See also* hypercalcaemia.

hypo- Prefix meaning below the normal range, or abnormally low.

hypocalcaemia Low blood *calcium, leading to vomiting and uncontrollable twitching of muscles if severe; may be due to underactivity of the parathyroid gland, kidney failure, or *vitamin D deficiency.

hypochlorhydria Partial deficiency of hydrochloric acid secretion in the *gastric juice. *See also* achlorhydria; anaemia, pernicious.

hypoglycaemia Abnormally low concentration of plasma glucose; may result in loss of consciousness, hypoglycaemic coma.

hypoglycaemic agents Drugs used to lower blood glucose concentrations in *diabetes mellitus.

hypokalaemia Abnormally low plasma potassium (Latin name *kalium*).

hypoproteinaemia Abnormally low total plasma protein concentration.

hyposite Little used word, from the Greek, for low-energy food.

hypothermia Low body temperature (normal is around 37 ˚C). Occurs among elderly people far more readily than in younger adults, often with fatal results. Also used in connection with deliberate reduction of body temperature to 28 ˚C to permit heart and brain surgery.

hypothyroidism Underactivity of the thyroid gland, leading to reduced secretion of *thyroid hormones and a reduction in *basal metabolic rate. Commonly associated with *goitre due to *iodine deficiency. In hypothyroid adults there is a characteristic moon-faced appearance, lethargy, and mental apathy. In infants, hypothyroidism can lead to severe mental retardation, *cretinism. *See also* thyrotoxicosis.

hypotonic A solution more dilute than the body fluids, *see* isotonic.

hypovitaminosis *Vitamin deficiency.

hypoxanthine A *purine, an intermediate in the metabolism of *adenine and *guanine to *uric acid.

hyssop Pungent aromatic herb, *Hyssopus officinialis*, used in salads, soups, and in making liqueurs.

iatrogenic A condition caused by medical intervention or drug treatment; iatrogenic nutrient deficiency is due to *drug-nutrient interactions.

Iberian moss *See* carrageenan.

iceberg lettuce Pale green variety of *lettuce with a crisp texture.

ice cream A frozen confection made from fat, milk solids, and sugar. Some European countries permit the use of non-milk fat and term the product ice cream, while if milk fat is used, it is termed dairy ice cream.

    According to UK regulations, contains not less than 5% fat and 7% other milk solids; according to US regulations, 10% milk fat and 20% other milk solids. Stabilizers such as carboxy methylcellulose, *gums, and alginates are included, and emulsifiers such as polysorbate and monoglycerides. Mono- and diglycerides bind the looser globules of water and are added in 'non-drip' ice cream.

    A 60-g portion of dairy ice cream is a *source of calcium and vitamin B_2; contains 6 g of fat of which 70% is saturated and 25% mono-unsaturated; supplies 115 kcal (480 kJ). A 60-g portion of non-dairy ice cream is similar, but the fat is about 50% saturated and 40% mono-unsaturated.

ice cream, Philadelphia Made from scalded cream, with no added thickening agents.

Iceland moss A lichen, *Cetraria islandica*, that can be boiled to make a jelly.

ice lolly (ice lollipop) A frozen ice cream or water-ice on a stick; known in the USA as a popsicle.

ice wine *See* Eiswein.

ichthyosarcotoxins Toxins in fish.

icing *See* frosting.

icing, royal Hard icing (*frosting) made from egg-white and icing sugar, and used to coat cakes that are to be decorated and kept for some time.

icing sugar *See* sugar.

IDDM Insulin-dependent *diabetes mellitus.

idli South-East Asian; small cakes made from a mixture of cooked rice and black gram, fermented with the aid of mould.

IHD Ischaemic heart disease, *see* heart disease.

ileitis Inflammation of the ileum. *See* gastro-intestinal tract.

ileostomy Surgical formation of an opening of the ileum on the abdominal wall, performed to treat severe ulcerative *colitis; *see* gastro-intestinal tract.

ileum Last portion of the small intestine, between the jejunum and the colon (large intestine); *see* gastro-intestinal tract.

ileus Obstruction of the intestines; *see* gastro-intestinal tract.

illipé butter *See* vegetable butters.

imam bayildi Turkish, Greek; dish of aubergines baked with olive oil, onions, tomatoes, and garlic; may be served hot or cold. There are two versions of the origin of the name, which means the 'imam (or priest) fainted': either he swooned in ecstasy when he tasted the dish or he fainted from fright at the cost of the large amount of olive oil used to prepare it.

imli Indian; sauce made from *tamarind.

immune system Series of defence mechanisms of the body. There are two major parts: humoral, mediated through antibodies secreted into the circulation (*immunoglobulins); and cell-mediated. *Lymphocytes produce antibodies against, and bind to, the antigens of foreign cells, leading to death of the invading organisms; other white blood cells are phagocytic and engulf the invading organisms.

immunoglobulins Specific antibodies produced in the blood in response to foreign proteins or other *antigens. Five classes, IgA, IgE, IgG, IgM, and IgI; present in circulating blood as a result of previous exposure to the antigens, and also present in breast milk to confer some (passive) immunity on the baby.

IMP 1 *Integrating motor pneumotachograph.
2 Inosine monophosphate, one of the *purine nucleotides.

impériale, à l' Dishes with a rich garnish of foie gras, truffles, cocks' combs, and kidneys.

imperial rolls *See* spring rolls.

improvers, flour *See* ageing.

inanition Exhaustion and wasting due to complete lack or non-assimilation of food; a state of starvation.

inborn errors of metabolism *See* genetic disease.

Incaparina A number of protein-rich dietary supplements developed by the Institute of Nutrition of Central America and Panama (INCAP), based on cottonseed flour, or soya and vegetables, with various nutrient supplements. All versions contain 27.5% protein.

index of nutritional quality (INQ) An attempt to provide an overall figure for the nutrient content of a food or a diet. It is the ratio between the percentage of the *reference intake of each nutrient and the percentage of the average requirement for energy provided by the food.

Indian corn *See* maize.

Indian fig *See* prickly pear.

Indian rice grass Perennial, growing wild in the USA, *Oryzopsis hymenoides*; tolerant to drought. The seeds, which resemble *millet, are small, round, and dark in colour, covered with white hairs.

Traditionally used by native Americans for flour, now used almost exclusively for forage.

Indian tonic water *See* tonic water.

indicação de proveniencia regulamentada (IPR) *See* wine classification, Portugal.

indigestion Discomfort and distension of the stomach after a meal, also known as dyspepsia, including *heartburn. Persistent indigestion may be a symptom of a digestive disorder such as *hiatus hernia or peptic *ulcer.

indigo carmine Blue food colour (E-132), derivative of indigotin, which comes from tropical leguminous plants *Indigofera* spp.

induction period The lag period during which a fat or oil shows stability to oxidation because of its content of *antioxidants, natural or added, which are oxidized preferentially. After this there is a sudden and large consumption of oxygen and the fat becomes rancid.

infant formula Modified milk products or milk substitutes for feeding infants in place of breast feeding. The nutritional composition is adjusted to approximate to that of breast milk, and is controlled by legal standards.

Special formula preparations are available for premature babies and those of very *low birth weight.

For infants intolerant of cow's milk, there are special formula preparations based on soya bean or other products. For those with *genetic diseases a range of special formulae are available.

infuse (infusion) To extract the flavour from herbs, spices, etc., by steeping them in a liquid, usually by pouring boiling liquid over them, covering them and leaving them to stand without further cooking or heating, as in making tea.

ingredient Any substance used in the manufacture or preparation of a foodstuff and still present in the finished product, even if in an altered form. Contaminants and adulterants are not considered to be ingredients.

inorganic Materials of *mineral, as distinct from animal or vegetable, origin. Apart from carbonates and cyanides, inorganic chemicals are those that contain no carbon.

inositol A carbohydrate derivative which is an essential nutrient for micro-organisms and many animals and sometimes classified as a vitamin, although there is no evidence that it is a dietary essential for human beings. Deficiency causes alopecia in mice and 'spectacle eye' (denudation around the eye) in rats. Obsolete names are inosite and meat sugar.

Chemically hexahydroxyclohexane $(CHOH)_6$; there are nine isomers, but only one, meso- or myo-inositol, is of physiological importance. It is a constituent of many *phospholipids (phosphatidyl inositols) involved in membrane structure and as part of the signalling mechanism for *hormones which act at the cell surface.

The insecticide gammexane is hexachlorocyclohexane, and appears to function by competing with inositol. The hexaphosphate ester of inositol is *phytic acid.

INQ *See* index of nutritional quality.

instant foods Dried foods that reconstitute rapidly when water is added, e.g. tea, coffee, milk, soups, precooked cereal products, potatoes, etc. The dried powders may be agglomerated to control particle size and improve solubility. 'Instant puddings' are formulated with pregelatinized starch and disperse rapidly in cold milk. (Instant coffee was first prepared in 1906 by an Englishman, G. Washington, living in Guatemala, and was marketed in 1909.)

insulin *Hormone secreted by the β-cells of the *pancreas which controls *carbohydrate metabolism. *Diabetes mellitus is the result of an inadequate supply of insulin or failure of its function. Since insulin is a protein it would be digested if taken by mouth so must be injected. Originally the hormone was prepared from beef or pork pancreas, but these differ slightly in structure from human insulin, and can lead to antibody formation after prolonged use. Most insulin for therapeutic use is now human insulin, the product of biosynthesis from the human insulin gene. *See also* diabetes mellitus; diet, diabetic; glucose tolerance.

integrating motor pneumotachograph (IMP) Apparatus for measuring *energy expenditure indirectly from oxygen consumption. It meters the expired air and removes a proportion for analysis. *See also* spirometer.

interesterification Fats are mixtures of *triacylglycerols consisting of various *fatty acids esterified with *glycerol. Interesterification is the result of heat treatment that causes an exchange of some of the fatty acids between the glycerol molecules and alters the properties of the fat. *Lard, for example, is not a good creaming agent for baked products until it has been so treated.

intermediate hydrogen carrier Most oxidation reactions in *metabolism involve the loss of hydrogen, which is transferred onto a *coenzyme, commonly derived from either *niacin or *vitamin B_2. The coenzyme is an intermediate hydrogen acceptor, and is reoxidized by transfer of the hydrogen to another substrate, or to oxygen, forming water.

intermediate moisture foods These are semi-moist with about 25% (15–50%) moisture but with some of the water bound (and so unavailable to *micro-organisms) by the addition of glycerol, sorbitol, salt, or certain organic acids, so preventing the growth of micro-organisms.

international units (iu) Used as a measure of comparative potency of natural substances, such as vitamins, before they were obtained in a sufficiently pure form to measure by weight. Still sometimes used (3.33 iu *vitamin A = 1 μg; 40 iu *vitamin D = 1 μg; 1 iu *vitamin E = 1 mg).

intestinal juice Also called succus entericus. Digestive juice secreted by the intestinal glands lining the small intestine. It contains a variety of *enzymes, including *enteropeptidase, the enzyme that converts trypsinogen to active *trypsin, *aminopeptidase, nucleases, and nucleotidases. *See also* gastro-intestinal tract.

intestine The *gastro-intestinal tract; more specifically the part after the stomach, i.e. the small intestine (duodenum, jejunum, and ileum) where the greater part of digestion and absorption take place, and the large intestine where water is absorbed.

intolerance (to foods) *See* adverse reactions to foods.

intravenous nutrition *See* parenteral nutrition.

intrinsic factor A protein secreted in the gastric juice which is required for the absorption of *vitamin B_{12}; impaired secretion results in *pernicious anaemia.

inulin Soluble but undigested polymer of *fructose found particularly in Jerusalem *artichoke, and, to a lesser extent, other root vegetables. Included with *non-starch polysaccharides (*dietary fibre). Also called dahlin and alant starch.

inversion Applied to *sucrose, means its hydrolysis to glucose and fructose (*invert sugar).

invertase Enzyme that splits *sucrose into glucose and fructose (*invert sugar); also called sucrase and saccharase.

invert sugar The mixture of glucose and fructose produced by hydrolysis of sucrose, 1.3 times sweeter than sucrose. So called because the *optical activity is reversed in the process. It is important in the manufacture of sugar confectionery, and especially *boiled sweets, since the presence of 10–15% invert sugar prevents the crystallization of sucrose.

in vitro Literally 'in glass'; used to indicate an observation made experimentally in the test-tube, as distinct from the natural living conditions, *in vivo.

in vivo In the living state, as distinct from *in vitro.

iodide A salt of the mineral *iodine.

iodine An essential mineral, a *trace element; the reference intake is about 140 µg per day. Iodine is required for synthesis of the *thyroid hormones, which are iodo-tyrosine derivatives. A prolonged deficiency of iodine in the diet leads to *goitre.

Iodine is plentifully supplied by sea foods and by vegetables grown in soil containing iodide. In areas where the soil is deficient in iodide, locally grown vegetables are also iodide deficient, and hence goitre occurs in defined geographical regions, especially inland upland areas over limestone soil. Where deficiency is a problem, salt may be *iodized to increase iodide intake.

iodine number (iodine value) Carbon-carbon double bonds in *unsaturated compounds can react with iodine; this provides a means of determining the degree of unsaturation of a fat or other compound by the uptake of iodine. *Drying oils (e.g. linseed oil) are highly unsaturated and have high iodine numbers. *See also* fatty acids, unsaturated.

iodine, protein-bound *See* thyroglobulin.

iodized salt Usually 1 part of iodide in 25,000–50,000 parts of salt, as a means of ensuring adequate *iodine intake in regions where deficiency is a problem.

ion An atom or group of atoms that has lost or gained one or more electrons, and thus has an electric charge. Positively charged ions are known as cations, because they migrate towards the cathode (negative pole) in solution, while negatively charged ions migrate towards the positive pole (anode) and hence are known as anions.

ion-exchange resin An organic compound that will adsorb ions under some conditions and release them under other conditions. The best-known example is in water-softening, where calcium ions are removed from the water by binding to the resin, displacing sodium ions. The resin is then regenerated by washing with a concentrated solution of salt, when the sodium ions displace the calcium ions. Ion-exchange resins are used for purification of chemicals, metal recovery, a variety of analytical techniques, and treatment of *hypercholesterolaemia.

ionization The process whereby the positive and negative *ions of a salt or other compound separate when dissolved in water. The degree of ionization of an *acid or *alkali determines its strength (*see* pH).

ionizing radiation Electromagnetic radiation that ionizes the air or water through which it passes, e.g. X-rays and γ-rays. Used for the sterilization of food, etc., by *irradiation.

IPR Indicação de proveniencia regulamentada, *see* wine classification, Portugal.

Irish cream Liqueurs prepared from Irish whiskey blended with other spirits and cream, sweetened, and sometimes flavoured with coffee or chocolate.

Irish moss A red seaweed, *Chondrus crispus*; source of the polysaccharide *carrageenan.

Irish stew *See* stew.

Irish whiskey *See* whisky.

iron An essential *mineral. The average adult has 4–5 g of iron, of which 60–70% is present in the blood as haem in the circulating *haemoglobin, and the remainder present in *myoglobin in muscles, a variety of enzymes, and tissue stores. Iron is stored in the liver as ferritin, in other tissues as haemosiderin, and as the blood transport protein transferrin.

   Iron balance: losses in faeces 0.3–0.5 mg per day, in sweat and skin cells 0.5 mg, traces in hair and urine, total loss 0.5–1.5 mg per day. Blood loss leads to a considerable loss of iron. The average diet contains 10–15 mg, of which 0.5–1.5 mg is absorbed. The haem iron of meat and fish is considerably better absorbed than the inorganic iron of vegetable foods. Reference intakes are 8.7 mg for adult men and 14.8 mg for women; women who have heavy menstrual blood losses may not be able to obtain enough from food, and supplements are necessary.

Absorption of iron is aided by *vitamin C taken at the same time as iron-containing foods, and reduced by phosphate and *phytic acid. Iron content of foods per 100 g: liver 6–14 mg, cereals up to 9 mg, nuts 1–5 mg, eggs 2–3 mg, meat 2–4 mg. Iron is added to flour so that it contains not less than 1.65 mg per 100 g. Fortified cereals provide 35% of the iron of British diets. Prolonged deficiency gives rise to *anaemia.

iron ammonium citrate *See* ferric ammonium citrate.

iron, reduced Metallic iron in finely divided form, produced by reduction of iron oxide. The form in which iron is sometimes added to foods, such as bread. Also known by its Latin name *ferrum redactum.*

iron storage Ferritin is the iron storage protein in the intestinal mucosa, liver, spleen, and bone marrow. It is a ferric hydroxide-phosphate-protein complex containing 23% iron. Haemosiderin is a long-term reserve (storage form) of iron in tissues; colloidal iron hydroxide combined with protein and phosphate, probably formed by agglomeration of *ferritin, the short-term storage form. Abnormally high levels of haemosiderin occur in *siderosis.

iron transport Iron is transported in blood plasma in combination with proteins, as transferrin or siderophilin.

irradiation *Ionizing radiation (X-rays or γ-rays from radioactive isotopes or the linear accelerator) kills micro-organisms and insects, and also inhibits sprouting of potatoes. *See also* microwave cooking; ultraviolet radiation.

irritable bowel syndrome Also known as spastic colon or mucous colitis. Abnormally increased motility of the large and small intestines, leading to pain and alternating diarrhoea and constipation; often precipitated by emotional stress.

ischaemic heart disease Or coronary heart disease. Group of syndromes arising from failure of the coronary arteries to supply sufficient blood to heart muscles; associated with *atherosclerosis of coronary arteries.

isinglass *Gelatine prepared from the swim bladder of fish (especially sturgeon). Used commercially to clear wine and beer, and sometimes in jellies and ice cream. Japanese isinglass is *agar.

islets of Langerhans The *endocrine parts of the *pancreas; *glucagon is secreted by the α-cells and *insulin by the β-cells of the islets.

isoascorbic acid *See* erythorbic acid.

isodesmosine *See* desmosines.

isoenzymes Enzymes that have the same catalytic activity, but different structures, properties, and/or tissue distribution.

isoflavones *See* flavonoids.

isoleucine An essential *amino acid, rarely limiting in food. It is one of the branched-chain amino acids, together with leucine and valine.

isomalt A bulk *sweetener, about half as sweet as sucrose, consisting of a mixture of two disaccharides, glucose-glucitol and glucose-mannitol. It is about 50% metabolized, yielding 9 kJ (2.4 kcal)/gram. It is thought to be less laxative than *sorbitol or *mannitol, and does not encourage tooth decay, so is used in *tooth-friendly sweets.

isomaltose A disaccharide composed of two glucose units, differing from *maltose only in the way in which the two glucose units are linked; unlike maltose it is not fermentable. Also known as brachyose.

Isomerose Trade name of high-fructose corn syrup: 70–72% solids, 42% fructose, 55% glucose, 3% polysaccharides. *See* fructose syrups.

isomers Molecules containing the same atoms but differently arranged, so that the chemical and biochemical properties differ. (1) In positional isomers the functional groups are on different carbon atoms; e.g. leucine and isoleucine, citric and isocitric acids. (2) D- and L-isomerism refers to the spatial arrangement of four different chemical groups on the same carbon atom (stereo-isomerism or optical isomerism). *R*- and *S*-isomerism is the same, but determined by a set of systematic chemical rules. *See* D-. (3) Cis- and trans-isomerism refers to the arrangement of groups adjacent to a carbon-carbon double bond; in the cis-isomer the groups are on the same side of the double bond, while on the trans-isomer they are on opposite sides.

isosyrups *See* fructose syrups.

isotonic Solutions with the same *osmotic pressure (concentration of solids); often refers to a solution with the same osmotic pressure as body fluids. Hypertonic and hypotonic refer to solutions that are more and less concentrated.

isotopes Forms of elements with the same chemical properties, differing in atomic mass because of differing numbers of neutrons in the atomic nucleus. Thus, hydrogen has three isotopes, of atomic masses 1, 2, and 3, generally written as ^1H, ^2H (deuterium), and ^3H (tritium). ^1H is the most abundant isotope of hydrogen; ^2H is stable, while ^3H is radioactive.

The incorporation of isotopes into compounds (labelled compounds or tracers) permits the metabolic fates of those compounds in the body to be followed easily.

isotopes, radioactive Some *isotopes are unstable, and decay to stable elements, emitting radiation in the process. This may be α-radiation, β-radiation (electrons), γ-radiation, or X-rays, depending on the particular isotope. Radioactive isotopes can readily be detected by the radiation emitted. The time taken for half the radioactive isotope to decay is the *half-life of the isotope, and can vary from a fraction of a second, through several days to years (e.g. the half-life of ^3H is $12^1/2$ years, that of ^{14}C is 5200 years).

isotopes, stable Some isotopes are stable, and can be detected only by their different atomic mass. Since they emit no radiation, they are considered completely safe for use in labelled compounds given to human beings. Examples of stable isotopes commonly used in nutrition research include ^2H, ^{13}C, ^{15}N, and ^{18}O.

isozymes *See* isoenzymes.

itai-itai disease *See* cadmium.

italienne, à l' Dishes made partly or wholly of pasta, often with cheese and tomato.

iu *See* international units.

izarra A herb-flavoured liqueur based on *armagnac, made in the Basque region of France; similar to chartreuse.

J

JACNE Joint Advisory Committee on Nutrition Education A UK working party that put nutritional guidelines into popular language. *See* nutritional recommendations.

Jägermeister German bitter-sweet herb liqueur.

jaggery 1 Coarse, dark sugar made from the sap of the coconut palm. **2** Raw sugar-cane juice, used in India as sweetening agent; also known as gur.

jaguar gum *See* guar gum.

jaiphal *See* mace.

jake paralysis *See* Jamaica ginger paralysis.

jak fruit (jack fruit) Large fruit, up to 30 kg, from tropical trees of *Artocarpus* species, related to breadfruit. Both pulp and seeds are eaten. A 100-g portion is a *source of vitamin C; supplies 70 kcal (295 kJ).

jam A conserve of fruit boiled to a pulp with sugar; sets to a *pectin jelly on cooling. (Known in the USA as jelly.) Standard jam, with certain exceptions, contains a minimum of 35 g of fruit per 100 g; extra jam, with certain exceptions, contains 45 g.

Jamaica ginger paralysis Polyneuritis caused by poisoning from an extract of Jamaica ginger ('jake', a variety of ginger grown in Jamaica) due to triorthocresyl phosphate.

Jamaican pepper *See* allspice.

jambalaya Southern USA; rice with pork, chicken, and/or shellfish, simmered with celery, peppers, and tomatoes.

jamón serrano Spanish; dry mountain *ham.

Japanese isinglass *See* agar.

jardinière, à la Dish prepared or served with a variety of vegetables.

jarmuz Polish; quartered white cabbage, stewed in stock, mixed with soured cream, and garnished with braised chestnuts.

jasmine tea A perfumed or scented tea made by adding petals of jasmine flowers to Chinese tea; not a *herb tea or tisane.

javatri Indian name for *nutmeg.

jejunostomy feeding *See* enteral nutrition.

jejunum Part of the small intestine, between the duodenum and the ileum; *see* gastro-intestinal tract.

jelabi Indian sweet; deep-fried spirals of dough served with syrup.

jello North American name for table *jelly.

jelly 1 Clear jam made from strained fruit juice by boiling with sugar. Also used in this sense in North America to mean any jam.

2 Table jelly is a dessert made from gelatine, sweetened and flavoured; known in North America as jello.

3 Savoury jelly made from calf's foot or gelatinous stock; *see* aspic.

jelly roll *See* Swiss roll.

jerked beef South American dried meat similar to *biltong; *see also* charqui.

jerky Jerked (dried) meat; *see* biltong; charqui.

Jesuit's bark Cinchona bark, source of quinine.

jésus French, Swiss; sausage made from pig's liver.

Jew's apple *See* aubergine.

jigger Measuring cup used by bar staff for spirits, etc., when the bottles do not have a dispenser fitted.

Job's tears *See* adlay.

jodbasedow *See* thyrotoxicosis.

jojoba oil Liquid wax of long-chain *fatty acids (eicosenoic and docosenoic (erucic) acids) esterified with long-chain alcohols (eicosanol and docosanol) from seeds of the shrub *Simmondsia chinensis*. Of interest in cosmetics as a replacement for sperm whale oil but also has food applications, e.g. coating agent for *dried fruits.

jonathan Calcined, ground oat chaff used as adulterant for maize and other cereals (mid-nineteenth century).

jonge Young Dutch *gin.

Joule The SI (Système Internationale) unit of *energy; used to express energy content of foods and energy expenditure of man and animals. Gradually adopted as a replacement for the *calorie from about 1970; 4.2 kilojoules (kJ) is equivalent to 1 kilocalorie (kcal).

jovennuevo Spanish; young wines.

jowar Indian name for *sorghum (*Sorghum vulgare*), also known as great millet, kaffir corn, guinea corn.

Judas goat Sheep cannot readily be driven to slaughter but will follow a goat. A Judas goat is used to lead the sheep to the killing pens.

jugged Food (especially hare) cooked in earthenware pot or jug.

jug-jug Caribbean (Barbadian); minced meat and pigeon peas cooked with *millet, served as an accompaniment to ham or roast chicken.

jujube 1 Sweet made from gum and sugar.

2 Shrub (*Ziziphus mauritania* or *Z. jujuba*), important fruit crop in India; the fruit is reddish-brown, up to 2 cm in diameter, with a single stone; a 100-g portion is a good *source of vitamin C.

julep Whisky or brandy flavoured with mint and served over ice.

julienne 1 Vegetables cut into thin, match-like strips.

2 A clear vegetable soup.

jumble Small rich biscuit flavoured with lemon or almond, formed into a letter S, or into tiny, rock-like heaps.

juniper The ripened berries of the bush *Juniperis communis*, used as a flavouring in *gin, and, together with other herbs, in stuffing or sauces, especially for *game.

junket Dessert made from milk by treating with *rennet to curdle the protein.

jus, au Dish served with the natural juices or gravy.

K

kabinett German and Austrian *wine classification, used for high-quality wines. In earlier years monastic wine producers used to set aside their best wine in a special cupboard or small room (the *kabinett*).

kabuní Albanian; rice sautéed in butter and stock with raisins, served with chicken or meat.

kaccavia Greek fish soup with tomatoes, vegetables, and garlic; the origin of *bouillabaisse. The name is derived from the *kakavia*, the earthenware pot in which fishermen cooked their fish in the middle of the boat.

kaffir beer See pombé.

kaffir corn See sorghum.

kaffir manna corn See millet.

kahlúa Mexican; coffee-flavoured liqueur.

kakdi See cucumber.

kaki See persimmon.

kale Scottish name for any type of cabbage; in England it means specifically open-headed varieties of cabbage with curly leaves, also known as curly kale or borecole. Distinct from sea kale or *Swiss chard.

kalia Polish; chicken broth flavoured with juice from pickled cucumbers and garnished with diced chicken, celery root, parsley root, and carrots.

kalonji Indian; wild black onion seeds (*Nigella indica*), used as a spice.

kalteszal Polish; soup made from egg yolk, sugar, cinnamon, and beer, served cold.

kamaboko Japanese; fish paste made from *surimi, sometimes with added starch.

kaoliang A drink made from the Chinese *sorghum, *Sorghum nervosum*; also used for the grain itself.

karaya gum Obtained from East Indian trees of the genus *Sterculia*. Used as a stabilizer, e.g. in frozen water ices; also used in combination with other stabilizers; sometimes used as a laxative. Also called sterculia gum.

kari phulia See nim.

Karo Syrup Trade name for a dextromaltose preparation made from maize starch, used as carbohydrate modifier in milk preparations for infant feeding. Consists of a mixture of dextrin, maltose, glucose, and sucrose.

kasha See buckwheat.

katadyn process See oligodynamic.

kataifi Greek; pastry in thin strands; the dough is squeezed through a perforated disc onto a hot metal plate, on which it is dried in long strands. Also the name for rolls made from these pastry strands, filled with chopped nuts and sugar, baked and served drenched with syrup.

katemfe The Sierra Leone name for an intensely sweet African fruit, *Thaumatococcus daniellii*; also known as the miraculous fruit of Sudan (not the same as *miracle berry). The active principle is a protein named *thaumatin.

kathepsins *See* cathepsins.

kcal Abbreviation for kilocalorie (1000 *calories), sometimes shown as Cal. *See also* Appendix I.

kebab Turkish for roast meat. Shishkebab is small pieces of mutton rubbed with salt, pepper, etc., and roasted on a skewer (*shish* in Turkish) sometimes interspaced with vegetables. Shashlik is a Georgian version.

   *Döner kebab is a Turkish speciality consisting of marinated mutton or lamb packed into a cylindrical mass and grilled on a vertical rotating spit (*shawarma* in Arabic).

kebobs Indian; slices of mutton or poultry dipped in egg and cooked on a skewer.

kedgeree Indian; dish of rice and pulses. Modified to Victorian breakfast dish of flaked fish with egg and rice.

kefir *See* milk, fermented.

keftethes Greek; minced meat rissoles.

keliweli (kellywelly) Ghanaian; spiced deep-fried banana or plantain.

Kellogg's Special K Trade name for an enriched breakfast cereal. A 40-g portion is a rich *source of vitamins B_1, B_2, niacin, B_6, B_{12}, folate, and iron; a source of protein and vitamin D; contains 1.2 g of dietary fibre; provides 150 kcal (630 kJ).

kelp Large brown seaweeds of the genus *Laminaria*. Occasionally used as food or food ingredient but mostly the ash is used as a source of alkali and iodine. Sometimes claimed as a *health food with unspecified properties.

kephalins Or cephalins; *phospholipids containing ethanolamine, hence *phosphatidylethanolamines. Found especially in brain and nerve tissue.

Kepler extract of malt Trade name for one of the earliest of the *malt extracts, intended as a dietary supplement and to aid the digestion, since it was rich in *diastase compared with ordinary malt extracts.

keratin The insoluble protein of hair, horn, hoofs, feathers, and nails. Not hydrolysed by digestive enzymes, and therefore nutritionally useless. Used as fertilizer, since it is slowly broken down by soil bacteria. Steamed feather meal is used to some extent as a supplement for ruminants.

kesari dhal A legume, *Lathyris sativus*; *see also* lathyrism.

Keshan disease *See* selenium.

keshy yena Caribbean; baked Edam or Gouda cheese with a variety of fillings. The name derives from the Spanish *queso relleno*, stuffed cheese.

Kesp Trade name for a textured vegetable protein product made by the spinning process.

ketchup (catsup or catchup) From the Chinese koechap or kitsiap, originally meaning brine of pickled fish. Now used for spicy sauce or condiment made with juice of fruit or vegetables, vinegar, and spices. Tomato ketchup is a common *sauce.

ketogenic amino acids *See* amino acids, ketogenic.

ketogenic diet A diet poor in carbohydrate (20–30 g) and rich in fat; causes accumulation of *ketone bodies in tissue; formerly used in the treatment of epilepsy.

ketonaemia High concentrations of *ketone bodies in the blood.

ketone bodies Acetoacetate, β-hydroxybutyrate and acetone; acetoacetate and acetone are chemically *ketones; although β-hydroxybutyrate is not, it is included in the term ketone bodies because of its metabolic relationship with acetoacetate.

In the fasting state (from about 4 hours after a meal), fatty acids are mobilized from adipose tissue as a metabolic fuel. Most tissues have only a limited capacity for fatty acid oxidation; however, the liver can oxidize more than is required for its own metabolic needs. Acetoacetate and β-hydroxybutyrate are formed from fatty acids in the liver, and are transported in the bloodstream for use as metabolic fuels by other tissues. Acetoacetate is chemically unstable and breaks down to *acetone, which is metabolically useless, and is excreted in the urine and on the breath.

ketones Chemical compounds containing a carbonyl group (C=O), with two alkyl groups attached to the same carbon; the simplest ketone is *acetone (dimethylketone, $(CH_3)_2$-C=O).

ketonic rancidity Certain moulds of the genera *Penicillium* and *Aspergillus* species attack fats containing short-chain fatty acids and produce *ketones with a characteristic odour and taste, so-called ketonic rancidity. Fats such as butter, coconut, and palm kernel are most susceptible.

Ketonil Trade name for protein-rich food low in *phenylalanine for feeding patients with *phenylketonuria.

ketonuria Excretion of *ketone bodies in the urine.

ketosis High concentrations of *ketone bodies in the blood.

khatta *See* clay.

kheer Or sheer, Indian creamed-rice dessert.

khira *See* cucumber.

khuri *See* clay.

khus-khus *See* poppy seed.

khush-khash *See* orange, bitter.

kibble To grind or chop coarsely.

kichals Middle-European (especially Jewish); spherical biscuits made from beaten egg, caster sugar, and self-raising flour.

kid Young goat (*Capra aegragus*) usually under 3 months old; similar to *lamb, but with a stronger flavour.

kidney (French: *rognon*; German: *Niere*.) Usually from lamb, ox, or pig; a 150-g portion is a rich *source of protein, niacin, iron, zinc, copper, selenium, vitamins A, B_1, B_2, B_{12}, and folate; a good source of vitamin B_6 and, unusually for a meat product, vitamin C; a source of iodine; contains about 9 g of fat of which one-third is saturated; supplies 150 kcal (630 kJ).

kidney failure *See* renal failure.

kieves Irish name for *mash tuns.

kilderkin Cask for beer (18 gallons = 80.1 L) and ale (16 gallons = 71.2 L).

kilo As a prefix for units of measurement, one thousand times (i.e. 10^3); symbol k. *See* Appendix I.

kimchi Korean; dish based on fermented cabbage with garlic, red peppers, and pimientos often with the addition of fish and other foods. Nutritional value depends on the ingredients but all preparations are good *sources of vitamin C.

king, à la Dish served in a rich cream sauce (often flavoured with sherry) and including mushrooms and green peppers.

kipper *Herring that has been lightly salted and smoked, by a process invented by John Woodger, a fish curer of Seahouses, Northumberland, in 1843. A 150-g portion of flesh (about 300 g including bones and skin) is an exceptionally rich *source of vitamins B_{12} and D, a rich source of protein, niacin, and iodine; a source of vitamin B_2, iron, and calcium; contains 1500 mg of sodium and 18 g of fat, of which about 20% is saturated and 60% mono-unsaturated; supplies 300 kcal (1260 kJ).

kir *See* cassis.

kirsch (kirschwasser) Brandy or *eau-de-vie distilled from fermented cherries, including the crushed stones, giving a pungent flavour; not sweet.

kitron Greek liqueur prepared by distillation of brandy with lemon leaves; sweetened.

kiwano The horned melon, a New Zealand fruit with a spiky yellow skin and green flesh.

kiwi Fruit of *Actinidia sinensis*, originally a native of China and also known as Chinese gooseberry. A 60-g portion (one fruit) is a rich *source of vitamin C; supplies 25 kcal (105 kJ).

kizel Russian, Baltic; cold dessert made from red fruit juice thickened with cornflour or arrowroot. Polish kiziel is similar.

Kjeldahl determination Widely used method of determining total nitrogen in a substance by digesting with sulphuric acid and a catalyst;

the nitrogen is reduced to ammonia which is then measured. In foodstuffs most of the nitrogen is *protein, and the term crude protein is the total 'Kjeldahl nitrogen' multiplied by a factor of 6.25 (since most proteins contain 16% nitrogen).

kleftiko Greek; clay oven. Also a joint of lamb baked in a clay oven. Originally a method of cooking meat in the embers of a fire in a pit in the ground.

kleik Polish; gruel made from barley and bouillon.

Klim Trade name for dried milk.

klipfish Salted and dried cod, mainly produced in Norway. The fish is boned, stored in salt for a month, washed, and dried slowly. It is known as bacalao in South America and Spain, bacalhau in Portugal.

kluski Polish; light dumplings or strips of noodles, used to garnish soups.

kneading Working dough by stretching and folding until it achieves the required consistency.

kneidl See knödeln.

knickerbocker glory Dessert made from layers of jelly of different colours, ice cream, and fruit, topped with whipped cream and served in a tall glass (a sundae glass).

knödeln, kneidl German; dumplings made from flour or *matzo meal; served like pasta or in soup. Nockerln are smaller; butternockerln are made with butter; lebernockerln contain finely chopped fried liver.

knuckle of veal Lower part of the leg of the calf furthest from the fillet or shoulder. See veal.

köche German; light steamed or baked pudding.

kofta Indian; spiced meat balls. Kofta may also be moulded over sweet-sour plums, minced dried apricots, and herbs or eggs (these latter are known as nargizi or narcissus).

kohlrabi (French: *chou-rave*.) Swollen stem of *Brassica oleracea gongylodes* (turnip-rooted cabbage, kale turnip (USA)); there are green and purple varieties. A 50-g portion is a rich *source of vitamin C and supplies 10 kcal (40 kJ).

koji See miso.

kokoh In the Zen *macrobiotic diet this is a mixture of ground seeds and cereals fed to young infants; it is deficient in a number of nutrients and can result in growth retardation unless supplemented.

kokoretsi Highly seasoned Greek *sausage made from lamb offal (heart, liver, kidneys, sweetbread) with the intestine wound around the coarsely chopped meat, skewered and grilled slowly.

komishbrot See mandelbrot.

konjac *Gum derived from tubers of *Amorphophallus konjac*; eaten in Japan as a firm jelly.

korma Indian; meat or vegetables braised with water, stock, yoghurt, or cream.

korn German spirit prepared by distillation of fermented maize, sometimes flavoured with juniper. Generally has a relatively low alcohol content; doppelkorn is 38% alcohol.

kosher The selection and preparation of foods in accordance with traditional Jewish ritual and dietary laws. Foods that are not kosher are traife.

The only kosher flesh foods are from animals that chew the cud and have cloven hoofs, such as cattle, sheep, goats, and deer; the hindquarters must not be eaten. The only fish permitted are those with fins and scales; birds of prey and scavengers are not kosher. Moreover, the animals must be slaughtered according to ritual before the meat can be considered kosher. From Hebrew *kosher*, right (Deut. 14: 3–21).

kosher for Passover *See* Passover.

koulouria Greek; sweet bread baked in a large ring, flavoured with sesame seeds.

koumiss *See* milk, fermented.

kourabiethes Greek; shortbread traditionally baked for Christmas and New Year.

kraftbruehe Austrian; soup made from minced beef, carrot, onion, leek, and Hamburg parsley root, cooked in consommé.

krapiva Russian; nettle soup.

kräuterbutter German; butter mixed with chopped herbs.

kreatopita Greek pie made with three kinds of meat (usually lamb, goat or kid, and chicken), together with cheese, onions, tomatoes, and raisins, with a pastry top.

Krebs' cycle Or citric acid cycle, a central pathway for the *metabolism of fats, carbohydrates, and proteins. Named for Sir Hans Krebs, who first described the pathway.

kreplach Jewish; *pasta envelopes filled with minced meat (similar to *ravioli) cooked in, and served with, soup.

krill Term that refers to many species of planktonic crustaceans but is mostly used for the shrimp *Euphausia superba*. This is the main food of whales, and some penguins and other seabirds; occurs in shoals in the Antarctic, containing up to 12 kg/m^3. Collected in limited quantities for use as human food: a 100-g portion is a rich *source of protein and niacin; a good source of calcium; a source of iron; supplies 100 kcal (420 kJ).

kromenski Russian or Polish; minced poultry, game, or meat, bound to a stiff paste with sauce, wrapped in bacon, coated in batter, and fried.

kryptoxanthin *See* cryptoxanthin.

kuban *See* milk, fermented.

kuchen dough Pastry dough, containing egg, margarine, and yeast.

kugelhopf German, Alsatian; cake made from yeast dough in the shape of an inverted flower pot, with a hole through the centre which is usually filled with raisins and currants.

kula *See* bananas.

kulfi Indian; ice cream containing rice flour or sesame seed and ground almonds.

kumiss *See* milk, fermented.

kümmel Liqueur flavoured with caraway seeds, fennel, and orris root; 40% alcohol.

kumquat A *citrus fruit of the genus *Fortunella*; widely distributed in S. China and now cultivated elsewhere; resembles other citrus fruits, but very small, of ovoid shape, with acid pulp and sweet, edible skin. A 50-g portion is a rich *source of vitamin C and supplies 30 kcal (125 kJ).

kvass (kwass) Russian and Eastern European; beer, normally home-brewed from rye, buckwheat, or wheat, with malt and yeast, often flavoured with mint; 2–4% *alcohol by volume, 1–5% carbohydrate, 60–150 kcal (250–630 kJ) per 300 mL.

kwashiorkor *See* protein-energy malnutrition.

L

L- *See* **D-**.

labelled substances To follow the metabolic fate of foodstuffs, etc., in the body, they can be labelled by introduction of an unusual chemical substituent or with a stable or radioactive *isotope, so that the products can readily be identified.

laberdan *Cod salted and packed in barrels immediately it is landed at port, rather than later at a factory.

laccase *Enzyme in bacteria, potato, and mushrooms that converts polyphenols to quinones.

lacquer With reference to canned foods, a layer of gum and gum resin coated on to tinplate and hardened with heat. The layer of lacquer protects the tin lining from attack by acid fruit juices.

lactalbumin One of the proteins of milk (casein 3%, lactalbumin 0.5%, lactoglobulin 0.25%). Not precipitated from acid solution as is casein; hence, during cheese making the whey contains lactalbumin and lactoglobulin. They are precipitated by heat and a whey *cheese can be made in this way.

lactase The enzyme that hydrolyses *lactose to glucose and galactose; normally present in the brush border of the intestinal mucosal cells; deficiency of lactase is *alactasia, leading to lactose intolerance.

lactates Salts of *lactic acid.

lactation The process of synthesizing and secreting milk from the breasts.

lactation, nutritional needs Lactating women have slightly increased energy and protein requirements compared with those who are not breast-feeding (although considerable reserves of fat are laid down in pregnancy to cope with the stress of lactation), and high requirements for iron and calcium. These increased needs are reflected in the increased *reference intakes for lactating women (*see* Appendices II–V).

lactein bread See bread, lactein.

lactic acid The acid produced by the anaerobic fermentation of carbohydrates. Originally discovered in sour milk, it is responsible for the flavour of fermented *milk and for the precipitation of the *casein curd in cottage *cheese. Also produced by fermentation in silage, *pickles, *sauerkraut, cocoa, and tobacco, its value here is in suppressing the growth of unwanted organisms.

It is formed in mammalian muscle under conditions of maximum exertion (*see* glucose metabolism) and by metabolism of glycogen in meat immediately after death of the animal. Lactic acid in muscle was at one time known as sarcolactic acid.

Used as an acidulant (as well as citric and tartaric acids) in sugar confectionery, soft drinks, pickles, and sauces. (E-270; salts of lactic acid are E-325–327.)

lactic acid, buffered A mixture of *lactic acid and sodium lactate used in sugar confectionery to provide an acid taste without *inversion of the sugar, which occurs at lower pH.

lactit *See* lactitol.

lactitol *Sugar alcohol derived from *lactulose. Not digested by digestive enzymes but fermented by intestinal bacteria to short-chain fatty acids, some of which are absorbed; it yields about 2 kcal/g and hence has a potential use as a low-calorie bulk sweetener; also retards crystallization and improves moisture retention in foods (E-966).

Because of the bacterial fermentation, it is also used to acidify the colon and hence prevent the absorption of ammonia in patients with liver failure. *Lactulose is used in the same way; lactitol is less sweet and is often preferred. Also known as lactit, lactositol, lactobiosit.

***Lactobacillus casei* factor** *See* folic acid.

lactobiose *See* lactose.

lactobiosit *See* lactitol.

lactochrome Pigment in *milk.

lactoferrin Iron-protein complex in human milk (only a trace in cow's milk), only partly saturated with iron; has a rôle inhibiting the growth of *E. coli* and other potentially pathogenic organisms.

lactoflavin Obsolete name for *riboflavin, so named because it was isolated from milk. *See* vitamin B$_2$.

lactogen A drug or other substance that increases the production and secretion of milk.

lactoglobulin *See* lactalbumin.

lactometer Floating device used to measure the specific gravity of milk (1.027–1.035).

Lac-tone Trade name; protein-rich baby food (26% protein) made in India from peanut flour, skim milk powder, wheat flour, and barley flour, with added vitamins and calcium.

lacto-ovo-vegetarian One whose diet excludes animal foods (i.e. flesh) but permits milk and eggs.

lactose The *carbohydrate of milk, sometimes called milk sugar. A *disaccharide of *glucose and *galactose. Used pharmaceutically as a tablet filler and as a medium for growth of micro-organisms. The fermentation of lactose to *lactic acid by bacteria is responsible for the souring of milk. Ordinary lactose is α-lactose, which is 16% as sweet as sucrose; if crystallized above 93 °C, it is converted to the β-form which is more soluble and sweeter.

lactose intolerance *See* disaccharide intolerance.

lacto-serum Grandiloquent word for *whey.

lactositol *See* lactitol.

lactostearin *See* glyceryl lactostearate.

lactulose A *disaccharide of galactose and fructose which does not occur naturally but is formed in heated or stored milk by isomerization of *lactose. About half as sweet as sucrose. Not hydrolysed by human digestive enzymes but fermented by intestinal bacteria to form *lactic and pyruvic acids. Thought to promote the growth of *Lactobacillus bifidus* and so added to some infant formulae; in large amounts it is laxative. Because of the bacterial fermentation, it is also used to acidify the colon and hence prevent the absorption of ammonia in patients with liver failure. *See also* lactitol.

ladies' fingers *See* okra; also a short kind of banana.

laetrile Name given to an extract of apricot kernels, amygdalin, a glucoside of benzaldehyde and cyanide. Claimed as a cancer cure, although there is no supporting evidence, and sometimes called vitamin B_{17}, although there is no evidence that it is a dietary essential or has any metabolic function.

laevorotatory *See* optical activity.

laevulose *See* fructose.

lager *See* beer.

lakerda (lakertha) Greek; pickled raw fish (usually *tuna or swordfish).

lamb (French: *agneau*; German: *Lammfleisch*.) Meat from sheep (*Ovis aries*) younger than 12–14 months. A 150-g portion is a rich *source of protein, niacin, iron, zinc, copper, and vitamin B_{12}; a good source of vitamins B_1, B_2, and B_6; different cuts contain up to 30 g of fat of which half is saturated; supplies 400–600 kcal (1700–2500 kJ).

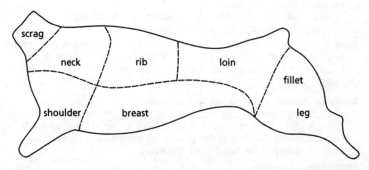

FIGURE 4.

lambrusco Italian; *wine with low alcohol content, lightly sparkling or *frizzante, made from the lambrusco variety of grape.

lamb's lettuce Or corn salad, a hardy annual plant, *Valerianella locusta* or *V. olitoria* used in salads in winter and early spring. A 50-g portion is a rich *source of vitamins A (as carotene) and C; supplies 5 kcal (20 kJ).

lamb's wool Old English drink made by pouring hot ale over pulped roasted apples and adding sugar and spices.

lampern *See* lamprey.

lamprey Cartilaginous fish resembling eels; sea lamprey is *Petromyzon marinus*, river lamprey or lampern is *Lampetra fluviatilis*.

Lancashire hotpot English (Lancashire) speciality; *see* hotpot.

Landwein *See* wine classification, Germany.

langouste *Shellfish, *Palinurus vulgaris*; *see* lobster.

langue de chat Thin, flat, crisp biscuit, shaped like a cat's tongue, sometimes with the edges dipped in chocolate.

lanolin The fat from wool. Consists of a mixture of cholesterol oleate, palmitate and stearate, and not useful as food; used in various cosmetics.

lapskaus Norwegian; boiled salted meat.

larch gum A *polysaccharide of galactose and arabinose (ratio of 1 : 6), found in the aqueous extract of the Western larch tree (*Larix occidentalis*); a potential substitute for *gum arabic, since it is readily dispersed in water.

lard Originally rendered fat from pig carcasses (sheep and cattle are also used). The best quality is from the fat surrounding the kidneys; neutral lard is the highest quality, prepared by agitating the minced fat with water at a temperature below 50 ˚C; kidney fat provides No. 1 quality; back fat provides No. 2 quality.

Leaf lard is made from the residue of kidney and back fat after the preparation of neutral lard by heating with water above 100 ˚C in an autoclave. Prime Steam Lard is fat from any part of the carcass, rendered in the autoclave.

Lard used to be stored in pig's bladder, hence the expression 'bladder of lard' for a grossly obese person.

lard compounds Blends of animal fats, such as oleostearin or *premier jus, with vegetable oils, to produce products similar to lard in consistency and texture. *See also* lard substitutes.

lardine *See* margarine.

larding Method of adding fat to lean meat so that it does not dry during long slow cooking. Narrow strips of bacon fat (lardoons) are threaded into the surface of the meat with a special 'larding needle' before cooking. Barding is the process of tying a thin sheet of bacon fat or a rasher of fat bacon over the meat.

lardoons *See* larding.

lard substitutes Vegetable shortenings made from mixtures of partially hardened vegetable fats with the consistency of *lard. *See also* lard compounds.

lardy cake West of England; made from bread dough, lard, sugar, and dried fruit.

lasagne Wide ribbons of *pasta; lasagne verdi is flavoured with spinach. Narrow ribbons are lasagnette.

lassam, lehsam *See* garlic.

lassi Indian; beverage made from yoghurt or buttermilk, mixed with water.

lathyrism Nerve damage associated with high intakes of *Lathyrus sativus* (Kesari dhal, chickling pea, chickling vetch). The crop is often grown in dry districts in Asia and North Africa together with wheat. Normally little is eaten, but when there is a drought and the wheat crop is poor, the dhal predominates and is eaten as a major food.

latkes Jewish; pancakes made from grated potatoes.

laung *See* cloves.

lauric acid A medium-chain saturated *fatty acid (12 carbons) in butter, coconut oil, and palm oil.

laver Edible seaweed. Laver bread is made from the seaweed *Porphyra* spp., by boiling in salted water and mincing to a gelatinous mass. It is made into a cake with oatmeal or fried. Locally known in S. Wales as bara lawr.

lax Scandinavian name for salmon; *see also* gravadlax; lox.

laxarinic acid *See* maltol.

laxative Or aperient, a substance that helps the expulsion of food residues from the body. If 'strongly' laxative it is termed purgative or cathartic. Dietary fibre and cellulose function because they retain water and add bulk to the contents of the intestine; *Epsom salts (magnesium sulphate) also retain water; castor oil and drugs such as aloes, senna, cascara, and phenolphthalein irritate the intestinal mucosa.

LD$_{50}$ An index of toxicity (lethal dose 50%), the amount of the substance that kills 50% of the test population of experimental animals when administered as a single dose.

LDL Low-density lipoproteins. *See* lipids, plasma.

lead A mineral of no nutritional interest, since it is not known to have any function in the body. It is toxic and its effects are cumulative. May be present in food from traces naturally present in the soil; as contamination of vegetables grown near main roads, which absorb volatile lead compounds from car exhaust fumes; from shellfish that have absorbed it from seawater; from lead glazes on cooking vessels; and in drinking water where lead pipes are used. Traces are excreted in the urine.

leaf lard *See* lard.

lean body mass Measure of body composition excluding adipose tissue, i.e. cells, extracellular fluid, and skeleton.

Lean Cuisine Trade name for a range of frozen meals prepared to a specified energy content.

leathers, fruit (Mango leathers, tomato leathers, etc.). Fruit purées dried in air in thin layers, 4–5 mm thick, then built up into thicker preparations.

leaven *Yeast, or a piece of dough kept to ferment the next batch.

leben *See* milk, fermented.

lebernockerln *See* knödeln.

lebkuchen German, Swiss; gingerbread, often baked in carved moulds, traditionally eaten at Christmas.

lecithin Chemically lecithin is phosphatidyl choline; a *phospholipid containing *choline. Commercial lecithin, prepared from soya bean, peanut, and maize, is a mixture of phospholipids in which phosphatidyl choline predominates. Used in food processing as an *emulsifier, e.g. in salad dressing, processed cheese, and chocolate, and as an anti-spattering agent in frying oils. Is plentiful in the diet and not a dietary essential.

leckeli Swiss; biscuit made with honey, almonds, candied peel, cloves, nutmeg, and ginger.

lectins Proteins from *legumes and other sources which bind to the carbohydrates found at cell surfaces. They therefore cause red blood cells to agglutinate *in vitro*, hence the old names haemagglutinins and phytoagglutinins.

Raw or undercooked beans of some varieties of *Phaseolus vulgaris* (red kidney beans) cause vomiting and diarrhoea within 2 hours of consumption due to the high level of lectins, but they are rapidly inactivated by boiling.

leek *Allium ampeloprasum*; a member of the onion family which has been known as a food for over 4000 years (eaten by the Israelites at the time of the Exodus from Egypt). The lower part is usually blanched by planting in trenches or earthing up, and eaten along with the upper long green leaves. A 125-g portion is a rich *source of vitamin C; a good source of folate; a source of iron; provides 3.1 g of dietary fibre; supplies 30 kcal (125 kJ).

legumes Members of the family Leguminosae eaten by man and domestic animals. Consumed as dry mature seeds (grain legumes or pulses) or as immature green seeds in the pod. On boiling, the dried seeds double in weight, so a 100-g cooked portion is approximately 50 g as a dried product.

Legumes include the groundnut, *Arachis hypogaea*, and soya bean, *Glycine max*, grown for their oil and protein, the yam bean *Pachyrrhizus erosus*, and African yam bean *Sphenostylis stenocarpa*, grown for their edible tubers as well as seeds.

legumin Globulin protein in legumes.

lekach Jewish; sponge cake made with ginger and honey.

lemon Sour yellow fruit of *Citrus limon*. A 100-g portion of fruit, or 100 ml of juice, is a rich *source of vitamin C; supplies 7 kcal (28 kJ).

lemonade Originally a beverage made from lemon juice with water and sugar; now also a wide variety of carbonated beverages.

lemon balm *See* balm.

lemon curd Cooked mixture of sugar, butter, eggs, and lemons. Legally (UK regulations) must contain 4% fat, 0.33% citric acid, 1% dried egg or equivalent, 0.125% oil of lemon or 0.25% oil of orange, and not less than 65% soluble solids.

lemon grass Lemon-scented grasses (*Cymbopogon* spp.), native to South East Asia, widely used in Thai, Indonesian, and Malay cooking.

lemon oil The peel oil of the lemon, 0.15–0.3% of the weight of the fruit.

lentils *Legumes; dried seeds of many varieties of *Lens esculenta*, they may be green, yellow, or orange-red. When ground, they are frequently used to thicken soup. A 120-g portion is a rich *source of copper and selenium; a good source of iron; a source of protein, vitamin B$_6$, folate, and zinc; contains 0.6 g of fat of which 20% is saturated; provides 4.8 g of dietary fibre; supplies 125 kcal (520 kJ).

lettuce Leaves of the plant *Lactuca sativa*; many varieties are grown commercially. A poor source of nutrients; an 80-g portion supplies 10 kcal (40 kJ).

leucine An essential *amino acid; rarely limiting in foods. Chemically, amino-isocaproic acid.

leucocytes White blood cells, normally 5000–9000/mm^3; includes polymorphonuclear neutrophils, lymphocytes, monocytes, polymorphonuclear eosinophils, and polymorphonuclear basophils. A 'white cell count' determines the total; a 'differential cell count' estimates the numbers of each type.
  Fever, haemorrhage, and violent exercise cause an increase (leucocytosis); starvation and debilitating conditions a decrease (leucopenia).

leucocytosis Increase in the number of *leucocytes in the blood.

leucopenia Decrease in the number of *leucocytes in the blood.

leucosin One of the water-soluble proteins of wheat flour.

leucovorin The synthetic (racemic) 5-formyl derivative of *folic acid; more stable to oxidation than folic acid itself, and commonly used in pharmaceutical preparations. Also known as folinic acid.

levans Polymers of *fructose (the principal one is *inulin) that occur in tubers and some grasses.

leveret A young *hare.

levitin One of the proteins of egg yolk; about one-fifth of the total, the remainder being vitellin. Rich in sulphur, it accounts for half of the sulphur in the yolk.

licoroso Portuguese; fortified sweet wines.

lieben German and Austrian classification for semi-sweet wines; *see* wine, sweetness.

Lieberkühn, crypts of Glands lining the small intestine which secrete the intestinal juice.

Liebfraumilch German sweet wine from the Rhine valley; originally from the vineyard beside the Liebfrauenkirche in Worms.

light (or lite) As applied to foods usually indicates: (1) a lower content of fat compared with the standard product (e.g. *breadspreads, sausages); (2) Sodium chloride substitutes lower in *sodium (*see* salt, light); (3) Low-alcohol *beer or *wine. US legislation restricts the term 'light' to modified foods that contain one-third less energy or half the fat of a reference unmodified food, or to indicate that the sodium content of a low-fat, low-calorie food has been reduced by half. *See also* fat-free; free from; low in; reduced.

lights Butchers' term for the lungs of an animal.

lignin (Or lignocellulose) indigestible part of the cell wall of plants (a polymer of aromatic alcohols). It is included in measurement of *dietary fibre, but not of *non-starch polysaccharide.

lignocellulose Alternative name for *lignin.

lillet French light *vermouth made from red or white Bordeaux wines in which fruit peel and herbs are steeped; aged in oak casks.

lima beans US term for flat, kidney-shaped bean, smaller ones are butter limas, called butter beans in the UK (*see* beans, butter), and larger ones are potato limas.

lime The fruit of *Citrus aurantifolia*, cultivated almost solely in the tropics, since it is not as hardy as other *citrus fruits. Used to prevent scurvy in the British Navy (replacing, at the time, lemon juice) and so giving rise to the nickname of 'Limeys' for British sailors and for British people in general. Contains about 10–20 mg vitamin C per 100 g fruit or fresh juice.

limit dextrin When a branched polysaccharide such as *glycogen or *amylopectin is hydrolysed enzymically, glucose units are removed one at a time until the branch point is reached. The hydrolysis then stops, leaving what is termed a limit dextrin; further hydrolysis requires a different enzyme.

limiting amino acid *See* amino acid.

Limmisax Trade name for *saccharin.

Limmits Trade name for a 'slimming' preparation composed of wholemeal biscuits with a methyl cellulose mixture as filling, containing some vitamins and minerals; intended as a meal replacement.

limonin The bitter principle in the albedo of the Valencia orange. Isolimonin is the bitter principle of the navel orange. Both are present as a non-bitter precursor which is liberated into the juice during extraction and is slowly hydrolysed, making the juice bitter.

limpet A *shellfish, *Patella vulgata*.

linamarin *Cyanogenic *glucoside found in *cassava (manioc) which may be a cause of neuropathies in areas where cassava is a major food; the cyanide is removed in traditional processing by grating and exposing to air.

linguini *See* pasta.

linie aquavit Norwegian *aquavit which is aged in oak casks that are shipped to Australia and back before bottling, thus crossing the equator (*linie*) twice.

linoleic acid An essential polyunsaturated *fatty acid (C18:2 ω6), predominant in most edible vegetable oils.

α-linolenic acid An essential polyunsaturated *fatty acid (C18:3 ω3).

γ-linolenic acid A non-essential polyunsaturated *fatty acid (C18:3 ω6) which has some pharmacological actions. Found in oils from the seeds of evening primrose, borage, and blackcurrant.

linseed oil Vegetable oil from the seeds of flax, *Linum usitatissimum*; rich in the essential *fatty acid α-linolenic acid.

Linzer torte Austrian; flan made with eggs, ground almonds, and mixed peel, with a covering of jam and a lattice of pastry on top.

liothyronine Alternative name for tri-iodothyronine (T3), the most potent of the *thyroid hormones.

lipaemia Increase in blood lipids, as occurs normally after a meal.

lipase Enzyme that hydrolyses fats to glycerol and fatty acids. Most lipases have low specificity and will attack any triglyceride or long-chain ester. Present in the pancreatic juice, liver, and *adipose tissue, and in many seeds and grains. Sometimes responsible for the development of rancidity in stored foods.

lipase, hormone-sensitive The *lipase of *adipose tissue; it is stimulated by the action of hormones such as *glucagon and *adrenaline, which are secreted when there is a need for release of free fatty acids from adipose tissue for use as a metabolic fuel.

lipectomy Surgical removal of subcutaneous fat.

lipidema Condition in which fat deposits accumulate in the lower extremities, from hips to ankles, with tenderness of the affected parts.

lipids (Also sometimes lipides, lipins.) A general term for fats and oils (chemically *triglycerides), waxes, *phospholipids, steroids, and terpenes. Their common property is insolubility in water and solubility in hydrocarbons, chloroform, and alcohols.

lipids, plasma *Triglycerides, free and esterified *cholesterol and *phospholipids, present as protein complexes in *blood plasma.
   Chylomicrons consist mainly of triglycerides and protein; they are the form in which lipids absorbed in the small intestine enter the bloodstream.
   Low-density lipoproteins (LDL) are assembled in the liver and exported to other tissues, where they are taken up and used as a source of cholesterol (and other lipids). High-density lipoproteins (HDL) are returned from tissues to the liver. *See also* hypercholesterolaemia; hyperlipidaemia.

lipins *See* lipids.

lipochromes Plant pigments soluble in fats and organic solvents, such as chlorophyll, carotenoids.

lipodystrophy Abnormality in the metabolism or deposition of fats; abnormal pattern of subcutaneous fat deposits.

lipofuscin A group of pigments that accumulate in several body tissues, particularly the myocardium, during life and are consequently associated with the ageing process.

lipoic acid Chemically, dithio-octanoic acid, a coenzyme (together with *vitamin B₁) in the oxidative decarboxylation reactions of *glucose metabolism and the citric acid cycle. Although it is an essential growth factor for various micro-organisms, there is no evidence that it is a human dietary requirement.

lipolysis The *hydrolysis (splitting) of fats to yield glycerol and fatty acids. *See* lipase.

lipolytic rancidity Spoilage of foods as a result of *hydrolysis of fats to free fatty acids on storage (by the action of *lipase, either bacterial lipase or the enzyme naturally present in the food). Since the enzyme is inactivated by heat, this type of rancidity occurs only in uncooked foods.

lipoproteins Complexes of protein and lipids; *see* lipids, plasma.

liposuction Procedure for removal of subcutaneous adipose tissue in obese people using a suction pump device.

lipovitellenin A lipoprotein complex in egg comprising about one-sixth of the solids of the yolk.

liquefied herring *Herring reduced to liquid state by enzyme action at slightly acid pH; used as protein concentrate for animal feed.

liqueurs Distilled, flavoured, and sweetened alcoholic liquors. For example, curaçao (30% (weight/volume, w/v) alcohol, 30% sugar); cherry brandy (19% alcohol, 33% sugar); advocaat (13% alcohol, 30% sugar, 0.75% nitrogen).

liquid diet Diet consisting of foods that can be served as liquids or strained purées, prescribed in acute inflammation of the *gastro-intestinal tract and for patients unable to consume normal foods, especially after surgery.

liquid paraffin *See* medicinal paraffin.

liquorice Used in confectionery and to flavour medicines; liquorice root and extract are obtained from the plant *Glycyrrhiza glabra*; stick liquorice is the crude evaporated extract of the root. The plant has been grown in the Pontefract district of Yorkshire since the sixteenth century; hence the name Pontefract cakes for the sugar confection of liquorice. *See also* glycyrrhizin.

liquorose Italian; high strength, often fortified, wines.

Listeria A genus of bacteria commonly found in soil of which the commonest is *Listeria monocytogenes*. They can cause *food poisoning (listeriosis). *Listeria* species are especially found in unwashed vegetables and some soft cheeses; they resist cold and the presence of salt and can multiply in a refrigerator. Symptoms of listeriosis are flu-like, with high fever and dizziness. Pregnant women, babies, and the elderly are especially at risk.

litchi *See* lychee.

lite *See* light.

lithium Metal not known to have any physiological function, although it occurs in food and water; lithium salts are used in the treatment of manic-depressive illness.

liver (French: *foie*; German: *Leber*.) Usually from calf, pig, ox, lamb, chicken, duck, or goose; a 150-g portion (fried or stewed) is an exceptionally rich *source of iron and vitamins A, D, B_2, B_6, and B_{12}; a rich source of protein, zinc, copper, selenium, niacin, and vitamin B_1; also, unusually for meat, a good source of vitamin C; contains 10 g of fat of which one-third is *saturated; supplies 300–380 kcal (1250–1600 kJ). The vitamin A content of liver is high enough for it to pose a possible hazard to unborn children, and pregnant women have been advised not to eat liver. *See* vitamin A toxicity. Fish liver is a particularly rich source of vitamins A and D, and fish liver oils (especially cod and halibut) are used as sources of these vitamins as nutritional supplements.

liver sausage *Sausage based on liver. A 150-g portion is an exceptionally rich *source of iron, vitamin A, protein, vitamin B_2, and niacin; a rich source of vitamin B_1; contains 40 g of fat of which 40% is saturated; supplies 450 kcal (1900 kJ).

livetin A water-soluble protein fraction of egg yolk.

lobio Russian (Georgian); bean salad.

lobscouse Sailor's stew of meat and vegetables, classically thickened with ship's biscuit.

lobster (French: *homard*; German: *Hummer*.) A crustacean, *Homerus vulgaris*. A 100-g portion (meat from half a dressed lobster) is a rich *source of protein, niacin, vitamin B_{12}, and copper; a source of zinc, vitamin B_1, niacin, folate, and calcium; contains 370 mg of sodium and 3.5 g of fat; supplies 130 kcal (550 kJ).

lobster, rock or spiny *See* crawfish.

Locasol Trade name for a low-calcium milk substitute.

lockshen Thin noodles.

locksoy Chinese; fine-drawn rice macaroni.

locoweed *Astralagus* and *Oxytropus* spp., common in arid areas of the western USA. Toxic to cattle, causing locoism: neurological damage, abortion, and birth defects. Apparently caused by an alkaloid, swainsonine, which is also found in mouldy hay.

locust bean 1 *Carob seed.
2 African locust bean, *Parkia* spp.

loempias Dutch, Indonesian; *see* spring rolls.

Lofenalac Trade name for food low in *phenylalanine for treatment of *phenylketonuria.

loganberry Cross between European raspberry and Californian blackberry, *Rubus ursinus* var. *loganobaccus,* named after L. H. Logan. An 80-g portion is a rich *source of vitamin C; a source of copper; provides 4.8 g of dietary fibre, and supplies 15 kcal (60 kJ).

loin The back portion of animals; *see* pork, lamb.

lollipop Boiled sweet or toffee on a small wooden stick. Ice lollipop (ice lolly; popsicle in the USA) is water-ice on a stick.

Lonalac Trade name for a milk preparation free from *sodium.

London broil American name for steak, broiled or grilled and sliced thinly against the grain.

London gin *See* gin.

longaniza *See* sobresada.

lonzo Corsican; boned fillet of pork, steeped in wine and herbs, then air dried, thinly sliced, and eaten raw.

loonzein Rice from which the husk has been removed; also known as brown rice, hulled rice, and cargo rice.

loquat The small pear-shaped fruit of *Eriobotyra japonica*, a member of the apple family, also known as Japanese medlar. A 100-g portion supplies 50 kcal (210 kJ) but only a trace of vitamin C.

lotus The sacred lotus of India and China, *Nelumbium nuciferum*, a water plant whose rhizomes and seeds are eaten. A 100-g portion of the rhizome is a rich *source of vitamin C, and supplies 50 kcal (210 kJ).

loukoum *See* Turkish delight.

lovage Herb of the carrot family, *Ligusticum scoticum*, with a strong musky scent of celery. The stems can be candied like *angelica or used as a vegetable, and the leaves and stems are used in soup. The seeds can also be used as a seasoning, with a flavour like dill or fennel seed.

love apple Old name for *tomato.

low birth weight Infants born weighing significantly less than normal are considered to be premature; their chances of survival and normal development are considerably improved if they are fed special formula preparations to meet their needs, rather than being breast-fed or fed normal *infant formula. The normal range of weight at birth is between 2.5 and 4.5 kg.

low in EU legislation (in preparation in 1995) states that for a food label or advertising to bear a claim that it is low in fat, saturates, cholesterol, sodium, or alcohol, it must provide less than half the amount of the specified nutrient of a reference product for which no claim is made. UK legislation (in force in 1995) and US legislation set precise (low) levels at which such claims may be made.

low-salt diets *See* 'salt-free' diets.

lox American (originally Yiddish) name for smoked salmon; *see also* lax.

lozenges Shapes stamped out of a mixture of icing sugar, glucose syrup, and gum arabic or gelatine with flavourings, then hardened at 32–43 °C.

LSM Trade name (USA) for a low-sodium milk containing 50 mg/L; ordinary milk contains 500 mg/L.

lucerne The plant, *Medicago sativa*; essentially a forage crop, but eaten by man to a small extent. Also known as alfalfa.

Lucozade Trade name for a glucose beverage: 17.9% carbohydrate, 67 kcal (280 MJ)/100 mL.

lumpfish Large sea-fish, *Cyclopterus lumpus*, the pink eggs of which are salted, pressed, and coloured, as Danish or German *caviare.

lunch (luncheon) The midday meal (but in northern England the main meal is traditionally eaten at midday and is known as dinner).

luncheon meat Precooked, canned meat, usually pork. A 150-g portion is a rich *source of protein, niacin; a good source of iron; a source of vitamins B_1 and B_2; contains 40 g of fat of which 40% is saturated; supplies 450 kcal (1900 kJ).

lupeose *See* stachyose.

lupins Legumes of *Lupinus* spp. The ordinary garden lupin contains toxic alkaloids (quinolizidines) and tastes bitter; varieties selected for animal feed and grain crop are low in alkaloids and known as sweet lupins; they are rich in protein and fat.

lutefisk Norwegian; dried salted cod preserved in potash lye.

lutfisk Swedish; fish pickled in wood ash, lime, and soda, and then dried.

luting Strip of pastry placed round a dish to seal on the lid or pastry cover, used when preparing potted game, etc., in covered dishes.

luxus konsumption *See* diet-induced thermogenesis.

Lycasin Trade name for hydrogenated glucose syrup, a bulk *sweetener.

lychee (litchi) The fruit of *Litchi chinensis*, native to China; the size of a small plum, with a hard case and translucent, white, jelly-like sweet flesh surrounding the seed. A 100-g portion is a rich *source of vitamin C, and supplies 70 kcal (290 kJ).

lycopene Red *carotenoid pigment found in tomato, pink grapefruit, and palm oil. It has no vitamin A activity. The synthetic material is sometimes used as a food colour (E-160(d)).

lye-peeling A method of removing skins from vegetables by immersion in hot caustic soda solution (lye) followed by 'tumbling' in a wash to remove the skin and chemicals.

lymph The fluid between blood and the tissues; the medium in which oxygen and nutrients are conveyed from the blood to the tissues, and waste products back to the blood. Similar to *blood plasma in composition.

Dietary fat is absorbed into the lacteals (lymphatic vessels of the intestinal villi) as *chylomicrons which are formed in the intestinal mucosa, and enters the bloodstream through the thoracic duct. After a fatty meal the lymph is rich in emulsified fat and is called chyle.

lymphatics Vessels through which the lymph flows, draining from the tissues and entering the bloodstream at the thoracic duct.

lymphocytes *See* leucocytes.

lyonnaise, à la Dish with fried shredded onion as a principal ingredient.

lyophilization *See* freeze-drying.

lysergic acid The toxin of *ergot.

lysine An essential *amino acid of special nutritional importance, since it is the *limiting amino acid in many cereals. Can be synthesized on a commercial scale, and when added to bread, rice, or cereal-based animal feeds, it improves the nutritive value of the protein.

lysozyme An enzyme that digests some high-molecular-weight carbohydrates which are a common constituent of bacterial cell walls, and so lyses ('dissolves') bacteria. Widely distributed (e.g. in tears); egg-white is especially rich.

MA Modified atmosphere. *See* gas storage, controlled.

maatjes Dutch; cured *herring made only from young female herrings.

macadamia nut Fruit of *Macadamia ternifolia*. A 60-g portion (thirty-six nuts), is a good *source of vitamin B₁; a source of protein, niacin, and iron; contains 45 g of fat of which 15% is *saturated and 80% mono-unsaturated; supplies 450 kcal (1900 kJ).

macaroni *See* pasta.

macaroon Cake made from ground almonds or coconut, sugar, and egg-white, baked on *rice paper. Originated in Italy, where it is known as amaretti.

macassar gum *See* agar.

maccaroncelli *See* pasta.

mace *See* nutmeg.

macedoine Mixture of fruits or vegetables, diced, or cut into small even-shaped pieces.

macerases A group of *enzymes (usually extracted from the mould *Aspergillus*) used to break down *pectin in fruits to facilitate maximum extraction of the juice.

mackerel An oily *fish, *Scomber scombrus*. A 150-g portion is a rich *source of protein, vitamins D, B₂, B₆, B₁₂, niacin, copper, iodine, and selenium; a source of vitamin B₁ and iron; contains 24 g of fat of which 20% is saturated; supplies 330 kcal (1390 kJ).

macon *Bacon made from mutton.

maconochie A canned meat stew much used in the First World War; made by Maconochie Brothers.

macrobiotic diet A system of eating associated with Zen Buddhism; consists of several stages finally reaching Diet 7 which is restricted to cereals. Cases of severe malnutrition have been reported on this 'diet'. It involves the Chinese concept of *yin* (female) and *yang* (male) whereby foods, and even different vitamins (indeed, everything in life) are predominantly one or the other and must be balanced.

macrocytes Large immature precursors of red *blood cells found in the circulation in *pernicious anaemia and in *folic acid deficiency, due to impairment of the normal maturation of red cells; hence macrocytic *anaemia.

mad cow disease Bovine spongiform encephalopathy, *see* BSE.

Madeira cake Rich cake containing no fruit and flavoured with lemon; traditionally decorated with strips of candied citron peel.

Madeira nuts *See* walnuts.

Madeira wines Fortified wines from the Island of Madeira: sercial (dry); verdelho (semi-dry); bual (semi-sweet); malmsey (sweet).

madeleine French; small fancy sponge cake baked in a *dariole mould (or sometimes a scallop-shaped mould). English version is victoria sponge mixture topped with jam and coconut.

Madras curry Pungent *curry sauce with a large amount of chilli, but less than *vindaloo.

Madrid stew *Olla podrida* or rotten pot; Spanish (Castilian) stew containing chickpeas, chicken, beef on the bone, smoked bacon, tocino (salted pork fat), *chorizo, *morcilla, onion, cabbage, carrots, turnips, and garlic.

madrilène, à la Dish flavoured with tomato.

magma Mixture of sugar syrup and sugar crystals produced during sugar refining.

magnesium An essential mineral; present in all human tissues, especially bone. Involved in the metabolism of *ATP. Present in chlorophyll and so in all green plant foods, and therefore generally plentiful in the diet. Deficiency in human beings leads to disturbances of muscle and nervous system; in cattle, to grass tetany. Magnesium-deficient plants are yellow (or chlorosed).

magnum Large wine bottle, 1.5 L (double old British bottle, called 'reputed quart').

mahleb Spice prepared from black cherry kernels, Syrian in origin, widely used in Greek baked goods.

maids of honour Small tartlets filled with almond-flavoured custard; said to have originated in the court of Henry VIII, where they were made by Ann Boleyn when she was lady-in-waiting to Catherine of Aragon.

maigre, au Dish without meat and therefore traditionally suitable for Lent or a fast day.

Maillard reaction Two processes in foods can produce a brown colour. One is the enzymatic oxidation of phenolic substances such as occurs at the cut surface of an apple. The other is a reaction between *lysine in proteins and sugars, and is variously known as the Maillard reaction, the browning reaction and non-enzymic browning. It takes place on heating or prolonged storage and is one of the deteriorative processes that take place in stored foods. It is accompanied by a loss in nutritive value, since the part of the protein that reacts with the sugar is not digested. *See also* availability; available lysine.

maître d'hôtel 1 Simply prepared dishes garnished with butter creamed with parsley and lemon juice (maître d'hôtel butter); literally 'in the style of the chief steward'.
2 Especially in the USA, the head waiter.

maize Grain of *Zea mays*, also called Indian corn and (in the USA) simply corn. Staple food in many countries, made into *tortillas in Latin America, into *polenta in Italy, and flaked as cornflakes commonly eaten as a breakfast cereal; various preparations in the southern states of the USA are known as hominy, samp, and cerealine.

Two varieties of major commercial importance are flint corn (*Zea mays indurata*), which is very hard, and dent corn (*Z. mays dentata*); there is also sweet corn (*Z. mays saccharata*), and a variety that expands on heating (*Zea mays everta, see* popcorn). The starch prepared from *Z. mays dentata* is termed corn flour; the ground maize is termed maize meal. There is a white variety; the usual yellow colour is partly due to cryptoxanthin (a vitamin A precursor).

Because of its low content of the amino acid *tryptophan (and available *niacin), diets based largely on maize are associated with the development of *pellagra.

A 60-g portion of sweetcorn kernels is a *source of vitamin C; contains 1.2 g of fat of which 10% is saturated; provides 2.4 g of dietary fibre; supplies 75 kcal (315 kJ).

maize, flaked Partly gelatinized maize used for animal feed. The grain is cracked to small pieces, moistened, cooked, and flaked between rollers.

maize flour Highly refined and very finely ground maize meal from which all bran and germ have been removed.

maize oil *See* corn oil.

maize rice Finely cut *maize with bran and germ partly removed, also called mealie rice.

maize starches, waxy *Starch obtained from hybrids of *maize consisting wholly or largely (99%) of *amylopectin, compared with ordinary maize starch with 26% *amylose and 74% amylopectin. The paste is semi-translucent, cohesive, and does not form a gel.

makhani Indian; buttered rice prepared by steaming with butter and aromatic spices.

malabsorption syndrome Defect of absorption of one or more nutrients; signs include diarrhoea, *steatorrhoea, abdominal distension, weight loss, and specific signs of nutrient deficiency.

malai Indian; cream prepared by boiling milk, leaving it to cool, and then skimming off the clotted cream.

malic acid Organic acid occurring in many fruits, particularly in apples, tomatoes and plums. Molecular formula $COOH-CHOH-CH_2-COOH$. Used as a food additive to increase acidity (E-296).

malmsey *See* Madeira wines.

malnutrition Disturbance of form or function arising from deficiency or excess of one or more nutrients. *See also* cachexia; obesity; protein-energy malnutrition; vitamin toxicity.

malo-lactic fermentation The conversion of the malic acid in grape juice (and other fruit juices) into lactic acid, especially in red wines and cider, causing them to mellow and become less acid.

malpighia *See* cherry, West Indian.

malt (malt extract) Mixture of starch breakdown products containing mainly *maltose (malt sugar), prepared from barley or wheat.

The grain is allowed to sprout, when the *enzyme diastase (*amylase) develops and *hydrolyses the starch to maltose. The mixture is then extracted with hot water, and this malt extract contains a solution of starch breakdown products together with diastase. Malt extract may remain as the concentrated solution or evaporated to dryness.

maltase *Enzyme that *hydrolyses *maltose to yield two molecules of glucose; present in the brush border of the intestinal mucosal cells.

malted barley *See* malt; malt extract.

malt flour Germinated barley or wheat, in dried form. As well as dextrins, glucose, proteins, and salts derived from the cereal, it is rich in diastase and is added to wheat flour of low *diastatic activity for bread making; used as an ingredient of 'malt' loaf.

Malthus T. R. Malthus (1766–1835), author of an essay in 1798 postulating that any temporary or local improvement in living conditions will increase population faster than the food supply, and that disasters such as war and pestilence, which check population growth, are inescapable features of human society.

malting *See* beer.

maltitol A *sugar alcohol produced by hydrogenation of maltose. Slowly hydrolysed in the digestive tract to *glucose and *sorbitol and fairly completely utilized, providing 4 kcal (16 kJ)/gram; sweeter than maltose, and 90% as sweet as sucrose (E-965).

maltobiose *See* maltose.

maltol Also called laxarinic acid, palatone, veltol; chemically 3-hydroxy-2 methyl-γ-pyrone. Found in the bark of young larch trees, pine needles, chicory, and roasted malt; synthesized for use as a fragrant, caramel-like flavour for addition to foods; imparts a 'freshly baked' flavour to bread and cakes.

maltonic acid *See* gluconic acid.

maltose Malt sugar, or maltobiose, a *disaccharide consisting of two glucose units linked 1–4. Hydrolysed by *maltase. Does not occur in foods (unless specifically added as *malt) but formed during the acid or enzymic digestion of starch. It is one-third as sweet as sucrose.

maltose figure *See* diastatic activity.

maltose intolerance *See* disaccharide intolerance.

malt sugar *See* maltose.

malt whisky *See* whisky.

malvasia A *grape variety widely used for *wine making, although not one of the classic varieties.

manche French; cutlet bone. Manchette is the paper frill used to decorate the bone.

mandarin (Also called Algerian tangerine.) Loose-skinned *citrus fruit, *Citrus reticulata* or *C. nobilio*. Varieties include satsumas and tangerines (although all three names are used indiscriminately) with various hybrids including tangelo, tangor, temple, clementine.

mandelbrot Middle-European (especially Jewish); sponge cake with almonds. Also known as komishbrot.

mandeln Middle-European (especially Jewish); small pieces of dough shaped like almonds, baked and added to soup before serving.

mandolin Vegetable slicer.

manganese An essential trace mineral which functions as the *prosthetic group in a number of *enzymes. Dietary deficiency has not been reported in man; in experimental animals manganese deficiency leads to impaired synthesis of *mucopolysaccharides. Requirements are not known; intakes greater than 1.4 mg/day are considered *safe and adequate.

mangelwurzel, mangoldwurzel A root vegetable used as cattle feed, *Beta vulgaris rapa*; a cross between red and white *beetroot.

mange-tout Immature pods and embryo seeds of *Pisum sativum* var. *macrocarpum* (or *macrocarpon*) eaten whole; also known as sugar pea or snap pea. The name is sometimes used for immature French beans, *Phaseolus vulgaris*. A 100-g portion is a rich *source of vitamin C; a source of vitamins A (as carotene), B$_1$, and B$_2$; supplies 25 kcal (105 kJ).

mango A fruit, originally of Indo-Burmese origin and now grown widely throughout the tropics, *Mangifera indica*. The fruit is ovoid, 3–5 in (75–120 cm) in diameter, with orange-coloured sweet aromatic flesh surrounding a central stone. A 150-g portion (one quarter slice) is a rich *source of vitamins C and A (as carotene); a source of copper; supplies 75 kcal (320 kJ).

mangosteen A fruit of Indian origin, *Garcinea mangostana*, the size of an orange with thick purple rind and sweet white pulp in segments. A 100-g portion supplies 75 kcal (320 kJ); little vitamin C.

manihot starch *See* cassava.

manioc *See* cassava.

manna Dried exudate from the manna-ash tamarisk tree (*Fraxinus ornus*). Abundant in Sicily and used as a mild laxative for children; it consists of 40–60% *mannitol, 10–16% mannotetrose, 6–16% mannotriose, plus glucose, mucilage, and fraxin. This is thought to be the food eaten by the Children of Israel in the wilderness (Exod. 16: 15).

manna bread A cake-like product made from crushed, sprouted wheat without yeast; said to be a recipe of the Essenes who lived by the Dead Sea around the beginning of the Christian era.

manna sugar, mannite *See* mannitol.

mannitol Mannite or manna sugar, a six-carbon *sugar alcohol found in beets, pumpkin, mushrooms, onions; 50–60% as sweet as sucrose. Extracted commercially from seaweed (*Laminaria* spp.) or made from the sugar *mannose (E-421).

mannosans *Polysaccharides containing *mannose.

mannose A 6-carbon (hexose) sugar found in small amounts in legumes, *manna, and some gums. Also called seminose and carubinose.

mannotetrose *See* stachyose.

Manucol Trade name for sodium *alginate.

manzanilla *See* sherry.

maple syrup Sap of the north American sugar maple tree, *Acer saccharum*. Evaporated either to syrup (63% sucrose, 1.5% invert sugar) or to dry sugar for use in confectionery.

maple syrup urine disease A rare *genetic disease affecting the metabolism of the amino acids leucine, isoleucine, and valine leading to accumulation of high concentrations of these three amino acids and the immediate products of their metabolism in the plasma and urine. The urine has a characteristic smell like that of *maple syrup.

maraschino 1 Sweetened spirit prepared by distillation of fermented maraschino cherries (both the juice and the crushed kernels).
   2 Cherries preserved in real or imitation maraschino liqueur, used to decorate cocktails, ice cream, or fruit salad.

marasmic kwashiorkor The most severe form of *protein energy malnutrition in children, with weight for height less than 60% of that expected, and with oedema and other symptoms of *kwashiorkor.

marasmus *See* protein-energy malnutrition.

marc French; spirit distilled from the fermented residue of grape skins, stalks, and seeds after the grapes have been pressed for wine making. The same as grappa (Italian), bagaciera (Portugal), and aguardiente (Spain). Often a harsh raw spirit, drunk young, although some varieties (especially marc de bourgogne) are matured and smooth.

marengo Chicken or veal sautéed in oil, and cooked in a sauce of white wine, tomatoes, mushroom, and garlic; said to have been invented in 1800 by Napoleon's chef after the battle of Marengo in Italy.

margarine (Butterine, lardine, oleomargarine.) Emulsion of about 80% vegetable, animal, and/or marine fats and 20% water, originally made as a substitute for butter. Usually contains emulsifiers, anti-spattering agents, colours, vitamins A and D (sometimes E), and preservatives. Ordinary margarines contain roughly equal parts of *saturated, mono-unsaturated, and polyunsaturated fatty acids; special soft varieties are rich in *polyunsaturates. The energy yield is the same as that of *butter.
   A 40-g portion (a medium thickness spread on four slices of bread) is a rich *source of vitamins A and D; contains 32 g of fat (the percentage of saturated fat depends on the oils used in manufacture); supplies 290 kcal (1220 kJ). A single caterer's pat is 10 g; contains 8 g of fat; supplies 72 kcal (300 kJ).
   Low-fat spreads are made with 20–60% fat and correspondingly higher contents of air and water and less energy. A 40-g portion of low-fat spread contains 16 g of fat (of which typically 27% is saturated); supplies 145 kcal (610 kJ). A single caterer's pat is 10 g; contains 4 g of fat; supplies 35 kcal (150 kJ).

margarine, kosher Made only from vegetable fats, since ordinary margarine can include animal fats that may not be *kosher. It is fortified with carotene (which is derived from vegetable sources) as the source of vitamin A, instead of retinol (which may be obtained from non-kosher sources).

margarita Mexican cocktail based on *tequila with lime or lemon juice; traditionally served in glasses frosted with salt around the rim.

margherita A variety of *pizza.

marinade Mixture of oil with wine, lemon juice, or vinegar and herbs in which meat or fish is soaked before cooking, both to give flavour and to make it more tender. Hence to marinate.

marine biotoxins Toxins in shellfish and marine fish, either produced naturally or accumulated by the fish from their diet (includes *ciguatera and paralytic shellfish poisoning).

marine oils *See* fish oils.

marinière, à la French; literally 'in the seaman's style'; fish dishes cooked in white wine and garnished with mussels.

marjoram Dried leaves of a number of aromatic plants of different species, used as seasoning for poultry, meats, and cheese dishes. The most widely accepted marjoram herbs are the perennial bush *Origanum majorana* and the annual sweet marjoram *Majorana hortensis*. Spanish wild marjoram is *Thymus mastichina*.

marmalade Defined by EU Directive as *jam made from citrus peel; what was known as ginger marmalade is now known as ginger preserve. The name comes from the Portuguese *marmalada*, the quince, which was used to make preserves. Used in French and German for jam or preserves in general.

marmite 1 The original form of pressure cooker used by Papin in 1681; it was an iron pot with a sealing lid.
　　2 Cookery term for a stock, or the pot in which stock is prepared.

Marmite Trade name for *yeast extract flavoured with vegetable extract.

marque nationale *See* wine classification, Luxemburg.

marquise French; chocolate mousse.

marron glacé Chestnuts preserved in syrup; semi-crystallized.

marrow 1 Bone marrow; contents of bone cavities which are the site of formation of red blood cells.
　　2 Varieties of the *gourd *Cucurbita pepo*. Grouped with courgettes, squashes, and pumpkins; 95% water. A 100-g portion provides 1 g of dietary fibre, with only traces of nutrients and only 9 kcal (36 kJ). Courgettes and zucchini are varieties that have been developed for cutting when small.

marsala Sicilian; fortified white wine.

marshmallow Soft sweetmeat made from an aerated mixture of gelatine or egg albumin with sugar or starch syrup. *Nougat is harder, containing less water, and usually incorporating dried fruit and nuts. Originally using the root of the marshmallow plant (*Althaea officinalis*), which provides a mucilaginous substance as well as starch and sugar.

Martini Trade name for a brand of *vermouth; now also the name for a cocktail based on *gin and vermouth. A sweet martini is made with Italian (sweet) vermouth; a dry martini with French (dry) vermouth; the proportion of gin may vary from 50 to 90%. A vodka martini (vodkatini) contains vodka rather than gin.

Marumillon 50 Trade name for mixture of the sweet glycosides extracted from stevia leaves. *See also* stevioside; rebaudoside.

Maryland, à la Dish with a butter and cream sauce, often containing wine. Chicken Maryland is deep-fried and has a garnish of sweet corn fritters, fried bananas, and fruit fritters.

marzipan *See* almond paste.

masala dosha *See* dosha.

mascarpone Italian; soft cream *cheese from the Lombardy region, usually eaten as a dessert flavoured with fruit; also used in *tiramisu.

mashing In the brewing of *beer, the process in which the malted barley is heated with water, to extract the soluble sugars and to continue enzymic reactions started during malting.

mash tun Vessel used for *mashing.

mashum *See* maslin.

mask To cover or coat a cooked meat dish with savoury jelly, glaze, or sauce; also to coat the inside of a mould with jelly.

maslin, mashlum 1 Old term, still used in Scotland, for mixed crop of beans and oats used as cattle food.
    2 In Yorkshire and the north of England, a mixed crop of 2–3 parts of wheat and 1 part of rye, used for bread making.

Mason jar Screw-topped glass jar for home bottling; patented 1858.

massecuite The mixture of sugar crystals and syrup (mother liquor) obtained during the crystallization stage of sugar refining.

mast *See* milk, fermented.

mastic (mastic gum) Resin from the evergreen shrub *Pistacia lenticus* and related species, with a flavour similar to liquorice, used in Greek and Balkan cookery.

mastication Chewing, grinding, and tearing foods with the teeth while it becomes mixed with saliva.

mastika Greek sweet, milky-white liqueur flavoured with *anise and *mastic.

matai Chinese water chestnut, *see* chestnut.

maté Also yerba maté, or Paraguay or Brazilian tea. Infusion of the dried leaves of *Ilex paraguayensis*. Contains caffeine and tannin.

matelote A rich, well-seasoned fish stew made with wine (French for 'sailors' dish').

matoké Steamed green *banana or *plantain.

matsutake Edible wild fungus, *Tricholoma matsutake*, widely collected in Japan and exported canned or dried; *see* mushrooms.

matzo, motza (matzoth is the plural) Unleavened bread or *Passover bread made as thin, flat, round or square water biscuits, and, according to the injunction in Exodus, eaten by Jews during the eight days of Passover in place of leavened bread.

maw Fourth stomach of the ruminant.

mawseed *See* poppy seed.

MaxEPA Trade name for a standardized mixture of long-chain marine *fatty acids, eicosapentaenoic (EPA, C20:5 ω3) and docosohexaenoic (DHA, C22:6 ω3) acids.

mayieritsa *See* Easter soup.

mayonnaise *See* salad dressing.

maysin Coagulable globulin protein of maize.

mazindol Anorectic (*appetite suppressing) drug used in the treatment of *obesity.

mazun *See* milk, fermented.

mazurki Russian; baked sweetmeat made from chopped raisins, almonds, walnuts, figs, prunes, candied fruit, flour, and eggs.

mazzard *See* gean.

mead A traditional wine made by fermentation of honey, sometimes flavoured with herbs and spices. One of the oldest alcoholic drinks.

mealie(s) *See* maize.

mealie pudding *See* skirlie.

mealie rice *See* maize rice.

meat Generally refers to the muscle tissue of animal or bird, other parts being termed *offal. 150-g portions of meat of all types (different cuts and different species including game and poultry), excluding bone, are rich *sources of protein and niacin; most are rich sources of vitamin B_2 and iron; sources or good sources of vitamin B_1.
*Venison, *horse meat, *goose, and *game birds are exceptionally rich in iron; *pork is exceptionally rich in vitamin B_1. The fat content and proportions of *fatty acids differ considerably between individual carcasses, species, and cuts of meat.
See also beef, lamb, veal, pork, rabbit, hare, goat, horse, venison, duck, chicken, goose, partridge, turkey, pheasant, grouse, quail, pigeon; and heart, kidney, liver, oxtail, sweetbread, tongue, tripe.

meat bar Dehydrated cooked meat and fat; a modern form of *pemmican; 50% protein and 40% fat; provides 560 kcal (2350 kJ)/ 100 g.

meat conditioning After an animal has been slaughtered, muscle glycogen breaks down and is metabolized to lactic acid, which tends to improve the texture and keeping qualities of the meat. Meat that has been left until these changes have occurred is 'conditioned'. *See also* DFD meat; rigor mortis.

meat, curing Pickling with the aid of sodium chloride (*salt), sodium nitrate (saltpetre), and some sodium nitrite, which permits the growth of only salt-tolerant bacteria and inhibits the growth of *Clostridium botulinum*. The nitrite is the effective preserving agent and the nitrate is converted into nitrite during the process. The red colour of cured meat is due to the formation of nitrosomyoglobin from the myoglobin of muscle.

meat extender Vegetable proteins (commonly textured soya protein) added to meat dishes to replace part of the meat.

meat extract The water-soluble part of meat that is mainly responsible for its flavour. Commercially it is made during the manufacture of *corned beef; chopped meat is immersed in boiling water, when the water-soluble extractives are partially leached out and concentrated. Rich in the B vitamins (particularly vitamins B_1, B_{12}, and niacin), meat bases, and potassium. Pavlov showed that meat extract is the most powerful oral stimulant of *gastric acid secretion.

meat factor Factor used to calculate the fat-free meat content of sausages and similar meat products from a *nitrogen estimation.

meat, reformed An artefact having the appearance of a cut slice or portion of meat, formed by 'tumbling' chopped meat, with or without the addition of finely comminuted meat, the soluble proteins of which bind the small pieces together.

meat speciation Identification of species of animal from which the meat originated.

meat sugar Obsolete name for *inositol.

meaux mustard *See* mustard.

medicinal paraffin Liquid paraffin, a mineral oil of no nutritive value since it is not affected by digestive enzymes and passes through the intestine unchanged. Used as a mild laxative because of its lubricant properties.

medlar The fruit of *Mespilus germanica*. Can be eaten fresh from the tree in Mediterranean areas but in colder climates, as in Britain, does not become palatable until it is half rotten (bletted).

medlar, Japanese *See* loquat.

Meeh formula *See* body surface area.

megavitamin therapy Treatment of diseases with very high doses of vitamins, many times the *reference intakes; little or no evidence for its efficacy; *vitamins A, D, and B_6 are known to be toxic at high levels of intake.

meio seco Portuguese; medium dry wines.

mejing *See* monosodium glutamate.

melampyrin *See* dulcitol.

melangeur Mixing vessel consisting of rollers riding on a rotating horizontal bed. Used to mix substances of pasty consistency (hence melangeuring).

melangolo Italian name for the bitter *orange.

melba Peach poached in vanilla syrup, set in vanilla ice cream with a purée of raspberries. Created by Escoffier, 1892, in honour of the Australian Soprano Dame Nelly Melba.

melba sauce Sweet sauce made from raspberries.

melba toast Originally a split slice of toasted bread, retoasted; now a thin slice of bread dried in the oven to a golden-brown colour. *See also* zwieback.

melegueta pepper *See* pepper, melegueta.

melena Black tarry faeces, containing digested blood, the result of bleeding in the upper gastro-intestinal tract.

melezitose Trisaccharide composed of two glucose and one fructose; hydrolysed to glucose plus the disaccharide turanose.

melibiose *Disaccharide of *glucose and *galactose.

melilot Sweet clover, a wild plant (*Melilotus officinalis*) which commonly grows in fields and on waste ground, especially on sandy soil; used as forage. The dried leaves have a sweet hay-like flavour.

melitose, melitriose *See* raffinose.

melitzane *See* aubergine.

melitzanosalata Greek; purée of *aubergine with onion, garlic, and olive oil, served cold as a dip.

mellorine US term for *ice cream made from non-butter fat.

melon *Gourds, sweet fruit of *Cucurmis melo*. A 200-g portion is a rich *source of vitamin C (melons with orange or yellow flesh are a rich source of carotene); a source of vitamin B_6; provides 2 g of dietary fibre; supplies 45 kcal (190 kJ). The water melon is *Citrullis vulgaris*.

melopita Greek; honey and cheese cake.

melting point The temperature at which a compound melts to a liquid. Often characteristic of a particular chemical and used as a means of identification. Particularly valuable as an index of purity, since impurities lower the melting point.

melts *See* spleen.

membrane, semi-permeable One that allows the passage of small molecules but not large ones: e.g. pig's bladder is permeable to water but not salt; collodion is permeable to salt but not protein molecules. *See* isotonic; osmotic pressure.

menadione, menaphthone, menaphtholdiacetate Synthetic compounds with *vitamin K activity; vitamin K_3, sometimes known as menaquinone-0.

menaquinones Bacterial metabolites with *vitamin K activity; vitamin K_2.

menarche The initiation of menstruation in adolescent girls, normally occurring between the ages of 11 and 15. The age at menarche has become younger in Western countries, possibly associated with a better general standard of nutrition, and is later in less-developed countries.

menhaden Oily *fish, *Brevoortia patronus*, *B. tyrannus*, from Gulf of Mexico and Atlantic seaboard of the USA, a rich source of *fish oils.

menu Commonly used to mean the list of foods and dishes served by a restaurant, but correctly a set meal (with options) or dish of the day, as opposed to à la *carte.

meringue Confection made from whisked egg-white and sugar, baked slowly in a cool oven; flavouring may be added, and the meringues may be filled with cream, ice cream, or fruit.

merlot One of the 9 'classic' *grape varieties used for *wine making; important in some of the great fragrant, rich, red wines; widely grown throughout the world.

merrythought *See* wishbone.

mersin Turkish; orange-flavoured liqueur.

mescal *See* tequila.

mesocarp *See* albedo.

meso-inositol *See* inositol.

mesomorph Description given to a well-covered individual with well-developed muscles. *See also* ectomorph; endomorph.

mesophiles Pathogenic micro-organisms that grow best at temperatures between 25 and 40 °C; usually will not grow below 5 °C.

MET *See* metabolic equivalent.

metabolic equivalent (MET) Unit of measurement of heat production by the body; 1 MET = 50 kcal/hour/m^2 body surface area.

metabolic rate Rate of utilization of *energy. *See* basal metabolic rate.

metabolic water Produced in the body by the oxidation of foods. 100 g of fat produces 107.1 g; 100 g of starch 55.1 g; and 100 g of protein 41.3 g of water. *See also* water balance.

metabolic weight *Energy expenditure and *basal metabolic rate depend on the amount of metabolically active tissue in the body, not the total body weight; body weight$^{0.75}$ is generally used to calculate the weight of active tissue.

metabolism The processes of interconversion of chemical compounds in the body. Anabolism is the process of forming larger and more complex compounds, commonly linked to the utilization of metabolic energy. Catabolism is the process of breaking down larger molecules to smaller ones, commonly oxidation reactions linked to release of energy. There is approximately a 30% variation in the underlying metabolic rate (*basal metabolic rate) between different individuals, determined in part by the activity of the *thyroid gland. *See also* energy.

metabolism, inborn errors *See* genetic disease.

metalloproteins Proteins containing a metal. For example, *haemoglobin, *cytochromes, peroxidase, ferritin, and siderophilin all contain iron; many enzymes contain copper, manganese, or zinc as a prosthetic group.

methaemoglobin Oxidized form of *haemoglobin (unlike oxy-haemoglobin, which is a loose and reversible combination with oxygen) which cannot transport oxygen to the tissues. Present in small quantities in normal blood, increased after certain drugs and after smoking; found rarely as a congenital abnormality (methaemoglobinaemia).

It can be formed in the blood of babies after consumption of the small amounts of nitrate found naturally in vegetables grown in certain areas and in some drinking water, since the lack of acidity in the stomach permits reduction of nitrate to nitrite.

methaglen (metheglin) A traditional British wine made from honey (and thus a form of *mead) to which herbs are added before fermentation. Originally for medicinal purposes.

methe *See* fenugreek.

methionine An essential *amino acid; one of the three containing sulphur; cystine and *cysteine are the other two. Cystine and cysteine are not essential, but can only be made from methionine, and therefore the requirement for methionine is lower if there is an adequate intake of cyst(e)ine. For this reason the sulphur amino acids are always considered together.

Methocel Trade name for methyl *cellulose.

méthode champenoise Sparkling *wines made by a second fermentation in the bottle, as for *champagne, but not in the Champagne region of north-eastern France.

Methofas Trade name for methyl hydroxypropyl *cellulose.

methylated spirits *See* alcohol, denatured.

methyl alcohol (methanol, wood alcohol). The first member of the alcohol series, chemically CH_3—OH. It is a highly toxic substance and leads to mental disturbance, blindness, and death when consumed over a period. It is added to industrial alcohol and *methylated spirits, to 'denature' the ethyl alcohol and render it undrinkable. *See* alcohol, denatured.

methyl cellulose *See* cellulose.

methylene blue dye-reduction test When the dye methylene blue or resazurin is added to milk, the bacteria present take up oxygen and change the colour of the dye; methylene blue loses its colour; resazurin changes from blue-purple to pink. The speed of the change indicates the bacterial content. *Pasteurized milk must not reduce dye in less than half an hour.

3-methyl-histidine Derivative of the amino acid, *histidine, found almost exclusively in the contractile proteins of muscle (myosin and actin). Useful, among other purposes, as an index of the lean meat content of prepared foods, since it is not present in collagen or other added materials.

metmyoglobin *See* nitrosomyoglobin.

metodo classico Italian; sparkling wines made by the *méthode champenoise.

meunière, à la Fish dredged with flour, fried in butter, and served with this butter and chopped parsley; literally, 'in the style of the miller's wife'.

mezethakia Also orekita; Greek; appetizers or hors d'œuvre; sometimes abbreviated to mezes or mezze.

micro In general use, very small; as a prefix for units of measurement, one millionth part (i.e. 10^{-6}); symbol μ (or sometimes mc). *See* Appendix I.

micro-aerophiles Micro-organisms that can grow in low concentrations of oxygen and so lead to spoilage of foodstuffs unless all oxygen is excluded.

microbiological assay Biological method of measuring compounds such as vitamins and amino acids, using *micro-organisms. The principle is that the organism is inoculated into a medium containing all the growth factors needed except the one under examination; the rate of growth is then proportional to the amount of this nutrient added in the test substance.

microcapsules *See* microencapsulation.

microencapsulation Preparation of small particles of solids, or droplets of liquids, inside thin coatings (e.g. beeswax, starch, gelatine, and polyacrylic acid). The microcapsules range from 1 to 100 nm in size. Used to prepare liquids as free-flowing powders or compressed solids, to separate reactive materials, reduce toxicity, protect against oxidation and control the rate of release; used for enzymes, flavours, nutrients, etc.

microfiltration Filtration under pressure through a membrane of small pore size (0.1–10 μm; larger pores than for ultrafiltration). Used for clarification of beverages and to sterilize liquids by filtering off organisms.

microgram One-thousandth part of a milligram, and hence 1 millionth part of a gram; symbol μg (occasionally mcg, and the obsolete symbol γ is sometimes used). *See* Appendix I.

micrometre (micron) One-thousandth of a millimetre, and hence one millionth of a metre; symbol μm. *See* Appendix I.

micronization Extremely rapid heating with infra-red radiation produced by heating propane on a ceramic tile or with nichrome wire elements. Suggested as an alternative to steam heating or toasting where the shorter heating time is less damaging to the foodstuff.

micronutrients *Vitamins and *minerals, which are needed in very small amounts (micrograms or milligrams per day), as distinct from fats, carbohydrates, and proteins which are macronutrients, since they are needed in considerably greater amounts.

micro-organisms Bacteria, yeasts, and moulds; can cause food spoilage, and disease (pathogens); used to process and preserve food by *fermentation and have been used as foodstuffs (single cell protein and mycoprotein). *See also* food poisoning.

microwave cooking Rapid heating by passing high frequency waves from a magnetron (in the UK 2450 or 896 MHz (million cycles/second)) through the food or liquid to be heated. Water absorbs the microwaves very well, so food with a high water content cooks more rapidly; fat absorbs the energy more slowly, so foods consisting of mixtures of fat and water cook unevenly. The cooking time is short and microwaves do not cause browning, so the food may not develop flavours associated with longer cooking times. Metal containers reflect the microwaves and cannot be used.

middlings *See* wheatfeed.

midori Japanese; pale-green liqueur made from melons.

mid-upper-arm-circumference (MUAC) A rapid way of assessing nutritional status, especially applicable to children. *See also* anthropometry.

mien (mi) Chinese; noodles made from wheat and ground dried beans.

mignardise Small, dainty dishes.

mignon Small or dainty; hence *filet mignon is small portions of beef fillet.

mignonette 1 Coarsely ground white pepper.
    2 *See* nouet.

milanaise, à la Dish garnished with spaghetti, tomato sauce, and ham or tongue. Also food dipped in egg and a mixture of breadcrumbs and cheese, then fried.

milchig Jewish term for dishes containing milk or milk products, which cannot be served with or after meat dishes. *See also* fleishig, pareve.

milfoil A common wild plant (*Achillea millefolium*, or yarrow) with finely divided leaves which can be used in salads or chopped to replace chervil or parsley as a garnish.

milk The secretion of the mammary gland of animals including cow, buffalo, goat, ass, mare, ewe, and camel, and of human beings. A 300-mL portion of cow's milk is a rich *source of vitamins B_2, B_{12}, calcium, and iodine; a source of protein, vitamin A, and vitamin B_1; full cream milk contains 11.4 g of fat of which 63% is saturated; supplies 200 kcal (840 kJ); skimmed milk contains 0.3 g of fat; supplies 100 kcal (420 kJ); Channel Islands milk contains 14.4 g of fat of which 68% is saturated; supplies 230 kcal (970 kJ).
    Ordinary milk contains 3.9% fat; Channel Islands milk, 5.1%; sheep's milk, 6.0%, buffalo milk, 7.5%; human milk contains 4.1% fat.
    A 280-mL portion of goat's milk is a rich source of vitamin B_{12} and calcium; a good source of vitamin B_2; a source of protein, vitamin A, zinc, and copper; contains 13.5 g of fat of which 51% is saturated; supplies 215 kcal (900 kJ).

milk, accredited Term not used after October 1954. Referred to milk untreated by heat, from cows examined at specific intervals for freedom from disease.

milk, acidophilus A preparation similar to cultured *buttermilk but soured by *Lactobacillus* spp. instead of acid-producing streptococci.

milk-alkali syndrome Weakness and lethargy caused by prolonged adherence to a diet rich in milk, i.e. more than about 1 L (2 pints) daily, and alkalis.

milk baby Infant with iron deficiency *anaemia caused by excessive ingestion of milk and delayed or inadequate addition of iron-rich foods to the diet.

milk, citrated Milk to which sodium citrate has been added to combine with the calcium and inhibit the curdling of *caseinogen which would normally occur in the stomach. Claimed, with little evidence, to be of value in feeding infants and invalids.

milk, designated Legally milk may be designated pasteurized or sterilized and also tuberculin tested.

milk, dried Milk that has been evaporated to dryness, usually by spray- or roller-drying. May be whole (full-cream) milk (26% fat), three-quarter cream (not less than 20% fat), half-cream (not less than 14% fat), quarter-cream (not less than 8% fat), or skim milk (1% fat).

milk, dye-reduction test *See* methylene blue dye-reduction test.

milk, evaporated, condensed Full-fat, skimmed, or partly skimmed milk, sweetened or unsweetened, that has been concentrated by partial evaporation; fat and total solids for each type defined by law (French: *lait demi-écrémé concentré* (4–4.5% fat); German: *kondensierte Kaffeesahne* (15% fat)).

milk fat test *See* Gerber test.

milk, fermented In various countries, milk is fermented with a mixture of bacteria (and sometimes yeasts) when the lactose is converted to lactic acid and in some cases to alcohol. The acidity (and alcohol) prevent the growth of potentially hazardous micro-organisms, and the fermentation thus acts to preserve the milk for a time.

   These fermented milks include busa (Turkestan), cieddu (Italy), dadhi (India), kefir (Balkans), kumiss (Steppes), laban Zabadi (Egypt), mazun (Armenia), taette (N. Europe), skyr (Iceland), masl (Iran), crowdies (Scotland), kuban, and yoghurt.

milk, filled Milk from which the natural fat has been removed and replaced with fat from another source. The reason may be economic, if the butter fat can be replaced by a cheaper one, or more recently, to replace a fat rich in saturated *fatty acids with a vegetable oil with a lower content of saturates.

milk, freezing-point test A test for the adulteration of milk with water. Milk normally freezes between −0.53 and −0.56 °C; when it has been adulterated the freezing point rises nearer to that of water. A freezing point above −0.53 °C is indicative of adulteration.

milk, homogenized Mechanical treatment breaks up and redistributes the fat globules throughout the milk to prevent the cream rising to the surface.

milk, humanized Cow's milk that has had its composition modified to resemble human milk, for infant feeding. The main change is a reduction in protein content, often achieved by dilution with carbohydrate and restoration of the fat content.

milk, irradiated Milk that has been subjected to ultraviolet light, when the 7-dehydrocholesterol naturally present is partly converted into *vitamin D.

milk, lactose-hydrolysed Milk in which the *lactose has been hydrolysed to glucose and galactose by treatment with the enzyme lactase, intended for infants who are lactase-deficient (lactose intolerant). *See also* disaccharide intolerance.

milk, long A Scandinavian soured milk which is viscous because of 'ropiness' caused by bacteria. *See* rope.

milk, Long-life Trade name for UHT milk.

milk, malted A preparation of milk and the liquid separated from a mash of barley malt and wheat flour, evaporated to dryness.

Milkman's syndrome Form of *osteomalacia with characteristic X-ray appearance of the bones; named after the American radiologist L. A. Milkman.

milk, methylene blue test *See* methylene blue dye-reduction test.

milk of magnesia Magnesium hydroxide solution used as an *antacid and *laxative.

milk, pasteurized *See* pasteurization.

milk, ropy *See* milk, long; rope.

milk-stone Deposit of calcium and magnesium phosphates, protein, etc., produced when milk is heated to temperatures above 60 °C.

milk shake Beverage made from milk whisked with fruit syrup and ice cream.

milk, sweetened, condensed Evaporated to less than one-third volume with sugar added as a preservative; may be full cream or skimmed. First patented in the USA and the UK by Borden in 1856.

milk teeth *See* deciduous teeth.

milk, toned Dried, skim milk added to a high-fat milk such as buffalo milk, to reduce the fat content but maintain the total solids.

milk, tuberculin tested (TT) Applied to milk from herd that has been attested free from bovine tuberculosis.

milk, UHT (ultra-high temperature). Milk sterilized for a very short time (2 seconds) at ultra-high temperature (137 °C).

milk weed *See* sow thistle.

milk, witches' *See* witches' milk.

mille-feuille Cake made of layers of puff pastry split and filled with cream and jam, and iced on top; also puff pastry savoury (literally, 'a thousand leaves').

millerator Wheat-cleaning machine consisting of two sieves, the upper one retaining particles larger than wheat, the lower one rejecting particles smaller than wheat.

miller's offal *See* wheatfeed.

millet Cereal of a number of species of *Gramineae* (grass family) smaller
than wheat and rice and high in fibre content. Common millet
(*Panicum* and *Selaria* spp.) also known as China, Italian, Indian, French
hog, proso, panicled, and broom corn millet, foxtail millet (*Setaria
italica*); grows very rapidly, 2–2¹/₂ months from sowing to harvest.
Protein 10%, fat 2.5%, carbohydrate 73%.

　　Red, finger, South Indian millet, coracan, or ragi is *Eleusine coracana*.
Protein 6%, fat 1.5%, carbohydrate 75%.

　　Bulrush millet, pearl millet, bajoa, or Kaffir manna corn is *Pennisetum
typhoideum* or *P. americanum*; the staple food in poor parts of India.
Protein 11%, fat 5%, carbohydrate 69%.

　　Other species are hungry rice (*Digitaria exilis*), jajeo millet (*Acroceras
amplectens*), Kodo or haraka millet (*Paspalum scrobiculatum*), teff (*Eragrostis
tefor*, *E. abyssinica*). *See also* sorghum.

milli As a prefix for units of measurement, one thousandth part
(i.e. 10^{-3}); symbol m. *See* Appendix I.

milling The term usually refers to the conversion of cereal grain into its
derivative, e.g. wheat into flour, brown rice to white rice.

　　Flour milling involves two types of rollers: (1) break rolls are
corrugated and exert shear pressure and forces which break up the
wheat grain and permit sieving into fractions containing varying
proportions of *germ, *bran, and *endosperm; (2) reducing rolls are
smooth and subdivide the endosperm to fine particles. *See also* flour,
extraction rate.

mills *See* ball mill; disc mill; querns; roller mill.

milt (melt) Soft roe (testes) of male fish. Also *spleen of animals.

miltone A toned milk (*see* milk, toned) developed in India in which
peanut protein is added to buffalo or cow's milk to extend supplies.

mimosa American name for a mixture of sparkling wine and orange
juice, known in the UK as buck's fizz.

Minafen Trade name for food low in *phenylalanine for treatment of
*phenylketonuria.

Minamata disease Poisoning by organic mercury compounds, named
after Minamata Bay in Japan, where fish contained high levels of
organic mercury compounds after waste water from mercury
processing was passed into the estuary.

minarine Name sometimes given to low-fat *spreads with less than the
statutory amount of fat in a *margarine.

mince 1 To chop or cut into small pieces with a knife or, more
commonly, in a mincing machine or electric mixer.

　　2 Meat which is finely divided by chopping or passing through a
mincing machine; known as ground meat in the USA.

mincemeat A traditional product made from apple, sugar, vine fruits,
and citrus peel with suet, spices, and acetic acid, coloured with
caramel. Preserved by the sugar content and acid. Also called fruit

mince. Originally a meat product; in the USA a spiced mixture of chopped meat, apples, and raisins.

mince pie Small pastry tarts, filled with *mincemeat, traditionally eaten at Christmas.

mineola A *citrus fruit.

mineralocorticoids A general term for the *steroid hormones secreted by the *adrenal cortex which control the excretion of salt and water. *See also* water balance.

mineral salts The inorganic salts, including sodium, potassium, calcium, chloride, phosphate, sulphate, etc. So called because they are (or originally were) obtained by mining.

minerals, trace Those *mineral salts present in the body, and required in the diet, in small amounts (parts per million): *copper, *chromium, *iodine, *manganese, *molybdenum, *selenium; although required in larger amounts, *zinc and *iron are sometimes included with the trace minerals.

minerals, ultra-trace Those *mineral salts present in the body, and required in the diet, in extremely small amounts (parts per thousand million or less); known to be dietary essentials, although rarely if ever a cause for concern since the amounts required are small and they are widely distributed in foods and water, e.g. *cobalt, *manganese, *molybdenum, *silicon, *tin, *vanadium.

mineral water Natural, untreated, spring waters, some of which are naturally carbonated, may be slightly alkaline or salty. Numerous health claims have been made for the benefits arising from the traces of a large number of minerals found in solution. They are normally named after the town nearest the source. Examples are Evian, Malvern, Apollinaris, Vichy, Vittel, Perrier.

Sparkling mineral water may either contain the gases naturally present at the source or may be artificially carbonated (*soda water, Seltzer water, or club soda). Carbonated beverages are sometimes called minerals.

miners' cramp Cramp due to loss of *salt from the body caused by excessive sweating. Occurs in tropical climates and with severe exercise; mining often combines the two. Prevented by consuming salt, perhaps in the form of salt tablets as used by athletes.

minestra Italian; vegetable soup, thinner than *minestrone.

minestrone Italian; thick mixed vegetable soup with pasta or rice.

mint Aromatic herbs, *Mentha* spp., including spearmint, *M. spicata*; peppermint, *M. piperita*. Garden mint is spearmint, *Mentha spicata*. Oil of peppermint is distilled from stem and leaves of *M. piperita*, and used both pharmaceutically and as a flavour.

mint jelly Apple jelly flavoured with spearmint (*Mentha spicata*), often eaten with lamb.

mint julep *See* julep.

mint sauce Mint (spearmint, *Mentha spicata*) chopped in vinegar, sometimes with sugar added; traditionally eaten with lamb in Britain.

mirabelle French spirit prepared by distillation of yellow-green mirabelle plums; strong fruity aroma, not sweetened. Similar to the German *quetsch.

miracle berry The fruit of the West African bush *Richardella dulcifica* (also known as *Synsepalum dulcificum*). It contains a taste-modifying glycoprotein (miraculin) that causes sour foods to taste sweet. Hence the name miracle berry.

miraculin The taste-modifying glycoprotein of the *miracle berry.

mirepoix Mixture of finely chopped carrots, celery, and onions, fried in butter and used to flavour meat dishes.

miso A Japanese sauce, prepared from autoclaved soya beans mixed with cooked rice and partly fermented with *Aspergillus oryzae* and *A. sojae* to form *koji. Salt is added to stop further mould growth, bacterial fermentation continues with the addition of *Lactobacillus* (1–2 months). Barley miso is an alternative to soya beans alone.

mistelles French; partially fermented grape juice.

mithi *See* clay.

mitochondrion (Plural mitochondria). The subcellular organelles in all cells apart from red blood cells in which the major oxidative reactions of *metabolism occur, linked to the formation of *ATP from ADP.

mixiria Process of preserving meat and fish by roasting them in their own fat and preserving in jars covered with a layer of fat.

mixograph American instrument for measuring the physical properties of a dough, similar in principle to the *farinograph.

mL Millilitre, one-thousandth of a litre. *See* Appendix I.

mocca Mixture of coffee and cocoa used in bakery and confectionery products.

mocha 1 Variety of arabica coffee.
   2 Flavoured with coffee.
   3 In the USA a combination of coffee and chocolate flavouring.
See also mocca.

mock brawn *See* head cheese.

mock fritters *See* French toast.

mock goose North of England; beef heart simmered in stock until tender, then stuffed, wrapped in fatty bacon, and roasted.

mock turtle soup Gelatinous soup made from calf's head, beef, bacon, and veal; similar to turtle soup, but without the *turtle; mock turtle is a calf's head dressed to resemble a turtle.

mode, à la Beef braised in the classic way; also (in America) fruit or other sweet pie served with ice cream.

modified atmosphere *See* gas storage, controlled.

molasses The residue left after repeated crystallization of sugar; it will not crystallize. Contains 67% sucrose, together with glucose and fructose and (if from beet) raffinose and small quantities of dextrans;

260 kcal (1100 kJ)/100 g; more than 500 mg iron per 100 g, with traces of other minerals.

mole Mexican; sauce made from sweet pepper, avocado, tomato, and sesame, flavoured with aniseed, garlic, coriander, cinnamon, cloves, chilli, and grated chocolate.

molluscs Marine bivalve shellfish with soft unsegmented bodies; most are enclosed in a hard shell; they include *abalone, *clams, *cockles, *mussels, *oysters, *scallops, *whelks, *winkles.

molybdenum A dietary essential mineral, required for a number of enzymes, including xanthine, aldehyde, and pyridoxal oxidases, where it forms the functional part of the coenzyme molybdopterin. Deficiency is unknown, and there are no estimates of requirements. Average intakes are between 50 and 400 µg/day, and are considered to be *safe and adequate.

molybdopterin *See* molybdenum.

mondogo Caribbean (Puerto Rico); tripe stew.

monellin The active sweet principle, a protein, from the serendipity berry, *Dioscoreophyllum cumminsii*, 1500–2000 times as sweet as sucrose.

monethanolamine *See* ethanolamine.

monkfish A white *fish, *Lophius piscatorius*.

monoacylglycerol *See* superglycerinated fats.

monocalcium phosphate *See* calcium acid phosphate.

monoglycerides *See* superglycerinated fats.

monophagia Desire for one type of food.

monosaccharides Group name of the simplest sugars, including those composed of three carbon atoms (trioses), four (tetroses), five (pentoses), six (hexoses), and seven (heptoses). Also known as monoses or monosaccharoses. These are the units from which *disaccharides, *oligosaccharides, and *polysaccharides are formed.

monosaccharose (monose) *See* monosaccharides.

monosodium glutamate (MSG) The sodium salt of *glutamic acid, used to enhance the flavour of savoury dishes and often added to canned meat and soups. Originally called Aginomoto. *See also* flavour potentiators; umami.

mono-unsaturates Commonly used short term for mono-unsaturated *fatty acids.

monstera Fruit of the Swiss cheese plant, *Monstera deliciosa*, also known as fruit salad fruit (Australia), and 'delicious fruit'.

montmorency, à la Sweet dishes and cakes which include cherries.

montmorillonite *See* fuller's earth.

mooli Long, white *radish; oriental variety of *Raphanus sativa* (same botanical group as ordinary red radish).

moonshine American name for illicit home-distilled spirit.

moorfowl (moorcock, moorgame) Scottish name for *grouse.

morcilla Spanish; *black pudding.

morel Edible fungus *Morchella esculenta*, much prized for its delicate flavour; *see* mushrooms.

Moreton Bay bug Or Bay lobster, a variety of sand lobster found in Australia.

mornay, à la Dish served with béchamel cheese sauce (mornay sauce).

mortadella *See* sausage.

mortoban *See* phyllo pastry.

morue French; *cod, especially salt dried cod.

moss, Irish *See* carrageenan.

mother of vinegar *See* vinegar.

mottled teeth In areas where the drinking water contains *fluoride at a level of several parts per million, dull, chalky patches, known as mottling, occur on the teeth. Also known as dental fluorosis. These teeth are relatively free from decay, and lower levels of fluoride, about 1 ppm, reduce decay without causing mottling.

motza *See* matzo.

mould bran A fungal *amylase preparation produced by growing mould on moist wheat bran; used as source of starch-splitting enzymes.

mould inhibitors *See* antimycotics.

moulds Fungi characterized by their branched filamentous structure (mycelium), including *mushrooms and smaller fungi.
(1) They can cause food spoilage very rapidly, e.g. white *Mucor*, grey-green *Penicillium*, black *Aspergillus*. Many also produce *mycotoxins. (2) Some are used for large-scale manufacture of citric acid (*Aspergillus niger*), ripening of cheeses (*Penicillium* spp.), and as sources of enzymes for industrial use. (3) A number of foods are fermented with moulds, e.g. *idli, *miso, and *tempeh. (4) The mycelium of *Fusarium* spp. is used as *mycoprotein. (5) Most of the antibiotics are mould products.

moule *See* mussel.

mountain chicken *See* crapaud.

moussaka Greek, eastern Mediterranean; minced lamb, potatoes, onions, and aubergine (and sometimes tomatoes), topped with *béchamel sauce and baked.

mousse Light frothy dish based on white or custard sauce or fruit purée to which eggs, whipped cream and sometimes gelatine are added. May be sweet or savoury, served hot or cold.

mousseline French; general term for light, fluffy dish. Mousseline sauce is Hollandaise sauce to which beaten egg-white or whipped cream is added just before serving, to give a frothy texture.

mozzarella Italian, now made elsewhere; soft white curd *cheese, originally made from buffalo milk, now normally from cow's milk. Mainly used outside Italy as a topping for *pizza, although in Italy it is also eaten uncooked.

MPD Modified *polydextrose.

MSG *See* monosodium glutamate.

MUAC *See* mid-upper-arm-circumference.

mucilages Soluble but undigested complexes of the sugars arabinose and xylose found in some seeds and seaweeds; used as thickening and stabilizing agents in food processing by virtue of their water-holding and viscous properties. The mucilage of ispaghula seeds serves as a laxative. *See also* gum.

mucin Naturally occurring complexes of protein and carbohydrates secreted in the saliva, intestinal tract, etc.; highly viscous.

muck hill *See* fat hen.

mucopolysaccharides *Polysaccharides containing an amino sugar and uronic acid; constituent of the mucoproteins of cartilage, tendons, connective tissue, cornea, heparin, and blood-group substances.

mucoproteins *Glycoproteins containing a sugar, usually chondroitin sulphate, combined with amino acids or peptides; occur in *mucin.

Mucor *See* mould.

mucosa Moist tissue lining, for example, the mouth (buccal mucosa), stomach (gastric mucosa), intestines, and respiratory tract.

mucous colitis *See* irritable bowel syndrome.

muesli Breakfast cereal; a mixture of raw cereal flakes (oats, wheat, rye barley, and millet) together with dried fruit, apple flakes, nuts, sugar, bran, and wheatgerm. Originated in Switzerland in the late nineteenth century.

   Although of variable composition, a 75-g portion is a good *source of vitamins B_1, B_2, niacin, and iron; a source of protein and dietary fibre; contains about 5 g of fat of which 20% is saturated; supplies 250 kcal (1050 kJ).

muffins *See* dough cakes.

mulberry Dark purple-red fruit of the tree *Morus nigra*, slightly sweet and acid, similar in shape and size to a raspberry or loganberry. There is also a white mulberry, *M. alba*. Of little commercial importance as a fruit; the leaves of the mulberry are the only food plant of the silk-worm.

mulled ale Beer that has been spiced and heated, traditionally by plunging a red-hot poker into the liquid.

mulled wine Wine mixed with fruit juice, sweetened and flavoured with spices (especially cinnamon, cloves, and ginger), served hot.

müller-thurgau A *grape variety widely used for *wine making, although not one of the classic varieties. The major variety in Rheinhessen and Pfalz in Germany.

mulligatawny Anglo-Indian; *curry-flavoured soup made with meat or chicken stock.

multiple sclerosis A slowly progressive disease involving nerve degeneration; it may take many years to develop to the stage of paralysis, and the disease is subject to random periods of spontaneous remission. There is some evidence that supplements of polyunsaturated *fatty acids slow the progression of the disease.

muscadet A *grape variety widely used for *wine making, although not one of the classic varieties; makes light, very dry wines; also known as melon de bourgogne.

muscat A *grape variety widely used for *wine making, although not one of the classic varieties; they mostly make perfumed, sweet, white wines.

muscle The contractile cellular unit of skeletal muscle is the cylindrical fibre, composed of many myofibrils. Chemically, muscle consists of three main proteins, actin, myosin, and tropomyosin, as well as structural proteins such as *collagen and *elastin. Contraction is achieved by formation of a complex between actin and myosin.

The muscle fibre is surrounded by a thin membrane, the sarcolemma; within the muscle fibre, surrounding the myofibrils, is the sarcoplasm. Individual fibres are separated by a thin network of *connective tissue, the endomysium, and bound together in bundles by thicker sheets of connective tissue, the perimysium.

mush American; cakes of boiled ground rice served cold or fried.

mushrooms Various edible fungi (botanically both mushrooms and toadstools); correctly the fruiting bodies of the fungi. Altogether some 300 species are sold, fresh or dried, in markets around the world; most of these are gathered wild rather than cultivated.

The common cultivated mushroom, including flat, cup, and button mushrooms is *Agaricus bisporus*, as is the chestnut or Paris mushroom. Other cultivated mushrooms include: shiitake (or Black Forest mushroom); oyster mushroom; Chinese straw mushroom.

Some wild species are especially prized, including field mushroom; horse mushroom; parasol mushroom; beefsteak fungus; blewits; wood blewits; cep or boletus; chanterelle; matsutake; puffballs; morels; truffles; wood-ears (or Chinese black fungus); yellow mushroom. Many other wild fungi are also edible, but many are poisonous, too.

A 50-g portion provides 1.5 g of dietary fibre and is a rich *source of copper; a source of vitamin B_2, niacin, folate, and selenium; supplies 6 kcal (25 kJ).

mussels (French: *moules*; German: *Miesmuscheln*.) Various marine bivalve molluscs, *Mytilus edulis, M. californianus*. A 100-g portion of boiled flesh (330 g with shell) is an exceptionally rich *source of iodine, a rich source of protein, iron, copper, and selenium; a good source of calcium, vitamin B_2, and niacin; a source of zinc, and contains 200 mg of sodium; supplies 90 kcal (380 kJ).

mustard Powdered seeds of black or brown mustard (*Brassica nigra* or *B. juncea*), or white or yellow mustard (*Sinapsis alba*), or a mixture. English mustard contains not more than 10% wheat flour and turmeric (still referred to in parts of England as Durham mustard, after Mrs Clements of Durham).

French mustard: made from dehusked seeds (the light-coloured

Dijon) or black or brown seeds with salt, spices, and white wine or unripe grape juice. Bordeaux (usually called French mustard) is black and brown seeds mixed with sugar, vinegar, and herbs. Meaux mustard is grainy and made with mixed seeds.

American mustard, mild and sweet, is made with white seeds, sugar, vinegar, and turmeric.

mutagenicity test *See* Ames test.

mutton (French: *mouton*; German: *Hammelfleisch*.) Meat from the fully grown sheep, *Ovis aries*. (*Lamb is from animals under 1 year old.) Depending on the cut, protein ranges are 12–18%; fat, 13–32%; energy, 195–380 kcal (820–1600 kJ). A 150-g portion of fillet (5% fat) is a rich *source of protein and niacin; a good source of vitamin B$_2$; a source of iron and vitamin B$_1$; supplies 180 kcal (750 kJ).

mycoprotein Name given to mould mycelium used as a food ingredient; *see* Quorn.

mycotoxins Toxins produced by fungi (moulds), especially *Aspergillus flavus* under tropical conditions and *Penicillium* and *Fusarium* species under temperate conditions. The problem is caused by storage of food under damp conditions which favour the growth of moulds. They include aflatoxin (on nuts and cereals), ochratoxin (on meat products and pulses), patulin (on fruit products), zearalenone, and stigmatocystin.

myo-inositol *See* inositol.

myristic acid A *saturated fatty acid consisting of fourteen carbon atoms.

N

naartje Afrikaans; a small tangerine; *see* citrus fruit.

NACNE National Advisory Committee on Nutrition Education (UK) An *ad hoc* working party that published a discussion paper on nutritional guidelines in 1983. *See* nutritional recommendations.

NAD, NADP Nicotinamide adenine dinucleotide and nicotinamide adenine dinucleotide phosphate, the coenzymes derived from *niacin. Involved as hydrogen acceptors in a wide variety of oxidation and reduction reactions.

nan Indian flat bread, an egg dough prepared with white flour and leavened with sodium bicarbonate, normally baked in a *tandoor.

nano As a prefix for units of measurement, one thousand-millionth part (i.e. 10^{-9}), symbol n; e.g. nanogram, ng. *See* Appendix I.

nantua, à la Dish garnished with crayfish.

naphthoquinone The chemical ring structure of *vitamin K; the various chemical forms of vitamin K can be referred to as substituted naphthoquinones.

napolitaine, à la Dish garnished with spaghetti, cheese, and tomato sauce.

nargizi *See* kofta.

naringenin *See* naringin.

naringin A *glycoside (chemically trihydroxyflavonone rhamnoglucoside) found in grapefruit, especially in the immature fruit. It is extremely bitter, and dilutions of 1 part in 10 000 parts of water can be detected. Sometimes found in canned grapefruit segments as tiny, white beads. Hydrolysed to the aglucone, trihydroxyflavonone (naringenin), which is not bitter.

nasi goreng Dutch, Indonesian; fried rice with chicken, prawns, etc., topped with strips of omelette.

nasogastric tube Fine plastic tube inserted through the nose and thence into the stomach for *enteral nutrition.

nasturtium Both the leaves and seeds of *Tropaeolum officinalis* can be eaten; they have a hot flavour. The seeds can be pickled as a substitute for *capers, and the flowers can be used to decorate salads.

national flour *See* wheatmeal.

natto Japanese; soya bean fermented using *Bacillus natto*.

natural foods A term widely used but with little meaning and sometimes misleading since all foods come from natural sources. No legal definition seems possible but guidelines suggest the term should be applied only to single foods that have been subjected only to mild processing, i.e. largely by physical methods such as heating, concentrating, freezing, etc., but not chemically or 'severely' processed.

natural water *See* mineral water.

nature-identical Term applied to food *additives that are synthesized in the laboratory and are identical with those that occur in nature.

naturel, au Plain; uncooked, or very simply cooked.

navarin French; ragoût of mutton with potatoes and onions or spring vegetables.

N balance (equilibrium) *See* nitrogen balance.

NCHS standards Tables of height and weight for age used as reference values for the assessment of growth and nutritional status of children, based on data collected by the US National Center for Health Statistics. The most comprehensive such set of data, and used in most countries of the world.

N conversion factor *See* nitrogen conversion factor.

NDpCal *See* net dietary protein energy ratio.

neapolitan ice Block of ice cream in layers of different colours and flavours.

neat's foot Ox or calf's foot used for making soups and jellies. Now called cow heels.

neat's-foot oil Oil obtained from the knucklebones of cattle; used in leather working and for canning sardines.

nebbiolo A *grape variety widely used for *wine making, although not one of the classic varieties.

nectarine Smooth-skinned peach (*Prunus persica* var. *nectarina*). One medium-sized fruit, 150 g weighed with stone, provides 3 g of dietary fibre and is a rich *source of vitamin A (as carotene); a good source of vitamin C; a source of copper; supplies 70 kcal (300 kJ).

neep Scottish name for root vegetables; now used for *turnip (and sometimes for *swede in England).

NEFA *See* non-esterified fatty acids.

negus Drink made from port or sherry with spices, sugar, and hot water.

NEL *See* No Effect Level.

nem Vietnamese; *spring rolls.

NEO-DHC *See* neohesperidin dihydrochalcone.

neohesperidin dihydrochalcone A non-nutritive *sweetener, 1000 times as sweet as sucrose; formed by hydrogenation of the naturally occurring *flavonoid neohesperidin.

neomycin *Antibiotic isolated in 1949 from *Streptomyces fradii*; has a broad spectrum of activity, and is not absorbed from the gut; commonly used to treat serious intestinal bacterial infections.

neroli oil Prepared from blossoms of the bitter orange by steam distillation. Yellowish oil with intense odour of orange blossom.

Nescafé Trade name for a dried, instant coffee. Contains more potassium than any other food, at 4%.

nesselrode, à la Implies the use of chestnuts; nesselrode pudding is made from chestnuts, custard cream, and candied fruit.

net dietary protein calories *See* net dietary protein energy ratio.

net dietary protein energy ratio (NDpE) A way of expressing the protein content of a diet or food taking into account both the amount of protein (relative to total energy intake) and the *protein quality. It is protein energy multiplied by *net protein utilization divided by total energy. If energy is expressed in kcal and the result expressed as a percentage, this is net dietary protein calories per cent, NDpCal%.

net protein ratio (NPR) A measure of *protein quality.

net protein utilization (NPU) A measure of *protein quality.

net protein value A way of expressing the amount and quality of the protein in a food; the product of *net protein utilization and protein content per cent.

nettle The young leaves of the stinging nettle, *Urtica dioica*, can be cooked as a vegetable and used to make nettle beer.

neural tube defect Congenital malformations of the spinal cord caused by the failure of the closure of the neural tube in early embryonic development. Supplements of *folic acid (400 µg/day) begun before conception reduce the risk.

new cocoyam *See* tannia.

New Zealand process Drying process applied to meat. It is immersed in hot oil under vacuum when it dries to 3% moisture in about 4 hours. The fat is removed from the dry meat in a hydro-extractor.

NFE *See* nitrogen-free extract.

niacin A *vitamin; one of the B complex without a numerical designation. It is sometimes (incorrectly) referred to as vitamin B_3, and formerly vitamin PP (pellagra preventative). Deficiency leads to *pellagra, photosensitive dermatitis resembling severe sunburn, a depressive psychosis, and intestinal disorders; fatal if untreated. Niacin is the *generic descriptor for two compounds in foods which have the biological activity of the vitamin: nicotinic acid (pyridine carboxylic acid) and nicotinamide (the amide of nicotinic acid). In the USA niacin is sometimes used specifically to mean nicotinic acid, and niacinamide for nicotinamide.

The metabolic function of niacin is in the *coenzymes NAD (nicotinamide adenine dinucleotide) and NADP (nicotinamide adenine dinucleotide phosphate), which act as intermediate *hydrogen carriers in a wide variety of oxidation and reduction reactions.

Nicotinamide can also be formed in the body from the amino acid *tryptophan; on average 60 mg of dietary tryptophan is equivalent to 1 mg of preformed niacin. The total niacin content of foods is generally expressed as mg niacin equivalents; the sum of preformed niacin plus one-sixtieth of the tryptophan. This means that most foods that are good sources of protein are also good sources of niacin: meat, fish, cheese, pulses, eggs. In cereals niacin is largely present as *niacytin, which is not biologically *available; therefore the preformed niacin content of cereals is generally ignored when calculating intakes. Free niacin is added to white flour and enriched breakfast cereals in many countries.

niacinamide American name for nicotinamide, the amide form of the vitamin *niacin.

niacinogens Name given to protein-niacin complexes found in cereals; *see* niacytin.

niacin toxicity High doses of nicotinic acid have been used to treat *hypercholesterolaemia; they can cause an acute flushing reaction, with vasodilatation and severe itching (nicotinamide does not have this effect, but is not useful for treatment of hypercholesterolaemia). Intakes of niacin above 500 mg/d (the reference intake is 17 mg/d) can cause liver damage over a period of months; the risk is greater with sustained-release preparations of niacin.

niacytin The bound forms of the vitamin *niacin, found in some foods, particularly cereals. Complexes of niacin with polysaccharides and peptides or glycopeptides; not hydrolysed by intestinal enzymes, so biologically unavailable, but can be liberated by acid or alkaline hydrolysis or by baking the cereal, especially with an alkaline baking powder.

nib *See* chocolate.

niceritol A derivative of the vitamin, *niacin (chemically penta-erythritol tetranicotinate) used in large doses (several grams) to reduce plasma *cholesterol levels.

nickel An ultra-trace *mineral; known to be essential for experimental animals, although its function is not known. There is no information on requirements. Metallic nickel is used as a catalyst in the *hydrogenation of fats.

niçoise 1 A garnish for meat with tomatoes, olives, and French beans.
    2 Soup garnished with tomato, flageolets, and diced potato.
    3 A sauce made from concentrated tomato purée blended with demi-glace.
    4 Salade niçoise contains tuna, anchovy, hard boiled egg, tomatoes, lettuce, and olives.

nicotinamide One of the vitamers of *niacin.

nicotinamide adenine dinucleotide (phosphate) *See* NAD.

nicotinate, sodium Sodium salt of *nicotinic acid; has been used, among other purposes, to preserve the red colour in fresh and processed meats.

nicotinic acid One of the vitamers of *niacin.

Nigerian berry *See* serendipity berry.

nigerseed *Guizotia abyssinica*, or nug; grown in India and Ethiopia as a food crop.

night blindness Nyctalopia. Inability to see in dim light as a result of *vitamin A deficiency. *See also* dark adaptation; vision.

nim leaf Sweet nim, an aromatic Indian herb with an aroma resembling that of *truffles.

ninhydrin test For proteins and amino acids (actually for the amino group). Pink, purple, or blue colour is developed on heating the amino acid or peptide with ninhydrin.

nioigome Perfumed rice.

nisin *Antibiotic isolated in 1944 from lactic streptococci group N; inhibits some but not all clostridia; not used medically. The only antibiotic permitted in Great Britain to preserve specified foods. It is naturally present in cheese, being produced by a number of strains of cheese starter organisms. Useful to prolong storage life of cheese, milk, cream, soups, canned fruits and vegetables, canned fish, and milk puddings. It also lowers the resistance of many *thermophilic bacteria to heat and so permits a reduction in the time and/or temperature of heating when processing canned vegetables.

nitrates Plant nutrient and natural constituent of plants; the inorganic form of nitrogen used by plants to synthesize protein; found in soils and included in inorganic fertilizer. Nitrate is a natural constituent of crops in amounts sometimes depending on the content of the soil. Also found in drinking water as a result of excessive use of fertilizers.

Health problems can arise because within a day or two of harvesting some crops nitrates are converted into *nitrites which can react with the *haemoglobin (especially foetal haemoglobin) in the blood to produce an oxidized form (*methaemoglobin) which cannot transport oxygen. Maximum levels have been established for nitrate levels in certain foods and drinking water (an upper limit of 45–50 mg nitrate/L drinking water has been recommended for infants).

Nitrate is also used, together with nitrite, for *curing meat products. *See also* nitrosamines.

nitrites Found in many plant foods, since they are rapidly formed by the reduction of naturally occurring *nitrate. Nitrite is the essential agent in preserving meat by pickling, since it inhibits the growth of clostridia; it also combines with the *myoglobin of meat to form the characteristic red *nitrosomyoglobin. *See also* nitrosamines.

nitrogen A gas comprising about 80% of the atmosphere; in nutrition the term 'nitrogen' is used to refer to ammonium salts and nitrates as plant fertilizers, to proteins and amino acids as animal nutrients, and to urea and ammonium salts as excretory products. In other words, all nitrogen-containing substances are loosely referred to as 'nitrogen'.

nitrogen balance (N balance) The difference between the dietary intake of nitrogen (mainly protein) and its excretion (as urea and other waste products). Healthy adults excrete the same amount as is ingested, and so are in N equilibrium.

During growth and tissue repair (convalescence) the body is in positive N balance, i.e. ingestion is greater than loss and there is an increase in the total body pool of nitrogen (protein). In fevers, fasting, and wasting diseases the loss is greater than the intake and the individual is in negative balance; there is a net loss of nitrogen from the body.

nitrogen conversion factor Factor by which total nitrogen content of a material (the factor measured chemically) is multiplied to determine the *protein; depends on the amino acid composition of the protein of the food. For wheat and most cereals it is 5.8; rice, 5.95; soya, 5.7; most legumes and nuts, 5.3; milk, 6.38; other foods, 6.25. Errors arise if part of the nitrogen is present as non-protein nitrogen. In mixtures of proteins, as in dishes and diets, the factor of 6.25 is used. 'Crude protein' is defined as N × 6.25. *See also* Kjeldahl determination.

nitrogen equilibrium *See* nitrogen balance.

nitrogen-free extract (NFE) In the analysis of foods and animal feedingstuffs, the fraction that contains the sugars and starches plus small amounts of other materials.

nitrogen, metabolic Nitrogen in the faeces derived from internal or endogenous sources, as distinct from nitrogen-containing dietary sources (exogenous nitrogen). This nitrogen consists of unabsorbed digestive juices, the shed lining of the gastrointestinal tract and bacteria from the intestine, and continues to be excreted on a protein-free diet.

nitrosamines Compounds bearing the nitroso group on the N of *amines. Found in trace amounts in mushrooms, fermented fish meal and smoked fish, and in pickled foods, where they are formed by reaction between *nitrite and secondary amines. They cause cancer in experimental animals, but it is not known whether the small amounts in foods affect human beings, especially since they have also been found in human gastric juice, possibly formed by reaction between amines and nitrites or nitrates from the diet.

nitrosomyoglobin The red colour of cured meat. It is formed by the reaction of nitric oxide from the pickling salts (saltpetre; a mixture of *nitrates and *nitrites) with *myoglobin in the meat. Fades in light to yellow-brown metmyoglobin.

nitrous oxide A gas used as a propellant in pressurized containers, e.g. to eject cream or salad dressing from containers.

NOAE With respect to food additives, No Adverse Effect Level, equivalent to *No Effect Level.

noble rot White grapes affected by the fungus *Botrytis cinerea*. It spoils the grapes if they are damaged by rain, but if they are ripe and healthy, and the weather is sunny, it causes them to shrivel and concentrates the sugar, so that top quality sweet wines can be made. *See also* wine classification, Germany.

nocino Italian; liqueur made from walnuts steeped in brandy or other spirit.

nockerln Austrian, German; small oval dumplings served with soups, stews, goulash, etc., known as noques in Alsace. Sometimes known as butternockerln since they are made with butter. Lebernockerln contain fried, finely chopped liver.

No Effect Level (NEL) With respect to food *additives, the maximum dose of an additive that has no detectable adverse effects. *See also* Acceptable Daily Intake.

noggin Traditional measure of volume of liquor = $1/4$ pint (140 mL); also known as a quartern.

N-oil *See* fat replacers.

noisette 1 Small round individual portions or slices of meat.
   2 French liqueur made from hazelnuts.
   3 Flavoured or made with hazelnuts.

non admis *See* wine classification, Luxemburg.

non-enzymic browning *See* Maillard reaction.

non-essential amino acids Those *amino acids that can be synthesized in the body and therefore are not dietary essentials.

non-esterified fatty acids (NEFA) Free *fatty acids in the blood, as opposed to *triacylglycerols, which are esterified fatty acids; about 10% of the total blood fatty acids, usually 0.5–2.0 mmol/L. The plasma concentration increases in fasting as fatty acids are released from *adipose tissue as a metabolic fuel. Also known as unesterified fatty acids (UFA) or free fatty acids (FFA).

non-nutritive sweeteners *See* sweeteners, non-nutritive.

non-pareils The silver beads used to decorate confectionery, made from sugar coated with silver foil or aluminium-copper alloy.

non-saponifiable fats *See* saponification.

non-starch polysaccharides (NSP) Those *polysaccharides (complex carbohydrates) found in foods other than *starches. They are the major part of dietary *fibre and can be measured more precisely than total dietary fibre; include *cellulose, *pectins, *glucans, *gums, *mucilages, *inulin, and *chitin (and exclude lignin). The NSP in wheat, maize, and rice are mainly insoluble and have a laxative effect, while those in oats, barley, rye, and beans are mainly soluble and have a blood-cholesterol lowering effect. In vegetables the proportions of soluble to insoluble are roughly equal but vary in fruits. It is recommended that the average UK adult intake of NSP should be increased from 13 to 18 g per day.

non-sugar sweeteners *See* sugar alcohols; sweeteners, non-nutritive.

noodles Type of *pasta made with flour and water, sometimes with added egg, the flour being made from various grains such as rice, wheat, buckwheat, and mung bean starch. Made into a vast range of shapes and sizes.

noodles, cellophane Chinese; transparent noodles.

noques *See* nockerln.

nor- Chemical prefix to the name of a compound, indicating: (1) one methyl (CH_3) group has been replaced by hydrogen (e.g. *noradrenaline can be considered to be a demethylated derivative of adrenaline); (2) an analogue of a compound containing one fewer methylene (CH_2) groups than the parent compound; (3) an isomer with an unbranched side-chain (e.g. norleucine, norvaline).

noradrenaline Hormone secreted by the *adrenal medulla together with *adrenaline; also a neurotransmitter. Physiological effects similar to those of adrenaline. Also known as norepinephrine.

norepinephrine *See* noradrenaline.

nori Edible seaweed, *Porphyra umbilicalis*.

norite Activated carbon used to decolorize solutions.

normande, à la Dish containing apples or (for fish) served with Normandy sauce and garnished with shrimps, truffles, crayfish, or mussels.

Normandy pippins Whole peeled and cored dried apples.

Normandy sauce White sauce made with fish stock, butter, and egg.

normocytes *See* blood cells, red.

Norwegian omelette *See* baked Alaska.

notatin *See* glucose oxidase.

nouet French; small muslin bag containing spices and herbs which is cooked in liquids to impart flavour without leaving solid particles. Also known as mignonette.

nougat Sweetmeat made from a mixture of gelatine or egg albumin with sugar and starch syrup, and the whole thoroughly aerated. Originated in Montellimar in southern France.

Novadelox Trade name for benzoyl peroxide used for treating (*ageing) flour.

novel foods Foods and food ingredients consisting of or containing chemical substances not hitherto used for human consumption to a significant extent in the locality in question (including micro-organisms, fungi, or algae and substances isolated from them, and organisms obtained using genetic modification techniques).

A food or ingredient to which has been applied a process not currently used for food manufacture or which has not been previously marketed and which gives rise to changes that affect its nutritional value or safety.

noyau Liqueur made from peach, apricot, plum, or cherry kernels, with a flavour of almonds.

NPR Net Protein Ratio, a measure of *protein quality.

NPU Net Protein Utilization, a measure of *protein quality.

NPV Net Protein Value, a measure of *protein quality.

NSP *See* non-starch polysaccharides.

nubbing Term used in the canning industry for 'topping and tailing' of gooseberries.

nucellar layer Of wheat, the layer of cells that surrounds the endosperm and protects it from the entry of moisture.

nucleic acids Polymers of *purine and *pyrimidine sugar phosphates; two main classes: ribonucleic acid (RNA) and deoxyribonucleic acid (DNA). Collectively the purines and pyrimidines are called bases. DNA is a double-stranded polymer (the so-called 'double helix') containing the five-carbon sugar deoxyribose. RNA is a single-stranded polymer containing the sugar ribose.

They are not nutritionally important, since dietary nucleic acids are hydrolysed to their bases, ribose and phosphate, in the intestinal tract; purines and pyrimidines can readily be synthesized in the body, and are not dietary essentials.

nucleoproteins The complex of proteins and *nucleic acids found in the cell nucleus.

nucleosides Compounds of purine or pyrimidine bases with a sugar, most commonly ribose. For example, *adenine plus ribose forms adenosine. With the addition of phosphate a nucleotide is formed.

nucleotides Compounds of purine or pyrimidine base with a sugar phosphate. Natural constituents of human milk, often used to supplement infant formulae.

nug *See* nigerseed.

nun's beads Scottish; small fried pastries filled with cheese.

nuoc mam Vietnamese, Cambodian; fermented fish sauce. The fish is digested by autolytic *enzymes in the presence of salt added to inhibit bacterial growth.

nutmeg Dried ripe seed of *Myristica fragrans*; mace is the seed coat (arillus) of the same species. Both mace and nutmeg are used as flavourings in meat products and bakery goods. Nutmeg contains myristicin, which is toxic in large amounts, and may cause vomiting and hallucinations in moderate excess.

nutraceuticals Term for compounds in foods that are not nutrients but have (potential) beneficial effects. *See also* functional foods.

Nutrasweet Trade name for *aspartame.

nutrient density A way of expressing the nutrient content of a food or diet relative to the energy yield (i.e. /1000 kcal or /MJ) rather than per unit weight.

nutrient enemata Rectal feeding can be carried out with nutrient solutions as the colon can absorb 1–2 litres of solution per day; maximum daily amount of glucose that can be given is 75 g (equivalent to 300 kcal, 1260 kJ), and 1 g of nitrogen, in the form of hydrolysed protein (equivalent to 6 g of protein). *See also* enteral nutrition; parenteral nutrition.

nutrients Essential dietary factors such as *vitamins, *minerals, *amino acids and *fatty acids. Metabolic fuels (sources of energy) are not termed nutrients so that a commonly used phrase is 'energy and nutrients' (calories and nutrients).

nutrification The addition of nutrients to foods at such a level as to make a major contribution to the diet.

nutrition The process by which living organisms take in and use food for the maintenance of life, growth, the functioning of organs and tissues, and the production of energy; the branch of science that studies these processes.

nutritional claim Any representation that states, suggests, or implies that a food has particular nutrition-related health properties. The extent of such claims on food *labelling and advertising are controlled by law in most countries.

nutritional disorder Any morbid process or functional abnormality of the body due to the consumption of a diet not conforming to physiological requirements, or to failure in absorption or utilization of the food after ingestion.

nutritional labelling Any information appearing on *labelling or packaging of foods relating to energy and nutrients in the food. The information which must or may be given, and the format in which it must appear, is governed by law in most countries.

nutritional melalgia *See* burning foot syndrome.

nutritional recommendations Recommendations comprising nutrient goals, food goals, and dietary guidelines. In addition to *reference intakes of nutrients, key recommendations in developed countries are reduction of total *fat intake to 30% of energy intake, with a more severe restriction of *saturated fats (to 10% of energy intake); increase of *carbohydrate intake to 55% of energy intake (with a reduction of sugars to 10% of energy intake); increased intake of *non-starch polysaccharides and reduced intake of *salt.

nutritional status The condition of the body in those respects influenced by the diet; the levels of nutrients in the body and the ability of those levels to maintain normal metabolic integrity.

nutritional status assessment For adults, general adequacy of nutrition is assessed by measuring weight and height; the result is commonly expressed as the *body mass index, the ratio of weight (kg) to height^2 (m). Body fat may also be estimated, by measuring *skinfold thickness, and muscle diameter is also measured.

For children, weight and height for age are compared with standard data for adequately nourished children. The increase in the circumference of the head and the development of bones may also be measured.

Status with respect to individual vitamins and minerals is normally determined by laboratory tests, either measuring the blood and urine concentrations of the nutrients and their metabolites, or by testing for specific metabolic responses. *See also* anthropometry; enzyme activation tests.

nutrition, enteral *See* enteral nutrition; nutrient enemata.

nutritionist According to the US Department of Labor, *Dictionary of Occupational Titles*, one who applies the science of nutrition to the promotion of health and control of disease, instructs auxiliary medical personnel, and participates in surveys. Not legally defined in the UK, but there is a Register of Accredited Nutritionists maintained by the Nutrition Society and Institute of Biology. *See also* dietitian.

nutrition, parenteral *See* parenteral nutrition.

nutrition policy (or planning) A set of concerted actions, based on a governmental mandate, intended to ensure good health in the population through informed access to safe, healthy, and adequate food.

nutrition surveillance Monitoring the state of health, nutrition, eating behaviour, and nutrition knowledge of a given population for the purpose of planning and evaluating *nutrition policy. Especially in developing countries, monitoring may include factors that may be potential causes of nutritional emergencies, in order to give early warning of such emergencies.

nutritive ratio In animal feeding a measure of the value of a feeding ration for growth (or milk production) compared with its fattening value. It is the sum of the digestible carbohydrate, protein, and 2.3 × fat, divided by digestible protein. (Energy yield of fat is 2.3 times that of carbohydrate and protein.) Value 4–5 for growth, 7–8 for fattening.

nutritive value index In animal feeding; intake of digestible energy expressed as energy digestibility multiplied by voluntary intake of dry matter of a particular feed, divided by *metabolic weight (weight$^{0.75}$), compared with standard feed.

nutro-biscuit Indian; biscuit baked from a mixture of 60% wheat flour and 40% peanut flour; contains 16–17% protein.

nutro-macaroni Indian; mixture of 80 parts wheat flour and 20 parts defatted peanut meal (total 19% protein).

nuts Hard-shelled fruit of a wide variety of trees, e.g. *almonds, *Brazil, *cashew, *peanut, *walnut: all have high fat content, 45–60%; high protein content, 15–20%; 15–20% carbohydrate. The *chestnut is an exception, with 3% fat and 3% protein, being largely carbohydrate, 37%. A number of nuts are grown specially for their oils; *see* oilseed.

nyctalopia *See* night blindness.

oats Grain from *Avena* spp., the three best-known being *A. sativa, A. steritis*, and *A. strigosa*. A 100-g portion (raw) is a rich *source of vitamin B_1; a good source of protein, iron, and zinc; a source of niacin; contains 9 g of fat of which 20% is saturated and 40% polyunsaturated, and 7 g of dietary fibre; supplies 375 kcal (1580 kJ).

Oatmeal is ground oats; oatflour is ground oats with the bran removed; groats are husked oats; Embden groats are crushed groats; Scotch oats are groats cut into granules of various sizes; Sussex ground oats are very finely ground oats; rolled oats are crushed by rollers and partially precooked.

obesity Excessive accumulation of body fat. A *body mass index (BMI, the ratio of weight (kg) to height^2 (m)) above 30 is considered to be obesity (and above 40 gross obesity). The desirable range of BMI for optimum life expectancy is 20–25; between 25 and 30 is considered to be *overweight rather than obesity. People more than 50% above *desirable weight are twice as likely to die prematurely as those within the desirable weight range. Overweight is often defined as 110–119% of standard, and obesity as 120% or more of standard range. *See* Appendix VII.

obesity drugs *See* anorectic drugs.

obstipation Extreme and persistent *constipation caused by obstruction of the intestinal tract.

octave A cask for wine containing one-eighth of a *pipe, about 13 imperial gallons (59 L).

octopus Marine creature (*Octopus* spp.) with beak-like mouth surrounded by eight tentacles bearing suckers.

oedema Excess fluid in the body; may be caused by cardiac, renal, or hepatic failure and by starvation (famine oedema).

oenin An anthocyanidin from the skin of purple grapes.

oestradiol, oestriol, oestrone *See* oestrogens.

oestrogens The female sex hormones; chemically they are *steroids, although non-steroidal compounds also have oestrogen activity, including the synthetic compounds stilboestrol and hexoestrol. These have been used for chemical caponization of cockerels and to increase the growth rate of cattle. *See also* capon.

Compounds with oestrogen activity are found in a variety of plants; collectively these are known as phyto-oestrogens.

offal Corruption of 'off-fall'. (1) With reference to meat, the term includes all parts that are cut away when the carcass is dressed, including liver, kidneys, brain, spleen, pancreas, thymus, tripe, and tongue. In the USA the term used is 'organ meats' or variety meat. (2) With reference to wheat, offal is the bran discarded when milled to white flour.

offal, millers' *See* wheatfeed.

offals, wheat *See* wheatfeed.

ohmic heating Sterilization by heat generated by passing an electric current through the food or mixture.

oil, frying, heavy duty Virtually any edible oil or fat can be used to fry foods; heavy duty oils can be used (commercially) for prolonged periods because they have been processed to resist breakdown by heat and air.

oilseed A wide variety of seeds are grown as a source of oils, e.g. cottonseed, sesame, groundnut, sunflower, soya, and nuts such as coconut, groundnut, and palm nut. After extraction of the oil the residue is a valuable source of protein, especially for animal feedingstuffs, as in oil-seed cake.

oils, essential *See* essential oils.

oils, fixed The *triacylglycerols (triglycerides), the edible oils, as distinct from the volatile or *essential oils.

oke *See* okolehao.

okolehao Hawaiian; liqueur made by distillation of fermented extract of the ti tree; also known as oke.

okra Also known as gumbo, bamya, bamies, and ladies' fingers; the edible seed pods of *Hibiscus esculentus*. Small ridged mucilaginous pods resembling a small cucumber, grown in South America, the West Indies, and India; used in soups and stews. There are two varieties: gomba are oblong, bamya are round. A 100-g portion (raw) is a rich *source of vitamin C; a good source of calcium; a source of carotene (500 µg), vitamin B_1, and folate; contains 4 g of dietary fibre; supplies 30 kcal (125 kJ).

okroschka Russian; sour, cold soup made from sour cream, soured milk, and *kvass (rye beer).

olallie berry Cross between *loganberry and *youngberry.

old clothes stew (Spanish: *Ropa vieja*.) Castilian; dish prepared from left-over cooked meat simmered with a *sofrito made from onions, red or green peppers, aubergines, tomatoes, and garlic.

old fashioned Alcoholic drink made from whisky, sugar, bitters, and soda water.

oleic acid Mono-unsaturated *fatty acid (C18 : 1 ω9); found to some extent in most fats; olive and rapeseed oils are especially rich sources. By far the most abundant of the unsaturated fatty acids, and beneficial in *heart disease.

oleomargarine *See* margarine.

oleo oil *See* premier jus; tallow, rendered.

oleoresins In the preparation of some spices such as pepper, ginger, and capsicum, the aromatic material is extracted with solvents which are evaporated off, leaving behind thick oily products known as oleoresins.

oleostearin *See* premier jus; tallow, rendered.

oleovitamin Preparation of fish liver oil or vegetable oil containing one or more of the fat-soluble *vitamins.

Olestra *See* fat replacers.

oligodynamic Sterilizing effect of traces of certain metals. For example, *silver at a concentration of 1 in 5 million will kill *Escherichia coli* and staphylococci in 3 hours.

oligopeptides Polymers of 4 or more amino acids; more than about 20–50 are termed polypeptides, and more than about 100 are considered to be proteins.

oligosaccharides Carbohydrates composed of 3–10 monosaccharide units (with more than 10 units they are termed *polysaccharides).

olive Fruit of the evergreen tree, *Olea europea*; picked unripe when green or ripe when they have turned dark blue or purplish, and usually pickled in brine. Olives have been known since ancient times. The tree is extremely slow-growing and continues to fruit for many years; there are claims that trees are still fruiting after 1000 years.

A 50-g portion (ten olives weighed with stones) contains 700 mg of sodium and 5 g of fat, of which 20% is saturated and 65% mono-unsaturated; supplies 40 kcal (170 kJ).

olive oil Pressed from ripe *olives, the fruit of *Olea europea*. Virgin olive oil is not refined and the flavour varies enormously with the locality where it is grown. Other types have been refined to varying extents. Used in cooking, as salad oil, for canning sardines, and for margarine manufacture. Apart from the special flavour of olive oil it is valued nutritionally because of its high content, 70%, of mono-unsaturates (mainly oleic acid) and its low content, 15%, of *saturates.

olives, beef *See* beef olives.

olla podrida *See* Madrid stew.

oloroso *See* sherry.

omasum *See* rumen.

omega-3, -6, or -9 (ω3, ω6, or ω9) fatty acids Three series of long-chain polyunsaturated *fatty acids derived respectively from linolenic, linoleic, and oleic acids. Omega (ω) or n being the position of the first double bond counting from the terminal methyl group. *See* Appendix X.

omega-3 (ω3) marine triglycerides A mixture of triacylglycerols (triglycerides) rich in two polyunsaturated *fatty acids, eicosapentaenoic acid (EPA, C20 : 5 ω3) and docosohexaenoic (DHA, C22 : 6 ω3).

omelette Egg whisked and fried. May be plain or filled with mushrooms, bacon, cheese, etc. Spanish omelette (*tortilla) is filled with potato. *See also* soufflé.

omelette, Norwegian *See* baked Alaska.

omophagia Eating of raw or uncooked food.

onglet French; cut of beef corresponding to the top of the skirt.

onion (French: *oignon*; German: *Zwiebel*.) Bulb of *Allium cepa*; there are many varieties with white, brown, and red (purple) skins. A 60-g portion, raw, supplies 20 kcal (80 kJ); boiled onions supply half of this.

onion, Egyptian (tree onion) *Allium cepa*, proliform group. A type that produces clusters of aerial bulbs which develop shoots to form a multi-tiered plant; the aerial bulbs are cropped.

onion, everlasting *Allium perutile*, similar to Welsh *onion.

onion, green *See* onion, spring; onion, Welsh.

onion, Japanese bunching *Allium fistulosum*, similar to Welsh onion, but larger.

onion, perennial *See* onion, Welsh.

onion, spring Young plants of *Allium cepa*, generally eaten whole (developing bulb and leaves) as a salad vegetable. Also known as salad onions or scallions. A 60-g portion (three onions) is a rich *source of vitamin C; a source of folate, calcium, and iron; contains 400 µg of carotene; provides 1.8 g of dietary fibre; supplies 15 kcal (65 kJ).

onion, Welsh The perennial onion, *Allium cepa perutile*, the leaves of which are cropped, leaving the plant to grow. Similar to, but smaller than, the Japanese bunching onion, *Allium fistulosum*. Also sometimes used as an alternative name for the *leek.

Oolong tea *See* tea.

opsomania Craving for special food.

optic Dispenser attached to bottles of spirits, etc., in bars to ensure delivery of a precise volume.

optical activity The ability of some compounds to rotate the plane of polarized light because of the asymmetry of the molecule. If the plane of light is rotated to the right, the substance is dextrorotatory and is designated by the prefix (+); if laevorotatory (rotated to the left), the prefix is (−). A mixture of the two forms is optically inactive and is termed racemic.

   Sucrose is dextrorotatory but is hydrolysed to glucose (dextrorotatory) and fructose, which is more strongly laevorotatory so hydrolysis changes optical activity from (+) to (−); hence, the mixture of glucose and fructose is termed invert sugar.

   (The obsolete notation for (+) was *d*- and for (−) was *l*-; this is separate from D- and L-, which are used to designate stereo-isomerism; *see* D-.)

optical rotation *See* optical activity.

opuntia *See* prickly pear.

orange *Citrus fruit, from the subtropical tree *Citrus sinensis*. Of nutritional value mainly because of its vitamin C content of 40–60 mg/100 g. Blood oranges are coloured by the presence of *anthocyanins in the juice vesicles. One medium orange (160 g) is a rich *source of vitamin C; a good source of folate; a source of vitamins A (as carotene) and B_1; contains 3.2 g of dietary fibre; supplies 60 kcal (250 kJ).

orangeade Carbonated beverage flavoured with orange juice and orange peel oil.

orange, bitter The fruit of the subtropical tree *Citrus aurantium*; known as Seville orange in Spain, bigaradier in France, melangol in Italy, and khush-khash in Israel.

It is used mainly as root stock, because of its resistance to the gummosis disease of citrus. The fruit is too acid to be edible, but is used in the manufacture of *marmalade; the peel oil is used in the liqueur *curaçao; the peel and flower oils (neroli oil) and the oils from the green twigs (petit-grain oils) are used in perfumery.

orange butter Chopped whole orange, cooked, sweetened, and homogenized.

orange Pekoe *See* tea.

orange, Seville *See* orange, bitter.

orcanella *See* alkannet.

oreganum Or Mexican sage; *see* marjoram.

orekita *See* mezethakia.

organic 1 Chemically the term means a substance containing carbon in the molecule (with the exception of carbonates and cyanide). Substances of animal and vegetable origin are organic; *minerals are inorganic.

2 The term organic foods refers to 'organically grown foods', meaning plants grown without the use of (synthetic) pesticides, fungicides, or inorganic fertilizers, and prepared without the use of preservatives. Foodstuffs must be grown on land that has not been treated with chemical fertilizers, herbicides, or pesticides for at least three years. Organic meat is from animals fed on organically grown crops without the use of growth promoters, with only a limited number of medicines to treat disease, and commonly maintained under traditional, non-intensive, conditions.

organic acids *Acids occurring naturally in foods that contain, as do all *organic compounds, carbon; e.g. *acetic, *citric, fumaric, *lactic, *malic acids. As distinct from the inorganic (mineral) acids such as hydrochloric and sulphuric acids, they can be metabolized in the body to provide 2.4–3.6 kcal (10.3–15 kJ) per gram for the various acids; for labelling purposes a value of 2 kcal (8 kJ/g) is used for all organic acids.

organ meat *See* offal.

organoleptic Sensory properties, i.e. those that can be detected by the sense organs. For foods, it is used particularly of the combination of *taste, texture, and astringency (perceived in the mouth) and aroma (perceived in the nose).

orientale, à l' Fish, eggs, or vegetables, cooked with tomatoes and flavoured with garlic and saffron.

ormer *See* abalone.

ornithine An *amino acid that occurs as a metabolic intermediate (e.g. in the synthesis of *urea), but not involved in protein synthesis. Of no nutritional importance, since it is not found in proteins and can be synthesized in adequate amounts in the body.

ornithine-arginine cycle The metabolic pathway for the synthesis of *urea.

orotic acid An intermediate in the biosynthesis of *pyrimidines; a growth factor for some micro–organisms and at one time called vitamin B$_{13}$. There is no evidence that it is a human dietary requirement.

ortanique A Jamaican *citrus fruit; a cross between orange and tangerine.

orthophenylphenol (OPP) A compound used for the treatment of *citrus fruit and *nuts after harvesting to prevent the growth of moulds (E-231). *Diphenyl (E-230) is also used.

ortolan Small wild song bird, *Emberiza hortulana*, still caught in the wild and eaten in parts of Europe, where it is prized for its delicate flavour.

oryzenin The major protein of *rice.

Oslo breakfast A breakfast requiring no preparation, introduced in Oslo, Norway, in 1929 for schoolchildren before classes started. It consisted of rye-biscuit, brown bread, butter or vitaminized margarine, whey cheese, and cod liver oil paste, $1/3$ litre of milk, raw carrot, apple, and half an orange.

osmazome Obsolete name given to an aqueous extract of meat regarded as the 'pure essence of meat'.

osmophiles Micro-organisms that can flourish under conditions of high *osmotic pressure, e.g. in jams, honey, brine pickles; especially yeasts (also called xerophilic yeasts).

osmosis The passage of water through a semi-permeable *membrane, from a region of low concentration of solutes to one of higher concentration. Reverse osmosis is the passage of water from a more concentrated to a less concentrated solution through a semi-permeable membrane by the application of pressure. Used for desalination of sea water, concentration of fruit juices, and processing of cheese whey. The membranes commonly used are cellulose acetate or polyamide of very small pore size, 10^{-4}–10^{-3} μm. *See also* osmotic pressure.

osmotic diarrhoea *See* diarrhoea.

osmotic pressure The pressure required to prevent the passage of water through a semi-permeable *membrane from a region of low concentration of solutes to one of higher concentration, by *osmosis.

ossein The organic matrix of the bone left behind when the mineral salts are removed by solution in dilute acid. Chemically similar to *collagen and hydrolysed by boiling water to gelatine; hence the manufacture of glue from bones, known as ossein gelatine.

osseomucoid Mucoid substance forming part of the structure of bone.

osso bucco Italian; veal stew.

osteocalcin A calcium-binding protein in bone, essential for the normal mineralization of bone. Its synthesis requires *vitamin K, and is controlled by *vitamin D.

osteomalacia The adult equivalent of *rickets; a bone disorder due to deficiency of *vitamin D, leading to inadequate absorption of calcium and loss of calcium from the bones.

osteoporosis Degeneration of the bones with advancing age due to loss of bone mineral and protein; this is largely a result of loss of *hormones with increasing age (oestrogens in women and testosterone in men). Although there is negative *calcium balance (net loss of calcium from the body) this is the result of osteoporosis, not its cause, and there is no evidence that calcium supplements affect the progression of the disease. A high calcium intake in early life may be beneficial, since this may result in greater bone density at maturity, but the most important factor is regular exercise to stimulate bone metabolism.

Vitamin D supplements do not improve osteoporosis, and may even exacerbate the condition. Nevertheless, an adequate intake of vitamin D is important for the elderly to prevent the development of *osteomalacia.

Ostermilk Trade name for dried milk for infant feeding. Ostermilk No. 1 is half-cream; No. 2 is full-cream.

oude Old (matured) Dutch *gin.

ouzo Greek; herb liqueur flavoured with *anise. Turkish equivalent is raki; Arabic arrack.

ovalbumin The albumin of egg-white; comprises 55% of the total solids.

Ovaltine Trade name for a preparation of *malt extract, milk, eggs, cocoa, and soya, for consumption as a beverage when added to milk. Fortified with thiamin, vitamin D, and niacin.

oven spring The sudden increases in the volume of a dough during the first 10–12 minutes of baking, due to increased rate of fermentation and expansion of gases.

overrun In ice cream manufacture, the percentage increase in the volume of the mix caused by the beating-in of air. Optimum overrun, 70–100%. To prevent excessive aeration US regulations state that ice cream must weigh 4.5 lb per gallon (0.48 kg/L).

overweight Excessive accumulation of body fat, but not so great as to be classified as *obesity.

ovomucin A carbohydrate-protein complex in egg-white, responsible for its firmness. Comprises 1–3% of the total solids.

ovomucoid A protein of egg-white, 12% of the total solids. It inhibits the digestive *enzyme *trypsin, but is inactivated by the stomach enzyme *pepsin.

oxalates Salts of *oxalic acid.

oxalic acid A dicarboxylic acid, chemically COOH—COOH. Poisonous in large amounts; present especially in spinach, chocolate, rhubarb, and nuts. The toxicity of rhubarb leaves is due to their high content of oxalic acid.

High concentrations of oxalates in the urine can form kidney stones; while most of these oxalates are of endogenous metabolic origin, patients with hyperoxaluria are advised to avoid dietary sources of oxalates.

oxidase, phenol *See* phenol oxidases.

oxidases (oxygenases) *Enzymes that oxidize compounds by removing hydrogen and reacting directly with oxygen to form water (or sometimes hydrogen peroxide). They thus differ from dehydrogenases, which transfer the hydrogen to an *intermediate hydrogen carrier.

oxidation The chemical process of removing electrons from an element or compound (e.g. the oxidation of iron compounds from ferrous to ferric); frequently together with the removal of hydrogen ions (H^+). The reverse process, the addition of electrons or hydrogen, is reduction.

In biological oxidation and reduction reactions, *cytochromes act to transfer electrons, while *coenzymes derived from the vitamins *niacin and *vitamin B_2 are intermediate hydrogen acceptors, transferring both electrons and H^+ ions.

Oxo Trade name for a dried preparation of hydrolysed meat, meat extract, salt, and cereal in cube form, used as a drink or gravy.

oxtail Classed as *offal; a 150-g portion of stewed lean meat is a rich *source of iron, vitamin B_2, protein, and niacin; contains 20 g of fat and supplies 360 kcal (1500 kJ).

oxycalorimeter Instrument for measuring the oxygen consumed and carbon dioxide produced when a food is burned, as distinct from the *calorimeter, which measures the heat produced.

oxygenases *See* oxidases.

oxyhaemoglobin *Haemoglobin combined with oxygen; the form in which oxygen is transported in the blood.

oxymel Medicinal syrup or beverage made from honey and vinegar.

oxymyoglobin Myoglobin is the muscle oxygen-binding protein; it takes up oxygen to form oxymyoglobin, which is bright red, while myoglobin itself is purplish-red. The surface of fresh meat that is exposed to oxygen is bright red from the oxymyoglobin, while the interior of the meat is darker in colour where the myoglobin is not oxygenated.

oxyntic cells Or parietal cells; glands in the stomach that produce the hydrochloric acid and *intrinsic factor of the *gastric juice.

oxytetracycline *See* tetracycline.

oyster (French: *huitre*; German: *Auster*.) Marine bivalve *mollusc, *Ostreidae* and *Crassostrea* spp. One dozen oysters (120 g of the edible portion) are an exceptionally rich *source of vitamin B_{12}; a rich source of iron, iodine, selenium, and vitamin D; a good source of protein and niacin; a source of vitamins A, B_1, and B_2, and supply 85 kcal (360 kJ).

oyster crabs American; small young crabs found inside oysters, cooked and eaten whole, including the soft shell.

oyster mushroom *Pleurotus ostreatus*, *see* mushrooms.

oyster plant (vegetable oyster) *See* salsify.

ozone Chemically composed of three atoms of oxygen, O_3. A powerful germicide, used to sterilize water and in antiseptic ice for preserving fish.

P.4000 A class of synthetic *sweeteners, chemically nitro-amino alkoxybenzenes. One member of the group, propoxy-amino nitrobenzene is 4100 times as sweet as saccharin, but these compounds are not considered harmless and are not permitted in foods. Dutch name is Aros.

PABA *See* para-amino benzoic acid.

pacificarins Compounds present in foods that resist micro-organisms; they may be of microbial origin or synthesized by the plant itself. Also known as phytoncides.

paddy *Rice in the husk after threshing; also known as rough rice.

paella Spanish (Valenciana) rice dish, seasoned with saffron, containing sea-food and chicken.

pain perdu *See* French toast.

pak hoy Chinese cabbage or Chinese leaves, *Brassica chinensis*.

pakora Indian; vegetables, shrimps, etc., deep-fried in batter made from chickpea flour.

PAL *See* physical activity level.

palak *See* spinach.

palatinose Isomaltulose. a *disaccharide of glucose and fructose.

palatone *See* maltol.

Palestine bee *See* bee wine.

Palestine soup English, nineteenth century, made from Jerusalem *artichokes and named in the mistaken belief that the artichokes came from Jerusalem.

palmier Cake made from puff pastry sandwiched with cream or jam. Also small sweet biscuits made from puff pastry.

palmitic acid A saturated *fatty acid with sixteen carbon atoms (C16 : 0), common in the triglycerides of many animal and vegetable fats.

palmitoleic acid A mono-unsaturated fatty acid with sixteen carbon atoms (C16 : 1 ω9), widespread in fats and oils.

palm kernel oil One of the major oils of commerce, widely used in cooking fats and margarines; oil extracted from the kernel of the nut of the oil palm, *Elaeis guineensis*, pale in colour in contrast with 'red' *palm oil from the outer part of the nut; about 80% saturates and 15% mono-unsaturates.

palm oil From outer fibrous pulp of the fruit of the oil palm, *Elaeis guineensis*. Coloured red because of very high content of α-carotene (30 mg per 100 g) and β-carotene (30 mg) (together with about 60 mg vitamin E), but these are usually removed to produce a pale oil; 45% *saturated and 40% mono-unsaturated, 10% polyunsaturated.

palm stew West African; prepared by stewing the entire head of nuts of the oil palm *Elaeis guineensis*, and skimming off the oil as it separates. Although most of the oil is removed, the final dish has a deep red colour because of the high content of carotenes of *palm oil.

palm, wild date *Phoenix sylvestris*, a relative of the true date palm, *P. dactylifera*, grown in India as a source of sugar, obtained from the sap.

palm wine Fermented sap from various palm trees, especially date and coconut palms.

palomino A *grape variety widely used for *wine making, although not one of the classic varieties.

pan *See* betel.

panada Mixture of fat, flour, and liquid (stock or milk) mixed to a thick paste; used to bind mixtures such as chopped meat, and also as the basis of soufflés and choux *pastry.

panage French; to coat food with breadcrumbs before frying or grilling. Food so treated is *pané*.

panary fermentation Yeast fermentation of dough in bread making.

pan broil American; to cook food in a pan on top of the stove, dry and with enough oil only to prevent it sticking.

pancake Batter fried on a lightly greased griddle. Served plain (with lemon and sugar) or filled with sweet or savoury mixture.

pancake rolls *See* spring rolls.

pancetta Italian; spiced pickled *bacon, rolled in the form of a long sausage.

pancreas A gland in the abdomen with two functions: the endocrine pancreas (the islets of Langerhans) secretes the *hormones *insulin and *glucagon; the exocrine pancreas secretes the *pancreatic juice. Known by the butcher as sweetbread or gut sweetbread as distinct from chest sweetbread which is thymus.

A 150-g portion (coated and fried) is a rich *source of protein, niacin, and iron; unusually for a meat product, a good source of vitamin C; contains about 20 g of fat of which one-third is saturated, and supplies 350 kcal (1470 kJ).

pancreatic juice The alkaline digestive juice produced by the pancreas and secreted into the duodenum. It contains the inactive precursors of a number of *protein digestive enzymes. Trypsinogen is activated to trypsin by *enteropeptidase in the intestinal lumen; in turn, trypsin activates the other enzyme precursors: chymotrypsinogen to chymotrypsin, pro-elastase to elastase, procarboxypeptidase to carboxypeptidase. Also contains *lipase, *amylase, and nucleases.

pancreatin Preparation made from the pancreas of animals containing the enzymes of *pancreatic juice. Used to replace pancreatic enzymes in *cystic fibrosis as an aid to digestion.

pancreozymin Hormone produced by the intestinal mucosa which, together with *secretin, stimulates the secretion of *pancreatic juice.

pan dowdy American; baked apple sponge pudding, served with the apple side up.

panettone Italian, half bread and half cake; sweet, with candied peel and sultanas; a speciality of Lombardy.

pangamic acid Chemically the N-di-isopropyl derivative of glucuronic acid. Claimed to be an *antioxidant, and to speed recovery from fatigue. Sometimes called vitamin B_{15}, but there is no evidence that it is a dietary essential, nor that it has any metabolic function.

panne French; the fat surrounding the pig's kidneys. See lard.

pannfisch German; large fried fishcake.

panoufle French; the underpart of the top of a sirloin of beef.

panperdy (pain perdu) See French toast.

panthenol The alcohol form of *pantothenic acid; biologically active.

pantothenic acid A vitamin of the B complex with no numerical designation. Chemically, the β-alanine derivative of pantoic acid. Required for the synthesis of *coenzyme A (and hence essential for the metabolism of fats, carbohydrates, and amino acids) and of acyl carrier protein (and hence essential for the synthesis of fatty acids).

Dietary deficiency is unknown; it is widely distributed in all living cells, the best sources being liver, kidney, yeast, and fresh vegetables. Human requirements are not known with any certainty; average intakes are between 3 and 7 mg/d, which is therefore considered to be a *safe and adequate level of intake.

Experimental deficiency signs in rats include greying of the hair (hence at one time known as the anti-grey-hair factor; there is no evidence that it affects greying of human hair with age). Experimental deficiency in human beings leads to fatigue, headache, muscle weakness, and gastro-intestinal disturbances. See also burning foot syndrome.

pao-tzu Chinese; see steamed buns.

papain *Proteolytic *enzyme from the juice of the *pawpaw (Carica papaya) used in tenderizing meat; sometimes called vegetable pepsin. The enzyme is obtained as the dried latex on the skin of the fruit by scratching it while still on the tree, and collecting the flow. In the tropics meat is often tenderized by wrapping in pawpaw leaves.

The rate of reaction is slow at room temperature, increasing to maximum activity at 80 °C and rapidly inactivated at higher temperatures; hence, the papain continues to tenderize the meat during the early stages of cooking.

papaw Purple fruit of Asiminia triloba, related to the *custard apple; distinct from the *pawpaw or papaya.

papaya See pawpaw.

papillote, en Made or served in a paper case.

Papin's digester Early version of the pressure cooker. Named after D. Papin, French physicist, 1647–1712; originally invented for the purpose of softening bones for the preparation of *gelatine. *See* autoclave.

papoutsakia Greek; stuffed aubergines (literally 'little shoes').

paprika *See* pepper.

PAR *See* physical activity ratio.

para-amino benzoic acid (PABA) Essential growth factor for micro-organisms. It forms part of the molecule of *folic acid and is therefore required for the synthesis of this vitamin. Mammals cannot synthesize folic acid, and PABA has no other known function; there is no evidence that it is a human dietary requirement.

Sulphanilamides (sulpha drugs) are chemical analogues of PABA, and exert their antibacterial action by antagonizing PABA utilization.

parabens Methyl, ethyl, and propyl esters of *p*-hydroxybenzoic acid used together with their sodium salts as antimicrobials in food (E-214–219). Effective over a wide range of *pH; more effective against moulds and yeast than against bacteria.

paracasein Obsolete name for milk *casein after precipitation.

paraffin, medicinal (liquid) *See* medicinal paraffin.

Paraflow Trade name for a plate heat exchanger used for pasteurizing liquids.

parakeratosis Disease of swine characterized by cessation of growth, erythema, seborrhoea, and hyperkeratosis of the skin; due to *zinc deficiency and possibly to changes in essential *fatty acid metabolism.

paralactic acid *See* sarcolactic acid.

paralytic shellfish poisoning Caused by shellfish that have accumulated toxins from the dinoflagellate plankton, *Gonyaulax* spp.

parasol mushroom *Macrolepiota procera*, *see* mushrooms.

paratha Indian whole-wheat unleavened bread; the dough is rolled and brushed repeatedly with melted butter before cooking on a buttered griddle. Frequently stuffed with spiced potato or other vegetables.

parathormone Commonly used as an abbreviation for the *parathyroid hormone; correctly a trade name for a pharmaceutical preparation of the hormone.

parathyroid hormone The hormone secreted by the parathyroid glands; four glands situated in the neck near to the thyroid gland but not connected with its function. The hormone is secreted in response to a fall in plasma calcium, and acts on the kidney to increase the formation of the active metabolite of *vitamin D (calcitriol), leading to an increase in plasma calcium by increasing intestinal absorption and mobilizing the mineral from bones. It also reduces urinary excretion of phosphate.

parboil Partially cook. Of special interest in nutrition is the parboiling of brown rice, i.e. steaming rice in the husk before milling. The water-soluble vitamins diffuse from the husk into the grain; when the rice is polished, it contains far more of these vitamins than polished raw rice.

parch To brown in dry heat.

parcha Indian; foods cooked en papillote; wrapped in parchment or banana leaf.

parchita *See* passion fruit.

pare To peel or trim.

parenteral nutrition Slow infusion of solution of nutrients into the veins through a catheter. This may be partial, to supplement food and nutrient intake, or total (TPN, total parenteral nutrition), providing the sole source of energy and nutrient intake for patients with major intestinal problems. Parenteral means not enteral, or through the intestinal tract; *see also* enteral nutrition; nutrient enemata.

pareve (parve) Jewish term for dishes containing neither milk nor meat. Orthodox Jewish law prohibits mixing of milk and meat foods or the consumption of milk products for 3 hours after a meat meal. *See also* milchig, fleishig.

parfait Frozen dessert, similar to a *mousse but lighter.

parietal cells *See* oxyntic cells.

parillin Highly toxic glycoside from *sarsaparilla root; consists of glucose, rhamnose and parigenin. Also known as smilacin.

parkin English (Yorkshire); oatmeal, ginger, and treacle cake.

parlies Scottish; ginger cakes, believed to be so named because they were eaten by members of the Scottish parliament.

parma ham (*Prosciutto do Parma, prosciutto crudo*), Italian; smoked, raw ham served in very thin slices.

parmentier French; made or served with potatoes, named after Parmentier, who popularized the potato in France in the eighteenth century. Pommes parmentier are diced and fried; parmentier soup is a leek and potato soup.

parmesan cheese English (and French) name for the hard Italian cheese parmigiana. Made from semi-skimmed cow's milk cooked with rennet, dried for six months, and then coated with a black substance to make the product airtight. When at least 2 years old it is called vecchio; stravecchio is 3 years old; stravecchione, 4 years old. It is hard and usually served on dishes grated; it cooks without becoming sticky. A 25-g portion is a rich *source of calcium, a good source of protein, a source of vitamin A and niacin, contains 8 g of fat and 250 mg of sodium, and supplies 110 kcal (460 kJ).

parmigiana Made or served with *parmesan cheese.

PARNUTS An EU term for foods prepared for particular nutritional purposes (intended for people with disturbed metabolism, or in special physiological conditions, or for young children). Also called dietetic foods.

parsley Leaves of the herb *Petroselinum crispum, P. hertense,* or *P. sativum.* Since it is largely used as a garnish and for flavouring, the nutrients per serving are negligible.

parsley, Hamburg Root of *Petroselinum crispum* var. *tuberosum*, grown for its root (also called turnip-rooted parsley); similar in appearance to *parsnip. A 100-g portion is a rich source of vitamin C and supplies 40 kcal (170 kJ).

parsnip Root of *Pastinaca sativa*, eaten as a vegetable. A 100-g portion, boiled, is a good *source of folate; a source of vitamin C; contains 5 g of dietary fibre; supplies 70 kcal (290 kJ).

parson's nose The small fatty joint holding the tail feathers of poultry. Also known as pope's nose.

partridge *Game bird, *Perdix perdix* and related spp. A 150-g portion is a rich *source of protein and iron; contains 10 g of fat of which one-third is saturated, and supplies 200 kcal (840 kJ).

parts per million (ppm) Method of describing small concentrations and means exactly what the term says. Mg per kg is also ppm. Usually used with regard to traces of contaminants and food additives.

pasendah *See* pursindah.

pashka Russian; dessert of curd cheese with cream, almonds, and dried fruit, an Easter speciality.

passion fruit Also known as parchita, granadilla, and water lemon; fruit of the tropical American vine, *Passiflora* spp. Purple or greenish-yellow when ripe, it contains watery pulp surrounding small seeds; used in fruit drinks. A 100-g portion (four fruits, 60 g of edible flesh and pips) is a good *source of vitamin C; supplies 20 kcal (85 kJ).

Passover The Jewish festival celebrating the Exodus from slavery in Egypt. There was no time to allow bread dough to rise, and unleavened bread was eaten. In commemoration, Jews abstain from leavened bread for the week of Passover, eating *matzo instead, and using matzo meal or potato flour for baking. Foods certified free from leavened bread are known as 'kosher for Passover'. *See also* kosher.

pasta (Alimentary paste); dried dough, traditionally made with hard wheat (semolina) but soft wheat may be added, sometimes with egg and milk. Spinach or tomato may be added to the dough to give a green or red colour. The dough is partly dried in hot air, then more slowly. Sold both completely dry, when it can be stored for a long period, or 'fresh', i.e. less dried and keeping for a week or so only. A 230-g portion (boiled) is a good *source of copper; a source of protein; contains 4.6 g of dietary fibre and 0.7 g of fat of which 33% is saturated; supplies 280 kcal (1180 kJ).

It is made in numerous shapes: spaghetti is a solid rod about 2 mm in diameter; vermicelli is about one-third this thickness; ravioli (envelopes stuffed with meat or cheese), fettucine, and linguini (ribbons), and a range of twists, spirals, and other shapes. Macaroni is tubular shaped, about 5 mm in diameter; at 10 mm it is known as zitoni, and at 15 mm fovantini or maccaroncelli. Cannelloni are tubes 1.5–2 cm wide and 10 cm long, stuffed with meat; penne are nib-shaped. Lasagne is sheets of pasta. Farfals are ground, granulated, or shredded.

pasteurization A means of prolonging the storage time of foods for a limited time, by killing the vegetative forms of many pathogenic organisms. This can be done by mild heat treatment, whereas destruction of all bacteria and spores (sterilization) requires higher temperatures for longer periods, often spoiling the product in the process.

In flash pasteurization, the product is held at a higher temperature than for normal pasteurization, but for a shorter time, so that there is less development of a cooked flavour.

Pasteurization of milk destroys all pathogens, and although it will sour within a day or two, this is not a source of disease. It is achieved either by heating to 63–66 °C for 30 minutes (holder method), followed by immediate cooling, or (the high-temperature short-time process) heating to 71 °C for 15 seconds. The efficacy of pasteurization is checked by either the *methylene blue dye reduction test or the *phosphatase test.

pasteurizer Equipment used to pasteurize liquids such as milk, fruit juices, etc. The material is passed continuously over heated plates, or through pipes, where it is heated to the required temperature, maintained for the required time, then immediately cooled.

pastille Round, flat sweet, often coated with sugar, sometimes medicated.

pastis French; spirit prepared by distilling anise and liquorice as opposed to *anise, which is prepared by steeping the herbs in spirit.

pastourma Greek and Turkish; black-rinded smoked bacon, highly flavoured with garlic; generally fried until crisp.

pastrami Middle-European (especially Romanian-Jewish); smoked and seasoned beef, also made from turkey. Known in Canada as smoked beef.

pastry Baked dough of flour, fat, and water. There are six basic types: shortcrust, in which the fat is rubbed into the flour; suet crust, in which chopped suet is mixed with the flour; puff and flaky, in which the fat is rolled into the dough; hotwater crust and choux, in which the fat is melted in hot water before being added to the flour (choux pastry also contains eggs and is whisked to a paste before cooking). *Phyllo pastry is made from flour and water only.

Suet pastry is raised using baking powder or self-raising flour; puff and flaky and choux pastry are raised by the steam trapped between layers of dough.

pasty Individual dish enclosed in pastry, folded over, and baked on a flat tray.

patatas bravas Spanish; fried slices of potato eaten with a *mayonnaise strongly flavoured with garlic.

pâte French for paste; used for pastry, dough, or batter, also for *pasta.

pâté Literally, French for a savoury pie, now used almost exclusively to mean a savoury paste of liver, meat, or fish.

patent flour Flour of 30–50% *extraction rate; mainly the endosperm of the grain.

pathogens Disease-causing bacteria, as distinct from those that are harmless.

pâtisserie French; ornate small cakes and pastries.

patri *See* clay.

patsa Greek tripe soup.

patty Small savoury pie, normally made with short-crust pastry; also (in the USA) small cakes of minced meat or poultry, like croquettes but not dipped in breadcrumbs before cooking.

patulin *Mycotoxin found in juice from fruits infected with one of a variety of moulds (*Penicillium expansum*, *Aspergillus clavatus*, *A. terreus*, and *Byssochlamys nivea*). Removed by fermentation and also pasteurization.

patum peperium *See* Gentleman's relish.

paunching To remove the entrails of rabbits, hares, etc.

paupiette Small, thinly cut piece of meat wrapped round a filling of forcemeat and braised.

pavé French; sweet or savoury cold dish made in a square or rectangular mould.

pavlova Australian; meringue cake topped with fruit and whipped cream; created in honour of the Russian ballerina Anna Pavlova on her visit to Australia in the 1920s.

pawpaw (papaya) Large green or yellow melon-like fruit of the tropical tree *Carica papaya*, widely grown in all tropical regions. The proteolytic enzyme, *papain, is derived from the fruit. A 150-g portion is a rich *source of vitamin C; a good source of vitamin A (as carotene); supplies 55 kcal (230 kJ).

paysanne, à la Peasant or simple country style. Meat or poultry, usually braised and accompanied by a garnish of mixed vegetables, bacon, etc.

payusnaya Russian, Eastern European; coarse, pressed *caviare including skins of ovaries.

PBI *See* protein-bound iodine.

PCM Protein-calorie malnutrition; *see* protein-energy malnutrition.

peanut Fruit of *Arachis hypogaea*, also known as groundnut, earth-nut, arachis nut, monkey nut. A 60-g portion (sixty nuts) is a rich *source of protein, niacin, and vitamins E and B_1, a good source of copper and zinc, and a source of protein, vitamin B_6, folate, and iron. When dry-roasted or roasted and salted some of the vitamin B_1 is damaged and the nuts are only a source of this vitamin; dry-roasted peanuts usually contain about 500 mg of sodium per 60-g portion, and roast and salted about 250 mg. All three types contain 30 g of fat per portion of which 20% is *saturated and 50% mono-unsaturated; and supply 350 kcal (1470 kJ).

peanut butter Ground, roasted peanuts; commonly prepared from a mixture of Spanish and Virginia peanuts, since the first alone is too oily and the second is too dry. Separation of the oil is prevented by partial *hydrogenation of the oil and the addition of *emulsifiers. A 20-g portion (as thickly spread on one slice of bread) is a *source of protein, copper, and niacin; contains 1.5 g of dietary fibre and 11 g of fat of which 20% is saturated; supplies 120 kcal (500 kJ).

peanut (groundnut, arachis) oil From the peanut or groundnut, *Arachis hypogaea*; 20% saturated, 50% mono-unsaturated, 30% polyunsaturated. *See* saturated fats.

pear Fruit of many species of *Pyrus*; cultivated varieties all descended from *P. communis*; The UK National Fruit Collection has 495 varieties of dessert and cooking pears, and a further 20 varieties of *perry pears. A 200-g portion (an average fruit) is a *source of vitamins B_6 and C and copper; contains 4–5 g of dietary fibre; supplies 80 kcal (340 kJ). *See also* poire williams.

pearl barley *See* barley.

pear, prickly *See* prickly pear.

pease pudding English; a dish prepared from dried peas which are soaked, boiled, mashed, and sieved, traditionally served with baked ham.

peas, garden or green Seeds of the *legume *Pisum sativum*. Widely available in frozen, dried, and canned forms. A 75-g portion, boiled, is a rich source of vitamin B_1; a good source of vitamin C; a source of protein, niacin, and folate; contains 3 g of dietary fibre; supplies 60 kcal (250 kJ). *See also* mange-tout.

peas, mushy Northern English; a dish prepared from processed peas, boiled and mashed to give a smooth texture. A 100-g portion is a *source of protein; supplies 80 kcal (340 kJ).

peas, processed Garden *peas (*Pisum sativum*) that have matured on the plant and are then canned. A 75-g portion is a *source of protein; contains 3.5 g of dietary fibre; supplies 75 kcal (320 kJ).

pecan nuts From the American tree *Carya illinoensis*, a species of hickory nut. A 60-g portion (ten nuts), is a rich *source of selenium, vitamin E, and niacin; a good *source of vitamin B_1 and zinc; a source of protein and iron; contains 40 g of fat of which 10% is *saturated and 60% mono-unsaturated; supplies 400 kcal (1700 kJ).

pecorino Italian; cheese made from ewe's milk.

pectase An *enzyme in the pith (albedo) of *citrus fruits which removes the methoxyl groups from *pectin to form water-insoluble pectic acid. The intermediate compounds, with varying numbers of methoxyl groups are pectinic acids. Also known as pectin esterase, pectin methyl esterase, and pectin methoxylase; distinct from *pectinase.

pectic acid Demethylated *pectin.

pectin Plant tissues contain hemicelluloses (chemically polymers of galacturonic acid) known as protopectins which cement the cell walls together. As fruit ripens, there is maximum protopectin present; thereafter it breaks down to pectin, pectinic acid, and, finally, pectic acid, and the fruit softens as the adhesive between the cells breaks down.

Pectin is the setting agent in *jam; it forms a gel with sugar under acid conditions. Soft fruits, such as strawberry, raspberry, and cherry, are low in pectin; plums, apples, and oranges are rich. Apple pulp and orange pith are the commercial sources of pectin. Added to jams, confectionery, chocolate, and ice cream as an emulsifier and stabilizer instead of agar; used in making jellies, and as an anti-staling agent in cakes. Included in *non-starch polysaccharides.

pectinase An enzyme present in the pith (albedo) of citrus fruits, which hydrolyses *pectin or pectic acids into smaller polygalacturonic acids, and finally galacturonic acid and its methyl ester. Used to clarify fruit juices. Also known as pectolase, pectozyme, and polygalacturonase.

pectinic acid Partially demethylated *pectin.

pectins, low-methoxyl Partially demethylated pectins which can form gels with little or no sugar and are therefore used in low-calorie jellies.

pectolase, pectozyme See pectinase.

pectosase, pectosinase See protopectinase.

Pekar test A comparative test of flour colour.

pekmez Turkish; thick jelly made by evaporating grape juice, the basis of *Turkish delight and other sugar confectionery. Also the general Balkan name for jam.

Pekoe See tea.

pelagic fish Fish that swim near the surface, compared with demersal fish, which live on the sea bottom. Pelagic fish are mostly of the oily type such as herring, mackerel, and pilchard, containing up to 20% oil.

pellagra The disease due to deficiency of the *vitamin *niacin and the *amino acid *tryptophan. Signs include a characteristic symmetrical photosensitive dermatitis (especially on the face and back of the hands), resembling severe sunburn; mental disturbances (a depressive psychosis sometimes called dementia); and digestive disorders (most commonly diarrhoea); fatal if untreated.

Most commonly associated with a diet based on *maize or *sorghum, which are poor sources of both tryptophan and niacin, with little meat or other vegetables.

PEM See protein-energy malnutrition.

pemmican Mixture of dried, powdered meat and fat, used as a concentrated food source, e.g. on expeditions. Analysis per 100 g: water, 3 g, protein, 40 g, fat, 45 g; 560 kcal (2.4 MJ).

penicillin The first of the *antibiotics; found in the culture fluid of the *mould Penicillium notatum in 1929. Active against a wide range of bacteria and of great value clinically. Not used as food preservative because of the danger that repeated small doses will increase the development of penicillin-resistant organisms.

Penicillium A genus of *moulds; apart from the production of *penicillin, several species are valuable in the ripening of *cheeses.

pentosans *Polysaccharides of five-carbon sugars (*pentoses). Widely distributed in plants, e.g. fruit, wood, corncobs, oat hulls. Not digested in the body, and hence a component of *non-starch polysaccharides and *dietary fibre.

pentose phosphate pathway *See* glucose metabolism.

pentoses *Monosaccharide *sugars with five carbon atoms. The most important is ribose.

pentosuria The excretion of *pentose sugars in the urine. Idiopathic pentosuria is an inherited metabolic disorder almost wholly restricted to Ashkenazi (North European) Jews, which has no adverse effects. Consumption of fruits rich in pentoses (e.g. pears) can also lead to (temporary) pentosuria.

pepper 1 Bell pepper, bullnose pepper, capsicum, paprika, sweet pepper, Spanish name *pimiento* (not the same as pimento or *allspice); fruits of the annual plant *Capsicum annuum*. Red, yellow, purple, or brown fruits, often eaten raw in salads when green and unripe; very variable in size and shape; some varieties can be spicy but most are non-pungent. One-quarter of a green pepper (45 g) is a rich *source of vitamin C; contains 0.4 g of dietary fibre and 0.2 g of fat; supplies 6 kcal (25 kJ).

2 Red pepper, chilli (or chili), small red fruit of the bushy perennial plant *Capsicum frutescens*. Usually sun-dried and therefore wrinkled. Very pungent, an ingredient of *curry powder, pickles, and *tabasco sauce. Cayenne pepper is made from the powdered dried fruits. Unripe (green) chillis are also very pungent.

3 Black and white pepper, fruit of the tropical climbing vine, *Piper nigrum*; the fruits are peppercorns. Black pepper is made from sun-dried, unripe peppercorns when the red outer skin turns black. White pepper is made by soaking ripe berries and rubbing off the outer skin. Usually ground as a condiment. Green peppercorns are dried or pickled unripe fruit. Pungency due to the alkaloids piperine, piperdine, and chavicine.

4 Japan pepper, black seeds of *Zanthoxylum piperitum* with a pungent, peppery flavour.

peppercorn *See* pepper.

pepper dulse Red aromatic seaweed (*Laurencia pinnatifida*), dried and used as a spice in Scotland.

peppergrass Peppery-tasting cress (*Lepidium sativum*), also known as pepperwort and (in the USA) peppermint.

pepper, guinea *See* pepper, melegueta.

pepper, Jamaican *See* allspice.

pepper, melegueta Seeds of the West African tree *Amomum melegueta*, also known as guinea pepper or grains of paradise.

peppermint A hybrid (Mentha × piperita) between *M. aquatica* and *M. spicata* (spearmint). Not used for flavouring dishes but grown for the essential oil which is used in confectionery (e.g. peppermints) and medicinally. *See also* mint.

pepperoni *See* sausage.

pepperpot Caribbean (originally native American); stew flavoured with *cassareep.

pepperwort *See* peppergrass.

Pepsi-Cola Trade name for a *cola beverage. Originally made in 1896 in the USA by Caleb Bradham, druggist.

pepsin An *enzyme in the *gastric juice which hydrolyses proteins to give smaller polypeptides, known as peptones; an endopeptidase. Active only at acid pH, 1.5–2.5. Secreted as the inactive precursor pepsinogen, which is activated by acid.

pepsin, vegetable *See* papain.

peptic ulcer *See* ulcer.

peptidases *Enzymes that hydrolyse proteins, and therefore important in *protein digestion. Endopeptidases cleave at specific points in the middle of protein molecules (between specific amino acids, depending on the enzyme); exopeptidases remove amino acids sequentially from either the amino terminal (aminopeptidases) or carboxy terminal (carboxypeptidases).

peptides Compounds formed when *amino acids are linked together through the —CO—NH— (peptide) linkage. Two amino acids so linked form a dipeptide, three a tripeptide, etc.; medium-length chains of amino acids (four up to about 20) are known as oligopeptides, longer chains are polypeptides or proteins.

peptones Small polypeptides that are intermediate products in the hydrolysis of proteins. The term is often used for any partial hydrolysate of proteins as, e.g., bacteriological peptone, which is used as a medium for the growth of micro-organisms.

PER Protein Efficiency Ratio, a measure of *protein quality.

pericarp The fibrous layers next to the outer husk of cereal grains and outside the testa; of low digestibility and removed from grain during milling. The major constituent of bran.

périgord, à la (Also à la périgueux, à la périgourdine); dish made or served with *truffles and sometimes *foie gras.

perillartine Non-nutritive *sweetener derived from perillaldehyde, extracted from shiso oil (commercially available in Japan); 2000 times as sweet as sucrose.

perimysium *See* muscle.

peristalsis The rhythmic alternating contraction and relaxation of smooth muscle that forces food through the intestinal tract in peristaltic waves.

periwinkle *See* winkle.

Permutit An *ion exchange resin.

pernicious anaemia *See* anaemia, pernicious.

Pernod Trade name for anise-flavoured liqueur: originated as a substitute for *absinthe.

peroxide Any compound with the peroxy (—O—O—) group; atmospheric oxidation of unsaturated *fatty acids produces peroxides. Also used to mean specifically hydrogen peroxide (H_2O_2).

peroxide number Or peroxide value; a measure of the oxidative rancidity of fats by determination of the lipid peroxides present.

Perrier water Aerated *mineral water from Vergèze, France.

perry Fermented pear juice (in the UK it may include not more than 25% apple juice) analogous to *cider from apples. Sparkling perry is sometimes known as champagne perry.

Persian apple See citron.

persimmon Fruit of *Diospyros virginiana* (American persimmon or Virginia date) and *D. kaki* (Japanese persimmon, date plum, or kaki). Kaki may be eaten raw or cooked; American persimmon develops a sour flavour if cooked.

pesto Italian; basil and garlic sauce.

PET Polyethylene terephthalate; clear plastic used in packaging, especially bottles for drinks.

petechiae (petechial haemorrhages) Small, pin-point bleeding under the skin; one of the signs of *scurvy.

pétillant French; lightly sparkling wines, equivalent to Italian frizzante.

petit pois Small *peas, picked when young; also French for green pea.

petit salé French; salted belly or flank of pork.

petits fours Small, rich, sweet cakes and biscuits served after a meal.

PGA Pteroylglutamic acid, see folic acid.

pH Potential hydrogen, method of measuring degrees of acidity or alkalinity on a logarithmic scale. Defined as the negative logarithm of the hydrogen-ion concentration. The scale runs from 0, which is very strongly acid, to 14, which is very strongly alkaline. Pure water is pH 7, which is neutral; below 7 is acid, above is alkaline. See also acid; buffer.

phaeophytin Brownish-green derivative of *chlorophyll, due to the loss of the *magnesium in acid conditions. The formation of phaeophytin accounts for the colour change when green vegetables are cooked.

phage See bacteriophage.

phagomania Morbid obsession with food; also known as sitomania.

phagophobia Fear of food; also known as sitophobia.

phase inversion *Cream is an emulsion of fat in water; *butter is an emulsion of water in fat. The change from cream to butter is termed phase inversion.

phaseolin Globulin protein in kidney or haricot *bean (*Phaseolus vulgaris*).

phaseolunatin *Cyanogenic (cyanide-forming) *glucoside found in certain *legumes (such as Lima bean, chick pea, common vetch), which hydrolyses to glucose, acetone, and hydrocyanic acid; not proven harmful when present in the diet.

phasin Originally the *lectin from the bean *Phaseolus vulgaris*, now used for non-toxic plant lectins in general.

PHB ester *See* parabens.

pheasant (French: *faizan*; German: *Fasan*.) *Game bird, *Phasianus colchicus* and related spp. Total weight 1.5 kg; traditionally sold as a brace, i.e. cock and hen, although now commonly available as single birds; usually hung for 3 days (up to 3 weeks in very cold weather) to develop flavour. A 150-g portion is an extremely rich *source of iron; a rich source of protein, niacin, and vitamin B_2; contains about 15 g of fat of which one-third is saturated, and supplies 330 kcal (1400 kJ).

phenetylurea *See* dulcin.

phenol oxidases Enzymes that oxidize phenolic compounds to quinones. For example, monophenol oxidase in mushrooms, polyphenol oxidases in potato and apple are responsible for the development of the brown colour when the cut surface is exposed to air; tyrosinase in plants and animals forms the brown and black pigment melanin.

phenylalanine An essential *amino acid; in addition to its role in protein synthesis, it is the metabolic precursor of the non-essential amino acid *tyrosine (and hence *noradrenaline, *adrenaline, and the *thyroid hormones). Tyrosine in the diet spares phenylalanine, so reducing the requirement.

phenylketonuria A *genetic disease affecting the metabolism of *phenylalanine. Phenylalanine is normally metabolized to *tyrosine, catalysed by phenylalanine hydroxylase. Impairment of this reaction leads to a considerable accumulation of phenylalanine in plasma and tissues (up to 100 times the normal concentration) and metabolism to phenylpyruvate, phenyllactate, and phenylacetate, collectively known as phenylketones, which are excreted in the urine.

The very high plasma concentration of phenylalanine causes disruption of brain development, and if untreated there is severe mental retardation. All infants are screened for phenylketonuria shortly after birth (by measurement of plasma phenylalanine); treatment is by very strict limitation of phenylalanine intake, only providing sufficient to meet requirements for protein synthesis. Once brain development is complete (between the ages of 8 and 12 years) dietary restriction can be relaxed to a considerable extent, since high concentrations of phenylalanine seem to have little adverse effect on the developed brain. There may, however, be benefits from continuing dietary restriction into adult life, and phenylketonuriac women require extremely careful dietary control through pregnancy to avoid damage to the foetus's developing brain.

phitosite High-calorie food.

phosphatase test A test for the adequacy of *pasteurization of milk. The enzyme phosphatase, normally present in milk, is denatured at a temperature slightly greater than that required to destroy the tubercle bacillus and other pathogens; therefore the presence of detectable phosphatase activity indicates inadequate pasteurization. The test can detect 0.2% raw milk in pasteurized milk.

phosphate additives *See* polyphosphates.

phosphates Salts of *phosphoric acid; the form in which the element *phosphorus is normally present in foods and body tissues. *See also* polyphosphates.

phosphatides *See* phospholipids.

phosphatidic acid Glycerol esterified to two molecules of fatty acid, with the third hydroxyl group esterified to phosphate; chemically diacylglycerol phosphate; intermediates in the metabolism of *phospholipids.

phosphatidylcholine A phospholipid containing *choline, *see* lecithin.

phosphatidylethanolamine A *phospholipid containing ethanolamine.

phosphatidylinositol A *phospholipid containing *inositol.

phosphatidylserine A *phospholipid containing *serine.

phospholipids (Also known as phosphatides and phospholipins). Glycerol esterified to two molecules of *fatty acid, one of which is commonly a polyunsaturated fatty acid. The third hydroxyl group is esterified to phosphate and one of a number of water-soluble compounds, including *serine (phosphatidylserine), ethanolamine (phosphatidylethanolamine), *choline (phosphatidylcholine, also known as *lecithin), and *inositol (phosphatidylinositol).

Cell membranes are a double layer of phospholipids with the fatty acid side-chains on the inside and the water-soluble compound esterified to the phosphate interacts with water. This is why phospholipids can be used to emulsify oils and fats in water and are commonly used in food manufacture as *emulsifiers.

From the energy point of view they can be regarded as being equivalent to simple fats (*triacylglycerols); they also provide a dietary source of choline and inositol, neither of which is a dietary essential.

phospholipins *See* phospholipids.

phosphoproteins Proteins containing phosphate, other than as *nucleic acids (nucleoproteins) or phospholipids (lipoproteins), e.g. *casein from milk, ovovitellin from egg yolk.

phosphoric acid May be one of three types: orthophosphoric acid (H_3PO_4), metaphosphoric acid (HPO_3), or pyrophosphoric acid ($H_4P_2O_7$). Orthophosphoric acid and its salts are E-338−341, used as *acidity regulators and in acid-fruit-flavoured beverages such as lemonade.

phosphorus An essential element, occurring in tissues and foods as phosphate (salts of *phosphoric acid), *phospholipids, and phosphoproteins. In the body most (80%) is present in the skeleton and teeth as calcium phosphate (hydroxyapatite); the remainder is in the *phospholipids of cell membranes, in *nucleic acids, and in a variety of metabolic intermediates, including *ATP. The *parathyroid glands control the concentration of phosphate in the blood, mainly by modifying its excretion in the urine.

Human dietary needs (about 1.3 g per day) are always met; a deficiency never occurs in man. The *calcium to phosphate ratio of infant foods is, however, important. Phosphate deficiency is common in livestock and gives rise to *osteomalacia (also known as sweeny or creeping sickness).

Phosphate is also essential for plant growth, hence the use of inorganic phosphate or bone-meal as fertilizer. Bone-meal (mainly calcium phosphate), is often used as a supplement in human foods but as a source of calcium rather than of phosphate.

photosynthesis The synthesis of carbohydrates from carbon dioxide and water by plants in sunlight, with the release of oxygen.

phrynoderma Blocked pores or 'toad-skin' (follicular hyperkeratosis of the skin) often encountered in malnourished people. Originally thought to be due to *vitamin A deficiency but possibly due to other deficiencies, and also occurs mildly in adequately nourished people.

phulka See chapatti.

phulouri Caribbean; fritters made from dried split peas.

phycotoxins Marine biotoxins that accumulate in fish and shellfish from their diet (causing *paralytic and *ciguatera poisoning when the fish are eaten), as distinct from toxins naturally present (*tetramine poisoning).

phyllo pastry (filo pastry) Plain paper-thin pastry made from flour and water, rolled into small balls then tossed in the air and stretched until it forms an extremely thin sheet. Multiple layers are used as the basis for Greek and Middle-Eastern pastry dishes (e.g. *baklava). Known as mortoban in South East Asia.

phylloquinone See vitamin K.

phylloxera An aphid which threatened to destroy the vineyards of Europe in the middle of the nineteenth century. They were saved by grafting susceptible varieties on to resistant American vine rootstock.

physalin A *carotenoid pigment in the fruits of the *Cape gooseberry, Physalis spp.; zeaxanthin dipalmitate.

physalis See Cape gooseberry.

physical activity level (PAL) Total *energy cost of physical activity throughout the day, expressed as a ratio of *basal metabolic rate. Calculated from the *physical activity ratio for each activity, multiplied by the time spent in that activity. A desirable PAL for health is considered to be 1.7; the average in the UK is 1.4.

physical activity ratio (PAR) *Energy cost of physical activity expressed as a ratio of *basal metabolic rate.

physin Name given to a growth factor in liver, needed by rats; found to be vitamin B_{12}.

phytase An *enzyme (a phosphatase) that hydrolyses *phytate to *inositol and phosphate. Present in yeast, liver, blood, malt, and seeds. If a high level of yeast is used in baking with high extraction flours, some of the phytate is broken down.

phytate (phytic acid) *Inositol hexaphosphate, present in cereals, particularly in the bran, in dried legumes and some nuts as both water-soluble salts (sodium and potassium) and insoluble salts of calcium and magnesium. Magnesium calcium phytate is phytin.

It can bind calcium, iron, and zinc to form insoluble complexes; it is not clear how far phytate reduces the availability of these minerals in the diet, especially since there are *phytase enzymes in yeast and legumes (and possibly in the human gut) which may liberate these minerals.

phytic acid See phytate.

phytin Magnesium calcium *phytate, approximately 12% calcium, 1.5% magnesium, and 22% phosphorus.

phytoalexins Substances, often harmful to human beings, which increase in plant tissues when they are stressed, as by physical damage, exposure to ultraviolet light, etc.

phytoncides See pacificarins.

phyto-oestrogens Compounds with oestrogen activity found in a variety of plants; see oestrogens.

phytoplankton Minute plants floating in the sea which serve as the basic food for all marine life, since they photosynthesize. The basis of the marine *food-chain.

phytosterol General name given to sterols occurring in plants, the chief of which is sitosterol.

phytylmenaquinone See vitamin K.

pica An unnatural desire for foods; alternative words are cissa, cittosis, and allotriophagy. Also a perverted appetite (eating of earth, sand, clay, paper, etc.).

piccalilli Mixture of chopped, brine-preserved vegetables in mustard sauce (mustard and vinegar, thickened with tapioca starch, plus turmeric and other spices, coloured yellow).

piccata Italian; small thin slices of veal.

pickles, dill Pickles fermented in a mixture of brine, *dill weed, mixed spices, and vinegar.

pickling Also called *brining. Vegetables immersed in 5–10% salt solution (brine) undergo lactic acid fermentation, while the salt prevents the growth of undesirable organisms. The sugars in the vegetables are converted to lactic acid; at 25 °C the process takes a few weeks, finishing at 1% acidity. See also curing of meat; halophilic bacteria.

picklizes Caribbean (esp. Haitian); pickled mixed vegetables; piccalilli.

picnic shoulder American name for hand of pork.

pico As a prefix for units of measurement, one million-millionth part (i.e. 10^{-12}); symbol p. *See* Appendix I.

pidan *Chinese eggs.

pie Food cooked in a dish and covered with pastry; may be sweet or savoury. Also savoury dishes with a crust of mashed potato.

piernik Polish; spiced honey cake.

pierogi Polish; envelopes of dough stuffed with minced meat, cheese, vegetables, or fruit; similar to *ravioli.

pigeon (French: *pigeon*; German: *Taube*.) *Columbia livia*; young about 4 weeks old is a squab. A 150-g portion is an extremely rich *source of iron, a rich *source of protein, niacin, and vitamins B_1 and B_2; contains 20 g of fat; supplies 350 kcal (1500 kJ).

pignoli (pignolias, pinoli) *See* pine kernels.

pignut *See* earth-nut.

pig's fry *See* haslet.

pig weed *See* fat hen.

pikelets *See* dough cakes.

pilafi Greek; rice dishes.

pilau (pilaf) Dish of rice cooked in stock, with vegetables, meat, or fish added.

pilchard Oily *fish, *Sardina (Clupea) pilchardus*; young is the *sardine. A 100-g portion (canned in tomato sauce) is an exceptionally rich *source of vitamins D and B_{12}; a rich source of protein, niacin, calcium, selenium, and iodine; a good source of copper; a source of iron and vitamins B_2 and B_6; contains 5 g of fat of which one-fifth is *saturated and a third is mono-unsaturated; supplies 125 kcal (500 kJ).

piles *See* haemorrhoids.

pils Pale type of lager originally made in Czechoslovakia. *See* beer.

pimento *See* allspice.

pimentón Spanish; powdered, dried red *pepper. Pimentón picante (hot) is cayenne; pimentón dulce (sweet) is paprika.

pimiento *See* pepper.

Pimms Trade name; a ready-mixed cocktail based on spirits and flavoured with herbs and liqueurs, normally served as a long drink with ice and soda or lemonade, garnished with fruit, cucumber, or mint. Originally there were four varieties: No. 1 based on gin, No. 2 on whisky, No. 3 on brandy, No. 4 on rum; only No. 1, now based on vodka, survives.

pimpernel *See* burnet.

piña colada A long drink made from rum, pineapple juice, and coconut milk; also the trade name for a sweet liqueur made from rum, pineapple, and coconut.

pineapple (French: *ananas*; German: *Ananas*.) Fruit of the tropical plant *Ananas sativus*, one of the bromeliad family. The fruit contains the proteolytic *enzyme bromelain, which has been used (like *papain) to tenderize meat. A 100-g portion is a rich *source of vitamin C; a source of copper; provides 0.8 g of dietary fibre; supplies 30 kcal (125 kJ).

pineau Mixture of grape must and cognac; about 17% alcohol.

pine nuts Or pine kernels, edible seeds of various species of pine cone, especially Mediterranean stone pine, *Pinus pinea*.

pink gin A cocktail; *gin with *angostura bitters.

pinnochio Pine kernels, *see* pine nuts.

pinot Three varieties of *grape used for *wine making; pinot noir is one of the 9 'classic' varieties, used especially in champagne; pinot blanc and pinot gris are also widely used.

pinotage A South African *grape variety used for *wine making, the result of a cross between the *cinsaut and *pinot noir varieties.

pint, reputed $13\frac{1}{3}$ fl oz = 285 mL; half a reputed *quart.

pinto bean *Phaseolus acutifolius*, also known as frijole, Mexican haricot, or tepary bean. Able to grow during drought.

piononos Caribbean (Puerto Rico); stuffed plantains.

pipe Cask for wine; the volume varies with the type of wine, e.g. port, 115 gallons (517 L); Tenerife, 100 gal (450 L); Marsala, 90 gal (418 L).

piping To force a smooth mixture (e.g. icing or mashed potato) through a narrow nozzle to form fancy shapes to decorate a dish.

pipis Edible *mollusc, *Plebidonas deltoides*, widely distributed around Australian coastline.

piri-piri Small red chillies (about 1 cm long), extremely pungent. *See* pepper.

piri-piri seasoning Portuguese; crushed chillies, citrus peel, onion, garlic, pepper, salt, lemon juice, bay leaves, paprika, pimiento, basil, oregano, and tarragon. *See also* pepper.

pirozhki Russian; small baked pasties of yeast dough filled with chopped fish, meat, etc.

pis-en-lit French name for *dandelion leaves, eaten raw or cooked. So called because of the diuretic effect of dandelion.

pisco South American (Chilean, Peruvian); brandy made from muscat grapes. A pisco sour is a mixture of pisco with 2 parts lime juice, sweetened to taste.

pissaladière French (Provençale); savoury tart similar to *pizza.

pistachio Fruit of *Pistacchio vera*; yellow-green coloured nut. May be roasted and salted or used as flavouring for ice cream and (Indian) hot, sweet, milk beverage. A 60-g portion (weighed with shells) is a *source of protein, vitamins B_1, E, and niacin; contains 18 g of fat of which 10% is saturated and 50% mono-unsaturated; supplies 200 kcal (840 kJ).

pisto manchego Spanish (Castilian); vegetable hash.

pita (pitta) Middle-Eastern; unleavened flat bread, baked as an oval or circle, which can be opened up as an envelope.

pitanga Surinam cherry, *Eugenia uniflora* or *E. michelii*; small, round fruit, deeply ribbed, cherry-like with a single stone. A 100-g portion is a rich *source of vitamin C.

pitch lake pudding Caribbean (Barbadian, Trinidadian); dark rum and chocolate mousse.

pith *See* albedo.

pits Stones from cherries, plums, peaches, apricots. Oil extracted from these pits is used in cosmetics, pharmaceuticals, for canning sardines, and as table oil. The press cake left behind contains *amygdalin.

pitting Removing the stones (pits) from cherries, olives, etc.

pitz Swiss; raw tomatoes stuffed with minced apple and celeriac.

pizza Originally Italian; savoury tart on a base of yeast dough, traditionally cooked in a wood-burning oven. The topping varies with the region and may contain tomatoes, cheese, salami, or seafood.

plaice Flat *fish, *Pleuronectus platessa*.

plaki Greek; fish baked or braised with vegetables.

plancha, a la Spanish; cooking 'on the plate'. The plancha is a thick iron or aluminium plate, traditionally incorporated into the stove, an oiled hot plate or griddle.

planking Cooking (and usually serving) meat or fish on a small board of oiled hardwood.

plankton Minute organisms, both plant (phytoplankton) and animal (zooplankton), drifting in the sea, which serve as the basic foodstuffs of marine life; the basis of the marine *food chain.

plansifter A nest of sieves mounted together so that material being sieved is divided into a number of fractions of different size. Widely used in flour milling.

plantago *See* psyllium.

plantain Adam's fig; variety of banana (*Musa* spp.) with higher starch and lower sugar content than dessert bananas, picked when the flesh is too hard to be eaten raw, and therefore cooked. Some varieties become sweet if left to ripen, others never develop a high sugar content. A 200-g portion is a rich *source of vitamins B_6 and C; a good source of folate and copper; a source of selenium; provides 12 g of dietary fibre; supplies 240 kcal (1000 kJ).

plaque, dental The growth of bacteria that adhere tightly to teeth, leading to the development of *caries.

plasma, blood *See* blood plasma.

plate count To estimate the number of bacteria in a sample, it is poured on to an *agar plate, when each bacterial cell multiplies to produce a colony of bacteria which is visible to the naked eye. A count of the number of colonies gives the number of bacteria in the portion of the sample that was taken. Pasteurized milk contains about 100,000 bacteria/mL; good quality raw milk contains less than 500,000/mL.

Plato *See* Balling.

Pliofilm Trade name for varieties of rubber hydrochloride, the first transparent wrapping paper (1934) that could be heat-sealed.

PLJ (Pure Lemon Juice) Trade name for lemon juice (containing 50 mg vitamin C per 100 mL).

plonk Colloquial term for cheap, indifferent wine; originated in Australia.

ploughman's lunch Basically cheese, bread, and pickle, now an English pub lunch; cheese (or sometimes pâté or ham) with salad and crusty bread.

pluck Butchers' term for heart, liver, and lungs of an animal.

plum (French: *prune*; German: *Plaume*.) Fruit of numerous species of *Prunus*. Common European plums are *P. domestica*; blackthorn or sloe is *P. spinosa*; bullace is *P. insititia*; damson is *P. damascena*; gages are *P. italica*. The UK National Fruit Collection contains 336 varieties of plum. A 200-g portion of dessert plums (four medium-size fruits weighed without stones) is a *source of vitamin C; provides 3 g of dietary fibre; supplies 100 kcal (420 kJ).

plumcote American fruit, a cross between plum and apricot.

plum sauce Chinese; chutney-like sauce made from plums, apricots, chilli, vinegar, and sugar.

Plymouth gin *See* gin.

pneumatic conveying Transfer of material in powder form by means of air currents. Applied to flour, sugar, etc.

pneumatic dryers The material is dried almost instantaneously in a turbulent stream of hot air, which also acts as a conveyor system. Applicable to powdered, granular, and flaky materials: used for starch, mashed potatoes, cereals, flour, and powdered soups.

poach To cook for a short time in a shallow layer of liquid kept at a temperature just below the boiling point.

POEMS (Polyoxyethylene monostearate) *See* crumb softener.

poire williams *Pear liqueur prepared by steeping Williams pears in pear brandy (eau de vie prepared by distillation of *perry).
Traditionally a bottle is placed over the developing fruit bud on the tree; when the fruit has ripened it is then steeped in pear brandy in the bottle in which it has grown.

poisoning, food *See* food poisoning.

polenta Traditional Italian porridge made from maize meal, often with cheese added. May be further cooked by baking or frying. Also the Italian word for coarsely ground maize meal, as hominy grits is the American term.

polished rice *See* rice.

pollards *See* wheatfeed.

polonaise, à la Dishes made with soured cream, beetroot, and red cabbage.

polony Italian smoked pork and veal sausage, ready to slice and eat; also known as bologna. A 150-g portion is a good *source of protein, vitamin B$_1$, and niacin; a source of iron; contains 30 g of fat and 1200 mg of sodium; supplies 320 kcal (1280 kJ).

polvorones Spanish (Andalusian); *shortbread.

polydextrose, modified Glucose polymer prepared by heating *glucose and *sorbitol with citric acid. It is more resistant to enzymic digestion than normal *polysaccharides and 60% is excreted in faeces undigested, so providing only about 1 kcal (4 kJ)/g; hence, termed 'non-sweetening sucrose replacement', or *bulking agent.

polygalacturonase *See* pectinase.

polyglucose *See* polydextrose.

polymorphism The ability to crystallize in two or more different forms. For example, depending on the conditions under which it is solidified, the fat tristearin can form three kinds of crystals, each of which has a different melting point, namely, 54, 65, and 71 ˚C.

polymyxins Antibiotics isolated from *Bacillus polymyxin* (*B. aerosporin*); polymyxin A is aerosporin. They are polypeptides, active against coliform bacteria; apart from clinical use, they are of value in controlling infection in brewing.

polyols *See* sugar alcohols.

polyose *See* polysaccharide.

polyoxyethylene *See* crumb-softener.

polypeptides *See* peptides.

polyphagia Excessive or continuous eating.

polyphosphates Complex *phosphates added to foods as *emulsifiers, *buffers, or *sequestrants. They prevent discoloration of sausages and aid mixing of the fat, speed penetration of the brine in curing, hold water in meat and fish products; E-450(a), (b), (c), and E-541, 544, 545.

polysaccharides Complex *carbohydrates formed by the condensation of large numbers of *monosaccharide units, e.g. *starch, *glycogen, *cellulose, *dextrins, *inulin. On hydrolysis the simple sugar is liberated. *See also* non-starch polysaccharides.

polysaccharose Alternative name for *polysaccharides.

polysorbates *See* crumb softeners.

polyunsaturated fatty acids Long-chain *fatty acids containing two or more double bonds, separated by methylene bridges: $-CH_2-CH=CH-CH_2-CH=CH-CH_2-$. *See* Appendix X.

polyunsaturates Commonly used short term for polyunsaturated *fatty acids.

pomace Residue of fruit pulp after expressing juice: also applied to fish from which oil has been expressed.

pombé African *beer prepared from millet; also known as kaffir beer. Commonly associated with *iron overload, since it is frequently brewed in iron drums, and alcohol greatly increases the absorption of iron.

pomegranate (French: *grenade*; German: *Granatapfel*.) The fruit of the subtropical tree *Punica granatum*. The juice is contained in a pulpy sac surrounding each of a mass of seeds; the outer skin contains tannin and is therefore bitter. The sweet juice is used to prepare *grenadine syrup for alcoholic and fruit drinks.

pomelo (pomeloe, pummelo) Fruit of *Citrus grandis*, from which the *grapefruit is descended; also called shaddock, after Captain Shaddock, who introduced it into Barbados in the sixteenth century. *See* citrus.

pomes Botanical name for fruits such as apple or pear, formed by the enlargement of the receptacle which becomes fleshy and surrounds the carpels.

pomfret *See* Pontefract cakes.

ponceau (ponceau 4R) Strawberry-red colour, E-124.

ponderal index An index of fatness, used as a measure of *obesity: the cube root of body weight divided by height. Confusingly, the ponderal index is higher for thin people, and lower for fat people. *See also* body mass index.

ponderocrescive Foods tending to increase weight: easily gaining weight; the opposite of ponderoperditive.

ponderoperditive Stimulating weight loss.

pone bread Colloquial name for corn bread in the southern states of the USA. (Corn pone are small corn cakes, a speciality of Alabama.)

Pontefract cake A round, flat sweetmeat made from *liquorice, originally in Pontefract in England; also called pomfret.

poonac The residue of *coconut after the extraction of the oil.

poor man's goose Casserole dish of liver and potatoes.

popcorn Variety of *maize (parch maize, *Zea mays everta*) that expands on heating, also the name of the fluffy white mass so formed.

pope's eye The small circle of fat in the centre of a leg of pork or mutton.

pope's nose *See* parson's nose.

popover Individual *batter pudding; small *Yorkshire pudding.

poppadom Indian; thin roasted or fried crisps made from lentil flour; may be spiced.

poppy seed Seeds of the opium poppy, *Papaver somniferum*, used mixed with honey in cakes, and as a flavouring on the crust of bread and rolls. Also called maw seed.

popsicle American name for *ice lolly.

Population Reference Intake, PRI *See* reference intakes; Appendices II–V.

pork (French: *porc*; German: *Schweinfleisch*.) Meat from the pig (swine, hog), *Suidae* spp., eaten fresh, as opposed to bacon and ham which are cured. By far the richest of all meat sources of vitamin B_1, a 150-g portion supplying more than the average daily requirement; a rich

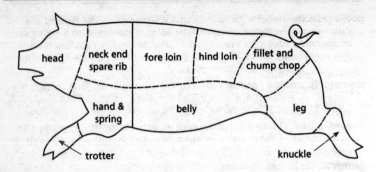

FIGURE 5.

*source of protein, niacin, vitamin B_{12}, copper, and selenium; a good source of vitamins B_2 and B_6, zinc, and iron; depending on the joint contains 30–45 g of fat of which one-third is saturated; supplies 430–500 kcal (1800–2100 kJ).

porphyra Red seaweed used to make *laverbread.

porridge Oatmeal cooked in water or milk as a breakfast dish; originally Scottish. Also similar thick soups made with other cereals. *See* oats.

port Fortified wines from the upper Douro valley of north-east Portugal. Mostly aged in wood and bottled when ready for drinking; vintage port is aged in wood for 2 years, then in the bottle for at least 10; late bottled vintage is aged less than 6 years. Crusted port is blended from quality vintages bottled young, and develops a sediment (crust) in the bottle. Ruby port is young; old tawny is aged for 10 or more years; fine old tawny is a blend of young and old wines. Tawny port is aged in wood, vintage in the bottle. White port is made from white grapes; generally served chilled as an aperitif. Around 16% alcohol by volume, 12% sugars; 160 kcal (670 kJ)/100 mL.

porter *See* beer.

porterhouse American term originally for large beef steak cut from the rear end of sirloin and including some fillet: served with beer (porter) in porterhouses. Now a thick slice cut from the wing-rib of *beef.

portuguese, à la Dishes made with tomato, onion, and garlic.

Poskitt index Index of fatness in children; per cent of expected weight for age.

posset Drink made from hot milk curdled with ale or wine, sometimes thickened with breadcrumbs and spiced. Formerly used as a remedy for colds; popular in the later Middle Ages.

Postum, Instant Trade name for a preparation of bran, wheat, and molasses consumed as a beverage.

potage French; thick soup.

potassium An essential mineral, widespread in nature; the human body contains about 125 g, mostly present inside the cells. *Reference

Nutrient Intake for adults is 3.5 g/day; abundant in vegetables, potatoes, fruit (especially bananas). One of the most important of the plant nutrients.

potassium nitrate *See* nitrate; saltpetre.

potassium sorbate Potassium salt of *sorbic acid (E-202).

potato crisps Flavoured, thin slices of potato, deep-fried and eaten cold, sometimes as an accompaniment to meals, more commonly as a snack. Called chips in the USA. A 30-g portion (1 oz bag) of conventional crisps, ten crisps, is a *source of niacin and vitamin C; contains 11 g of fat, of which 30% may be saturated and 40% mono-unsaturated; 180–450 mg of sodium; supplies 165 kcal (700 kJ). The same portion of low-fat crisps is a *source of niacin; may contain 6 g of fat; 180–450 mg sodium; supplies 145 kcal (610 kJ). A large bag of conventional crisps (75 g) is a rich source of vitamin C; a good source of niacin; a source of iron; contains 20 g of fat; provides 4 g of dietary fibre; 450–1100 mg of sodium; supplies 410 kcal (1700 kJ). The same portion of low-fat crisps is a good source of niacin; a source of vitamins B_1 and C, and iron; contains 16 g of fat; provides 5 g of dietary fibre; 450–1100 mg of sodium; supplies 360 kcal (1500 kJ).

potatoes, straw *See* allumettes.

potato, fairy *See* earth nut.

potato flour Dried potato tuber.

potato, Irish The 'ordinary' potato, tuber of *Solanum tuberosum*. A 200-g portion is a rich *source of vitamin B_6; a good source of vitamins B_1 and C (new potatoes are a rich source of vitamin C), and folate; a source of niacin; provides 2.5 g of dietary fibre, 560 mg of potassium; supplies 140 kcal (590 kJ).

potato starch Also called farina. Prepared from potato tuber and widely used as a stabilizing agent when gelatinized by heat.

potato, sweet Tubers of the herbaceous climbing plant *Ipomoea batatas*, known in Britain before the Irish potato. The flesh may be white, yellow, or pink (if carotene is present); the leaves are also edible. A 200-g portion is a rich *source of vitamins A (as carotene if pink) and C; a source of iron and vitamin B_1; provides 4.5 g of dietary fibre; contains 0.4 g of fat of which 16% is saturated; supplies 170 kcal (700 kJ).

pot-au-feu French; large deep earthenware casserole or *marmite; also a traditional dish of meat and vegetables.

poteen Irish name for illicit home-distilled spirit.

pot herbs Herbs for culinary use. Originally vegetables such as cabbage whose leaves were boiled for food.

pot roasting A method of cooking joints of meat in a saucepan or casserole with fat and a small amount of liquid.

pottage Thick, well-seasoned meat or vegetable soup, usually containing barley or other cereal or a pulse (e.g. lentils).

pottle Traditional English wine measure; $1/2$ gallon (= 2.25 L).

poularde A neutered hen bird.

poulette, à la Fricassée of cooked meat or poultry in rich white sauce, garnished with onions or garlic.

poultry General term for farmyard birds (as opposed to wild *game birds) kept for eggs and/or meat; *chicken, *duck, *goose, *guinea fowl, *pigeon, and *turkey.

poultry, New York dressed Poultry that have been slaughtered and plucked but not eviscerated.

pound cake American name for Madeira cake; rich cake containing a pound, or equal quantities, of each of the major ingredients: flour, sugar, and butter, with added eggs.

poussin Young *chicken, 4–6 weeks old.

PP factor or vitamin *See* niacin.

ppm Parts per million (= mg/kg).

prairie chicken American *game bird, *Tympanuchus cupido* and *T. pallidicinctus*.

prairie oyster Traditional cure for a hangover; a raw egg with *Worcestershire sauce and brandy; the egg is swirled with the liquid but the yolk remains intact.

praline 1 Confection of nuts and partially caramelized sugar, often used as a centre for chocolates.
2 In France, a sugar-coated almond.

prawns Shellfish of various tribes of suborder *Macrura*. Large fish of species of Palaemonidae, Penaeidae, and Pandalidae are prawns; smaller ones are shrimps. A 100-g portion (250 g with shell) is a rich *source of protein, niacin, and selenium; a good source of calcium; contains 1600 mg of sodium; supplies 110 kcal (460 kJ).
   The deep-water prawn is *Pandalus borealis*; common pink shrimp is *Pandalus montagui*; brown shrimp is *Crangon* spp. *See also* Dublin bay prawn; lobster; scampi.

PRE Protein Retention Efficiency, a measure of *protein quality.

prebiotics Non-digestible *oligosaccharides that support the growth of colonies of certain bacteria in the colon. They include derivatives of *fructose and *galactose, and lead to the growth of bifidobacteria, so changing and possibly improving the colonic flora. *Probiotics and prebiotics are sometimes termed synbiotics. They are considered to play a role as *functional foods.

precursors, enzyme Inactive forms of enzymes, activated after secretion; also called pro-enzymes or zymogens.

pregnancy, nutritional needs Pregnant women have slightly increased energy and protein requirements compared with their needs before pregnancy, although there are metabolic adaptations in early pregnancy which result in laying down increased reserves for the great stress of the last trimester, and high requirements for iron and calcium. These increased needs are reflected in the increased *reference intakes for pregnancy (*see* Appendices II–V).

premier cru *See* wine classification, Luxemburg.

premier jus Best-quality *suet prepared from oxen and sheep kidneys. The fat is chilled, shredded, and heated at moderate temperature. When pressed, premier jus separates into a liquid fraction (oleo oil or liquid oleo) and a solid fraction (oleostearin or solid tallow).

pré-salé French; mutton or lamb from sheep raised on salt marshes; prized for its flavour.

preservation Protection of food from deterioration by micro-organisms, enzymes, and oxidation: by cooling, destroying the micro-organisms and enzymes by heat treatment or *irradiation, reducing their activity through dehydration or the addition of chemical *preservatives, and by smoking, *salting, and *pickling.

preservatives Substances capable of retarding or arresting the deterioration of food; examples are *sulphur dioxide, *benzoic acid, specified *antibiotics, *salt, acids, and essential oils. *See* Appendix VIII.

preserving sugar *See* sugar.

pressed beef *See* beef, pressed.

pressure cooking By cooking under pressure, it is possible to achieve a higher temperature, and therefore boil or steam foods faster than in an open pan. *See also* autoclave.

pressure, blood *See* hypertension.

pressure, osmotic *See* osmotic pressure.

pretzels German; hard, brittle biscuits in the shape of a knot, made from flour, water, shortening, yeast, and salt. Also called bretzels.

PRI Population Reference Intake of nutrients; *see* Reference Intakes; Appendices II–VI.

prickly pear Fruit of the cactus *Opuntia* spp., also called Indian fig, barberry fig, and tuna; an important part of the diet in certain areas of Mexico. A 150-g portion is a rich *source of vitamin C; supplies 60 kcal (245 kJ).

primeurs French; early forced vegetables and fruits. Also used for young, early wine (e.g. *Beaujolais nouveau).

princesse, à la Dish with a garnish of asparagus tips and truffles or noisette potatoes.

printanière, à la Spring-style dish containing, or garnished with, small, young vegetables.

prion The infective agent(s) believed to be responsible for Kreutzfeld-Jacob disease, kuru and possibly other degenerative diseases of the brain in human beings, scrapie in sheep, and bovine spongiform encephalopathy (*BSE). They are simple proteins, and unlike viruses do not contain any nucleic acid. Transmission occurs by ingestion of infected tissue.

probiotics Preparations of live micro-organisms added to food (or used as animal feed), claimed to be beneficial to health by restoring microbial balance in the intestine. The organisms commonly involved are lactobacilli, bifidobacteria, streptococci, and some yeasts and moulds, alone or as mixtures. *See also* prebiotics.

Procea Trade name of a white bread with slightly increased protein content.

processing Any and all processes to which food is subjected after harvesting for the purposes of improving its appearance, texture, palatability, nutritive value, keeping properties, and ease of preparation, and for eliminating micro-organisms, toxins, and other undesirable constituents.

pro-enzymes Inactive precursors of enzymes, activated after secretion; also called zymogens.

profiterole Originally a light cake baked on hot ashes and filled with cream; now a small case of *choux pastry, baked, filled with cream, and served with chocolate sauce. Also small rounds of choux pastry used as a garnish for clear soups or consommés.

progoitrins Substances found in plant foods which are precursors of *goitrogens.

proline A non-essential *amino acid.

Promega Trade name for mixture of long-chain marine *fatty acids: eicosapentaenoic (EPA, C20 : 5 ω3) and docosohexaenoic (DHA, C22 : 6 ω3) acids. *See* Appendix X.

Pronutro Protein-rich baby food (22% protein) developed in South Africa; made from maize, skim-milk powder, groundnut flour, soya flour, and fish protein concentrate with added vitamins.

proof spirit An old method of describing the *alcohol content of *spirits; originally defined as a solution of alcohol of such strength that it will ignite when mixed with gunpowder. Proof spirit contains 57.07% alcohol by volume or 49.24% by weight in the UK. In the USA it contains 50% alcohol by volume. Pure (absolute) alcohol is 175.25 ° proof UK or 200 ° proof USA.

Spirits were described as under or over proof; a drink 30° over proof means that 100 volumes contains as much alcohol as 130 volumes of proof spirit; 30° under proof means that 100 volumes contains as much alcohol as 70 volumes of proof spirit.

Nowadays alcohol content is usually measured as % alcohol by volume.

propionates Salts of propionic acid, CH_3CH_2COOH, a normal metabolic intermediate. The free acid and salts are used as mould inhibitors, e.g. on cheese surfaces, and to inhibit *rope in bread and baked goods (E-280–283).

propyl gallate An *antioxidant, E-310.

prosciutto Italian for *ham; in English it means specifically smoked, spiced, Italian ham, eaten thinly sliced.

Prosparol Trade name for an emulsion containing 50% vegetable fat, 405 kcal (1.7 MJ)/100 g; used as a concentrated source of energy.

prosthetic group Non-protein part of an *enzyme molecule; either a coenzyme or a metal ion. Essential for catalytic activity. The enzyme protein without its prosthetic group is the apo-enzyme and is catalytically inactive. With the prosthetic group, it is known as the holo-enzyme. *See also* enzyme activation tests.

proteans Slightly altered proteins that have become insoluble, probably an early stage of denaturation.

protein All living tissues contain proteins; they are polymers of *amino acids, joined by *peptide bonds. There are twenty main amino acids in proteins, and any one protein may contain several hundred or over a thousand amino acids, so an enormous variety of different proteins occur in nature, i.e. in foods and our bodies.

Generally a polymer of relatively few amino acids is referred to as a peptide (e.g. di-, tri-, and tetrapeptides); oligopeptides contain up to about 50–100 amino acids; larger molecules are polypeptides or proteins.

The sequence of the amino acids in a protein determines its overall structure and function: many proteins are *enzymes; others are structural (e.g. *collagen in connective tissue and *keratin in hair and nails); many *hormones are polypeptides.

Proteins are constituents of all living cells and are dietary essentials. Chemically they are distinguished from fats and carbohydrates by containing nitrogen. They are composed of carbon, hydrogen, oxygen, nitrogen, sulphur, and sometimes phosphorus.

proteinases Enzymes that hydrolyse proteins, also known as peptidases. *See also* endopeptidases; exopeptidases.

protein-bound iodine The *thyroid hormones, tri-iodothyronine and thyroxine are transported in the blood-stream bound to proteins; measurement of protein-bound iodine, as opposed to total plasma iodine, was used as an index of thyroid gland activity before more specific methods of measuring the hormones were developed.

protein-calorie malnutrition *See* protein-energy malnutrition.

protein calories per cent *See* protein-energy ratio.

protein conversion factor *See* nitrogen conversion factor.

protein, crude Total *nitrogen multiplied by the *nitrogen conversion factor = 6.25. *See also* Kjeldahl determination.

Protein Efficiency Ratio (PER) A measure of *protein quality.

protein-energy malnutrition (PEM) A spectrum of disorders, especially in children, due to inadequate feeding. Marasmus is severe wasting and can occur in adults; it is the result of a food intake inadequate to meet energy expenditure. Kwashiorkor affects only young children and includes severe oedema, fatty infiltration of the liver, and a sooty dermatitis; it is likely that deficiency of *antioxidant nutrients and the stress of infection may be involved. The name kwashiorkor is derived from the Ga language of Ghana to describe the illness of the first child when it is weaned (on to an inadequate diet) on the arrival of the second child.

Emaciation, similar to that seen in marasmus, occurs in patients with advanced cancer and AIDS; in this case it is known as *cachexia.

protein-energy ratio The protein content of a food or diet expressed as the proportion of the total energy provided by protein (4 kcal, 17 kJ/ gram). The average requirement for protein is about 7% of total energy intake; average Western diets provide about 14%.

protein equivalent A measure of the digestible nitrogen of an animal feedingstuff in terms of protein. It is measured by direct feeding or calculated from the digestible pure protein plus half the digestible non-protein nitrogen.

protein, first class An obsolete system of classifying proteins into first and second class, to indicate their relative nutritional value or *protein quality. Generally, but not invariably, animal proteins were considered 'first class' and plant proteins 'second class', but this classification has no validity in the diet as a whole.

protein intolerance An *adverse reaction to one or more specific proteins in foods, commonly the result of an allergy. General protein intolerance may be due to a variety of *genetic diseases affecting amino acid metabolism. Treatment is normally by severe restriction of protein intake. *See also* amino acid disorders; hyperammonaemia.

protein milk Partially skimmed lactic acid milk plus milk curd (prepared from whole milk by *rennet precipitation); richer in protein and lower in fat than ordinary milk, and supposed to be better tolerated in digestive disorders. Also known as albumin milk and eiweiss milch.

protein quality A measure of the usefulness of a protein food for maintenance and repair of tissue, growth and formation of new tissues and, in animals, production of meat, eggs, wool, and milk. It is only important if the total intake of protein barely meets the requirement. Furthermore, the quality of individual proteins is relatively unimportant in mixed diets, because of *complementation between different proteins.

Two types of measurement are used to estimate protein quality: (a) biological assays and (b) chemical analysis.

(a) Biological Value (BV) is the proportion of absorbed protein retained in the body (i.e. taking no account of digestibility). A protein that is completely useable (e.g. egg and human milk) has BV = 0.9–1.0; meat and fish have BV = 0.75–0.8; wheat protein, 0.5; gelatine, 0.

Net Protein Utilization (NPU) is the proportion of dietary protein that is retained in the body under specified experimental conditions (i.e. it takes account of digestibility; NPU = BV × digestibility). By convention NPU is measured at 10% dietary protein (NPU_{10}) at which level the protein synthetic mechanism of the animal can utilize all of the protein so long as the balance of *essential amino acids is correct. When fed at 4% dietary protein, the result is NPU standardized. If the food or diet is fed as it is normally eaten, the result is NPU operative (NPU_{op}).

Protein Efficiency Ratio (PER) is the gain in weight of growing animals per gram of protein eaten.

Net Protein Retention (NPR) is the weight gain of animals fed the test protein, minus the weight loss of a group fed a protein-free diet, divided by the protein consumed.

Protein Retention Efficiency (PRE) is the NPR converted into a percentage scale by multiplying by 16: it then becomes numerically the same as Net Protein Utilization.

Relative Protein Value (RPV) is the ability of a test protein, fed at various levels of intake, to support *nitrogen balance, relative to a standard protein.

(b) Chemical Score is based on chemical analysis of the protein; it is the amount of the limiting *amino acid compared with the amount of the same amino acid in egg protein.

Protein Score is similar to Chemical Score, but uses an amino acid mixture as the standard, also known as amino acid score.

Essential amino acid index is the sum of all the essential amino acids compared with those in egg protein or the amino acid target mixture.

protein rating Used in Canadian Food Regulations to assess the overall protein quality of a food. It is Protein Efficiency Ratio multiplied by the protein content of food (per cent) multiplied by the amount of food that is reasonably consumed. Foods with a rating above 40 may be designated excellent dietary sources; foods with a rating below 20 are considered to be insignificant sources; 20–40 may be described as good sources.

protein, reference A theoretical concept of the perfect protein which is used with 100% efficiency at whatever level it is fed in the diet. Used as a means of expressing recommended intakes. The nearest approach to this theoretical protein are egg and human milk proteins, which are used with 90–100% efficiency (BV = 0.9–1.0) when fed at low levels in the diet (4%), but not when fed at high levels (10–15%).

Protein Retention Efficiency (PRE) A measure of *protein quality.

protein score A measure of *protein quality based on chemical analysis.

protein, second class *See* protein, first class.

protein turnover *See* half-life.

proteins, conjugated Proteins that include a non-protein prosthetic group, e.g. *haemoglobin and *cytochromes contain *haem; many oxidative *enzymes contain a prosthetic group derived from *vitamin B_2; many proteins are conjugated (combined) with carbohydrates (glycoproteins) or fatty acids.

proteolysis The hydrolysis of proteins to their constituent *amino acids, catalysed by alkali, acid, or enzymes.

proteoses Partial degradation products of proteins; soluble in water. The stages of breakdown are protein → proteoses → peptones → polypeptides → oligopeptides → amino acids.

prothrombin Protein in plasma involved in coagulation of *blood.

prothrombin time An index of the coagulability of *blood (and hence of *vitamin K nutritional status) based on the time taken for a citrated sample of blood to clot when calcium ions and thromboplastin are added.

protogen *See* lipoic acid.

protopectin *See* pectin.

protopectinase The enzyme in the pith of citrus fruits which converts protopectin into *pectin with the resultant separation of the plant cells from one another. Also known as pectosinase and pectosase.

provençale, à la Containing olive oil, garlic, and often tomato. Normally flavoured with mixed provençale herbs.

proving The stage in bread making when the dough is left to rise.

provitamin A substance that is converted into a vitamin, such as 7-dehydrocholesterol, which is converted into *vitamin D, or those *carotenes that can be converted to *vitamin A.

proximate analysis Analysis of foods and feedingstuffs for *nitrogen (for protein), ether extract (for fat), crude *fibre and *ash (mineral salts), together with soluble carbohydrate calculated by subtracting these values from the total (*carbohydrate by difference). Also known as Weende analysis, after the Weende Experimental Station in Germany, which in 1865 outlined the methods of analysis to be used.

prunelle French name for *sloe; also a liqueur made from sloes, similar to sloe gin.

prunes *See* dried fruit.

prunin *See* naringin.

Prunus Genus of plants including *plums, *peaches, *nectarines, *cherries, and *almonds.

Pruteen Trade name for microbial protein produced by growing bacteria, *Methylophilus methylotrophus*, on methanol (derived from methane or natural gas); 70% protein on dry weight.

P/S ratio The ratio between polyunsaturated and saturated *fatty acids. In Western diets the ratio is about 0.6; it is suggested that increasing it to near 1.0 would reduce the risk of atherosclerosis and coronary heart disease.

psychrophilic organisms Bacteria and fungi that tolerate low temperatures. Their preferred temperature range is 15–20 °C, but they will grow in cold stores at or below 0 °C; the temperature must be reduced to about −10 °C before growth stops, but the organisms are not killed and will regrow when the temperature rises.

Bacteria of the genera *Achromobacter, Flavobacterium, Pseudomonas*, and *Micrococcus; Torulopsis* yeasts; and moulds of the genera *Penicillium, Cladosporium, Mucor*, and *Thamnidium* are psychrophiles.

psyllium *Plantago psyllium*, also known as plantago or flea seed. Small, dark reddish-brown seeds which form a mucilaginous mass with water, taken medicinally to assist the passage of intestinal contents.

pteroylglutamic acid (pteroylglutamate), pteroylpolyglutamic acid (pteroylpolyglutamate) *See* folic acid.

ptomaines Loosely used name for amines formed by decarboxylation of amino acids during putrefaction of proteins: putrescine from arginine, cadaverine from lysine, muscarine in mushrooms, neurine formed by dehydration of choline. They have an unpleasant smell and were formerly thought to cause food poisoning.

ptyalin Obsolete name for salivary *amylase.

ptyalism Excessive flow of *saliva.

puberty, delayed The normal onset of puberty in boys is between the ages of 12–15; a number of factors may delay this, especially deficiency of *zinc. Severely zinc-deficient boys of 20 are still prepubertal.

puchero Spanish, Latin American; stew of beans, meat, and sausages.

pudding A baked or steamed sponge or suet dish, usually sweet and served as a dessert, but also savoury suet puddings (e.g. steak and kidney). Also milk puddings, made by baking rice, semolina, or sago in milk.

pudding, black *See* black pudding.

pudding, hasty *See* hasty pudding.

pudeena *See* mint.

PUFA Polyunsaturated fatty acids, *see* fatty acids.

puff pastry Prepared from alternating layers of fat and dough; upon baking steam accumulates between the dough layers and causes them to expand, forming large spaces between thin layers of *pastry.

puffballs Edible wild fungi; mosaic puffball *Calvatia (Lycoperdon) caelata*, and giant puffball *C. gigantea* (may grow to 30 cm in diameter), are normally eaten while still relatively small and fleshy. Much prized for their delicate flavour. *See* mushrooms.

Puffed Wheat Trade name of a breakfast cereal prepared by heating wheat grains under pressure and then rapidly releasing the pressure, when the superheated steam in the grain suddenly expands, so puffing or 'exploding' the grain. A 40-g portion is a good *source of copper; a source of protein, niacin, and iron; provides 2 g of dietary fibre; supplies 130 kcal (550 kJ).

puffer fish *See* tetrodontin poisoning.

pulpeta Caribbean (Cuban); meat loaf, served hot or cold.

pulque Sourish beer produced in Central and South America by the rapid natural fermentation of aquamiel, the sweet, mucilaginous sap of the agave (American aloe or century plant, *Agave americana*). Contains 6% alcohol by volume.

pulses Name given to the dried seeds (matured on the plant) of *legumes such as *peas, *beans, and *lentils. In the fresh, wet form they contain about 90% water, but the dried form contains about 10% water and can be stored.

pumpernickel Dense, sour-flavoured black bread made from rye, originating from Germany. Name said to be derived from Napoleon's remark that it was 'pain pour ma Nicole' (his horse). A 100-g portion is a *source of protein; contains 1 g of fat; provides 10 g of dietary fibre; supplies 200 kcal (850 kJ). Also used in the USA for any rye bread.

pumpkin A *gourd, fruit of *Cucurbita pepo*; a 90-g portion provides 1.8 g of dietary fibre and is a rich *source of vitamin A (as carotene); supplies 15 kcal (65 kJ).

punch A drink, hot or cold, made from wine and spirit, lemons and other fruit, spices and sugar.

punchnep Welsh; mashed potato and turnip with small holes punched into the top, into which cream is poured.

Punt-e-mes Trade name; Italian *vermouth with added quinine to give a bitter-sweet flavour.

purée Fruit, vegetable, meat, or fish that has been pounded or sieved (usually after cooking) to give a smooth, finely divided pulp. Also a soup made by sieving vegetables with the liquor in which they were cooked.

purgative *See* laxative.

puri (poori) Indian; unleavened whole-wheat bread prepared from a butter-rich dough, shaped into small pancakes and deep-fried in hot oil.

Purim fritters Traditional Jewish fritters eaten at Purim, similar to *French toast.

purines Nitrogenous compounds (bases) that occur in *nucleic acids (adenine and guanine) and their precursors and metabolites; inosine, caffeine, and theobromine are also purines. They are not dietary essentials; both dietary and endogenously formed purines are excreted as *uric acid.

Sweetbread (pancreas) is rich in purines, as is fish roe; there are moderate amounts in sardines and anchovies, lesser amounts in other fish and meat; little in vegetables, fruits, and cereals.

purl Old English winter drink; warmed ale with bitters and brandy or milk, sugar and spirit.

pursindah (pasendah) Indian; roast tender fillets of meat, cut into thin strips and beaten flat; normally cooked on skewers over charcoal.

putromaine Any toxin produced by the decay of food within the body.

pyridine nucleotides Obsolete name for the *coenzymes *NAD and NADP.

pyridoxal, pyridoxamine, pyridoxine *See* vitamin B$_6$.

pyrimidines Nitrogenous compounds (bases) that occur in *nucleic acids: cytosine, thymidine, and uracil.

pyrocarbonate *See* diethyl pyrocarbonate.

pyruvate Salts of *pyruvic acid.

pyruvic acid An intermediate in the metabolism of carbohydrates, formed by the anaerobic *glycolysis of *glucose. It may then either be converted to acetyl CoA, and oxidized through the *citric acid cycle, or be reduced to lactic acid. The oxidation to acetyl CoA is *thiamin dependent, and blood concentrations of pyruvate and lactate rise in thiamin deficiency.

Q

QbA Qualitätswein bestimmer Anbaugebeite; *see* wine classification, Germany.

QmP Qualitätswein mit Prädikat; *see* wine classification, Germany.

quahog American bivalve *shellfish, *Venus mercenaria*.

quail (French: *caille*; German: *Wachtel*.) Formerly a *game bird, now so endangered in the wild that shooting is prohibited, but farmed to some extent. Two main species, *Bonasa umbellus* and *Colinus virginianus*; Californian quail is *Lophortyx californica*. The small eggs are much prized as a delicacy. A 150-g portion (whole bird) is a rich *source of protein and niacin; a good source of vitamins B_1 and B_2; contains 3 g of fat and supplies 180 kcal (760 kJ).

qualitätswein *See* wine classification, Germany.

quamash Or camash; starchy roots of *Camassia quamash*, the staple food of West Coast native Americans.

quark (quarg) (French: *fromage blanc*; German, *Speisequark mage*.) When made from skim milk this is a very low-fat cheese originating from Germany; contains 80% water; a 100-g portion is a good *source of protein and vitamin B_{12}, a source of vitamin B_2, with only a trace of fat, contains 40 mg of sodium and 90 mg of calcium and supplies 80 kcal (325 kJ). Also available in some countries as '20% fat on dry matter' (5% fat); '40% fat on dry matter' (11% fat), being a good source of protein and a source of vitamin B_2; supplies 170 kcal (700 kJ) per 100-g portion.

quart Imperial measure of volume, equal to $^1/_4$ imperial gallon or 2 pints (i.e. 1.1 L).

quart, reputed The traditional 'bottle' of wine or spirits; approximately $^2/_3$ imperial quart, or $26^2/_3$ fl oz (730 mL). Reputed pint is $13^1/_3$ fl oz.

quartern *See* noggin.

queen cake Individual, small, light, rich cakes containing dried fruit.

queen of puddings Pudding made from custard and breadcrumbs, flavoured with lemon rind and vanilla, topped with jam or sliced fruit and meringue.

queen substance *See* royal jelly.

quenelle Dumplings made from finely pounded meat or fish.

quercitin A *flavone, found in onion skins, tea, hops, and horse chestnuts. Not known to be a dietary essential or to have any function in the body, but sometimes called *vitamin P.

quercitol *See* acorn sugar.

quercitron *See* flavin.

querns Pair of grinding stones used for pulverizing grain (from about 4000–2000 BC). The lower stone was slightly hollowed and the upper stone was rolled by hand on the lower one.

Quetelet's index *See* body mass index.

quetsch German plum brandy, prepared by distillation of fermented plums. Similar to *slivovitz and *mirabelle. Sometimes called zwetschgenwasser or zwetschenwasser.

quiche Savoury egg custard tart in a pastry case containing a wide variety of vegetable, meat, or fish fillings. Speciality of Alsace and Lorraine in France.

quick breads Baked goods such as biscuits, muffins, popovers, griddles, cakes, waffles, and dumplings, in which no yeast is used, but the raising is carried out quickly with baking powder or other chemical agents.

quick freezing Rapid freezing of food by exposure to a blast of air at a very low temperature. Unlike slow freezing, very small crystals of ice are formed which do not rupture the cells of the food and so the structure is relatively undamaged.

A quick-frozen food is commonly defined as one that has been cooled from a temperature of 0 °C to −5 °C or lower, in a period of not more than 2 hours, and then cooled to −18 °C.

quillaja (quillaia) Or soapbark; the dried bark of the shrub *Quillaja saponaria*, which contains *saponins and *tannins. Used to produce foam in soft drinks, shampoos, and fire extinguishers.

quince Pear-shaped fruit of *Cydonia oblongata*, with flesh similar to that of the apple; sour but strong aromatic flavour when cooked; rich in pectin and used chiefly in jams and jellies; used to be known as 'the apple and the vine'.

quince, Japanese Fruit of the ornamental shrub *Chaenomeles lagenaria*, hard, sour and aromatic, used in preserves and jellies.

quinine Bitter *alkaloid extracted from the bark of the cinchona tree (*Cinchona officinalis*), used to treat or prevent malaria and in aperitif wines, *bitters, and *tonic water.

quinoa Glutinous seeds of the South American plant *Chenopodium album*, used in Chile and Peru to make bread. A 100-g portion is a rich *source of iron and vitamin B_1; a good source of protein; a source of calcium, vitamin B_2, and niacin; supplies 350 kcal (1470 kJ).

quinquina French; bitter *vermouths based on partially fermented grape juice (mistelles) and *quinine; trade names include Byrrh, Dubonnet, and St Raphaël.

quintal 100 kg (220 lb).

Quorn Trade name for *mycoprotein from the mould *Fusarium graminearum*. A 150-g portion is a good *source of protein and niacin; a source of vitamin B_2; contains 4 g of fat, of which a quarter is saturated and half polyunsaturated; provides 7 g of dietary fibre; supplies 130 kcal (550 kJ).

R

R- and S- Prefixes to chemical names to denote the three-dimensional arrangement of the molecule based on rigorous chemical rules. *See* D-.

rabbit 1 (French: *lapin*; German: *Kaninchenfleisch*.) *Lepus cuniculus*; both wild and farmed rabbits are eaten. A 150-g portion is a rich *source of protein, niacin, vitamins B_2, B_6, and B_{12}, selenium and iron; a source of vitamin B_1, zinc, and copper; contains about 12 g of fat of which about 40% is *saturated and 20% mono-unsaturated; supplies 270 kcal (1100 kJ).
   2 Original form of rarebit, *see* Welsh rarebit.

racemic The mixture of the *D- and L-isomers of a compound, commonly shown as DL-.

rack Rib chops of lamb or mutton, left in one piece for roasting.

raclette Swiss; cheese melted over a fire, eaten with boiled potatoes.

racuszki Polish; deep-fried puffs made from mashed potato, served with sugar and sour cream.

radicchio Red *chicory.

radio frequency heating *See* microwave cooking.

radioallergosorbent tests (RAST) Tests for food allergy. *See* adverse reactions to foods.

radish The root of *Raphanus* spp. An 80-g portion is a good *source of vitamin C; supplies 10 kcal (40 kJ).

raffinade Best-quality refined sugar.

raffinose Trisaccharide of fructose, glucose and galactose, found in cotton seed, sugar-beet molasses, and Australian manna; also known as melitose or melitriose. Has 23% of the sweetness of sucrose. It is not digested.

ragi *See* millet.

ragoût Stew of meat or poultry and vegetables, browned in a little fat then gently simmered.

rainbow sugar Crystals of coffee *sugar, coloured.

raisin Dried seedless grapes of several kinds. Valencia raisins from Spanish grapes; Thompson seedless raisins produced mainly in California from the sultanina grape (the skins are coarser than the sultana). Raisins are also produced in Australia and South Africa. A 20-g portion provides 1.4 g of dietary fibre and supplies 50 kcal (210 kJ). *See also* currants, dried; dried fruit; sultanas. Raisin oil is extracted from the seeds of muscat *grapes, which are removed before drying them to yield raisins. The oil is used primarily to coat the raisins to prevent them sticking together, to render them soft and pliable and less subject to insect infestation.

raising powder *See* baking powder.

raita Indian; yoghurt with chopped cucumber, onion, garlic, and spices.

raki *See* ouzo.

Ralston Trade name; American breakfast cereal; whole wheat plus added wheat germ.

rambutan Fruit of *Nephelium lappaceum*; covered with yellowish-red, soft spines with large seed surrounded by white juicy flesh, similar to *lychee. The name means 'hairy man of the jungle' in Bahasa-Malay, reflecting the appearance of the fruit.

ramekin 1 Porcelain or earthenware mould in which mixture is baked and then brought to the table, or the savoury served in a ramekin dish. Paper soufflé cases are called ramekin cases.
 2 Formerly the name given to toasted cheese; now tarts filled with cream cheese.

rancidity The development of unpleasant flavours in oils and fats as a result of oxidation.

randomization of fats *See* interesterification.

rape *Brassica napus*, also known as cole, coleseed, or colza. Grown for its seed, as source of oil for both industrial and food use. Varieties low in erucic acid are termed '0' or single low; varieties also low in glucosinolates are termed '00' or double low, both these being undesirable constituents of ordinary rapeseed. Oil is very rich in mono-unsaturates (60%), contains 33% polyunsaturates, and only 7% saturates.

rarebit *See* Welsh rarebit.

rasgulla Indian; dessert of small balls of milk curd, ground almond, and semolina boiled in syrup.

rasher Slice of *bacon or *ham.

raspberry Fruit of *Rubus idaeus*. An 80-g portion is a rich *source of vitamin C; a source of folate and copper; supplies 6.4 g of dietary fibre; 20 kcal (85 kJ). Black raspberry is *Rubus occidentalis*, native of eastern USA.

raspings Finely ground breadcrumbs, used for coating rissoles, fishcakes, etc.

RAST Radioallergosorbent tests for food allergy. *See* adverse reactions to foods.

rastrello Sharp-edged spoon used to cut out the pulp from halved oranges or other *citrus fruit.

ratafia 1 Flavouring essence made from bitter almonds.
 2 Small macaroon-like biscuits flavoured with almonds.
 3 Almond-flavoured liqueur.

ratatouille Casserole or stew of aubergine, onions, peppers, courgettes, and tomatoes, originally from Provence in southern France.

ravigote butter *See* butter.

ravigote sauce 1 French; *salad dressing containing pounded hard-boiled egg, highly flavoured with garlic and chopped herbs.

2 Sauce made from ravigote butter melted in wine and vinegar added to a *velouté sauce; served with boiled poultry.

ravioli Square envelope of *pasta stuffed with minced meat or cheese.

raw sugar Brown unrefined sugar, 96–98% pure, as imported for refining. Contaminated with mould spores, bacteria, cane fibre, and dirt.

ray Cartilaginous *fish, *Raja* spp.

RD Região demarcada, *see* wine classification, Portugal.

RDA Recommended daily (or dietary) allowance (or amount) of nutrients; *see* reference intakes.

Ready Brek Trade name for instant, hot, oatmeal breakfast cereal. A 30-g portion made up to 200 g of porridge is a rich *source of vitamin B_1; a good source of vitamin B_6; a source of niacin, iron, and copper; contains 2.1 g of dietary fibre; 2.7 g of fat of which 13% is saturated; supplies 120 kcal (500 kJ).

rebaudioside Very sweet substance extracted from the leaves of *Stevia rebaudiana* (same source as *stevioside); 400 times as sweet as sucrose.

réchauffé Made-up dish of reheated food; literally 'reheated' (French).

reciprocal ponderal index An index of adiposity; height divided by cube root of weight. *See also* ponderal index.

Recommended Daily Amount (or Allowance), RDA *See* reference intakes; Appendices II–VI.

recommended intakes (of nutrients) *See* reference intakes; Appendices II–VI.

rectal feeding *See* nutrient enemata.

red blood cells *See* blood cells.

red colours *Amaranth (E-123), *carmoisine (E-122), *cochineal (E-120), *erythrosine (E-127), *poncho 4R (E-124), red 2G (E-128).

red cooking Chinese method of cooking; meat or poultry is first *stir fried, then simmered in broth or water with *soy sauce, herbs, and spices.

redcurrants Fruit of *Ribes sativum* (same species as whitecurrants); the UK National Fruit Collection contains 78 varieties. An 80-g portion is a rich *source of vitamin C; a source of copper; supplies 5.6 g of dietary fibre; 15 kcal (65 kJ).

red herrings *Herrings that have been well salted and smoked for about ten days. Bloaters are salted less and smoked for a shorter time; kippers lightly salted and smoked overnight. Also called Yarmouth bloaters.

red pepper *See* pepper.

red tide Sudden, unexplained increase in numbers of toxic organisms (dinoflagellates) in the sea which cause fish and shellfish feeding on them to become seasonally toxic.

reduce The process of boiling a mixture (especially when making a sauce, soup, or syrup) in an uncovered pan to evaporate surplus liquid and give a more concentrated product.

reduced EU legislation (in preparation in 1995) and US legislation state that for a food label or advertising to bear a claim that it contains a reduced amount of fat, saturates, cholesterol, sodium, or alcohol it must contain 25% less of the specified nutrient than a reference product for which no claim is made. A food may not claim to have a reduced content of a nutrient if it is already classified as *low in or *free from that nutrient.

reducing sugars *Sugars that are chemically reducing agents, including *glucose, *fructose, *lactose, *pentoses, but not *sucrose.

reduction The opposite of *oxidation; chemical reactions resulting in a gain of electrons, or hydrogen, or the loss of oxygen.

reduction rolls *See* milling.

reference intakes (of nutrients) Amounts of nutrients greater than the requirements of almost all members of the population, determined on the basis of the average requirement plus twice the standard deviation, to allow for individual variation in requirements and thus cover the theoretical needs of 97.5% of the population.

Reference intakes for energy are based on the average requirement, without the allowance for individual variation. Used for planning institutional catering and assessing the adequacy of diets of groups of people, but not strictly applicable to individuals. Tables of reference intakes published by different national and international authorities differ because of differences in the interpretation of the available data; see Appendices II–VI.

Variously called in different countries and by different expert committees: RDA, the Recommended Daily (or Dietary) Amount (or Allowance); RDI, Recommended Daily (or Dietary) Intake; RNI, Reference Nutrient Intake; PRI, Population Reference Intake; safe allowances.

Levels of intake below that at which health and metabolic integrity are likely to be maintained are generally taken as the average requirement minus twice the standard deviation. Variously known as Minimum Safe Intake (MSI), Lower Reference Nutrient Intake (LRNI), and Lowest Threshold Intake.

reference man An arbitrary physiological standard; defined as a man aged 25, weighing 65 kg, living in a temperate zone of a mean annual temperature of 10 °C, performing medium work, and assumed to require an average daily intake of 3200 kcal (13.5 MJ).

Reference Nutrient Intake, RNI *See* reference intakes.

reference protein *See* protein, reference.

reference woman An arbitrary physiological standard; defined as a woman aged 25, weighing 55 kg, living in a temperate zone of a mean annual temperature of 10 °C, engaged in general household duties or light industry, and assumed to require an average daily intake of 2300 kcal (9.7 MJ).

reformed meat *See* meat, reformed.

reform sauce *Espagnole sauce enriched with port and *redcurrant jelly; originated at the Reform Club in London as an accompaniment for breaded and fried lamb cutlets.

refractive index Measure of the bending or refraction of a beam of light on entering a denser medium (the ratio between the sine of the angle of incidence of the ray of light and the sine of the angle of refraction). It is constant for pure substances under standard conditions. Used as a measure of sugar or total solids in solution, purity of oils, etc.

refractometer Instrument to measure the *refractive index.

refreshing A process used by cooks when preparing vegetables. After the vegetables have been cooked, cold water is poured over them to preserve the colour; they are then reheated before serving.

refried beans *See* frijoles.

refrigerants Cooling agents in refrigerators and freezers, originally ammonia or carbon dioxide were used, subsequently replaced by chlorofluorocarbons (CFCs), trade names Freon and Arcton. Because of the persistence of CFCs in the upper atmosphere, where they destroy the protective ozone layer, they are considered an environmental hazard, and alternative refrigerants are being developed.

refrigeration *See* preservation.

região demarcada (RD) *See* wine classification, Portugal.

regional enteritis *See* Crohn's disease.

Register of Accredited Nutritionists A register of those with approved qualifications in nutrition maintained by the British Nutrition Society and Institute of Biology.

Rehfuss tube A small-diameter tube with a slotted metal tip for removing samples of food from the stomach after a test meal. *See also* Ryle tube.

Reichert-Meissl value Measure of the volatile fatty acids in fats.

reine, à la Dish based on chicken.

relative humidity *See* humidity.

Relative Protein Value A measure of *protein quality.

release agents Substances applied to tinned or enamelled surfaces or plastic films to prevent the food adhering, e.g. fatty acid amides, microcrystalline waxes, petrolatums, starch, methyl cellulose.

relish Culinary term for any spicy or piquant preparation used to enhance flavour of plain food. In the UK, a thin pickle or sauce with a vinegar base; in the USA it includes finely chopped fruit or vegetables with a dressing of salt, sugar, and vinegar, sometimes eaten as a first course (termed apple, garden, or salad relish).

relish, Gentleman's *See* Gentleman's relish.

rémoulade sauce Mayonnaise with added mustard and finely chopped capers, gherkins, parsley, chervil, and anchovy fillet. *See also* salad dressing.

remove Obsolete term for the main course of dinner.

renal failure Inability of the kidneys to excrete waste, as a result of kidney disease. Especially in advanced cases, as well as haemodialysis, treatment includes feeding a very low protein diet, so as to minimize the amount of nitrogenous waste that must be excreted.

rendering The process of liberating the fat from the cells that constitute the adipose tissue. Dry rendering, heating the fat dry, or wet rendering, when water is present.

rennet Extract of calf stomach; contains the enzyme *chymosin (rennin) which clots milk. Used in cheese making and for *junket.

rennet, vegetable The name given to proteolytic enzymes derived from plants, such as bromelain (from the pineapple) and ficin (from the fig), as well as biosynthetic *chymosin. Used for the preparation of 'vegetarian' cheeses.

rennin See chymosin.

rentschlerizing Sterilizing by treatment with ultraviolet light, named after Dr H. C. Rentschler, who developed the lamp.

renversé Turned out of a mould, as for a cream or jelly.

resazurin test See methylene blue dye-reduction test.

resins, ion-exchange See ion-exchange resins.

resistant starch See starch, enzyme resistant.

respiratory quotient (RQ) Ratio of the volume of carbon dioxide produced when a substance is oxidized, to the volume of oxygen used. The oxidation of carbohydrate results in an RQ of 1.0; of fat, 0.7; and of protein, 0.8.

respirometer See spirometer.

restoration The addition of nutrients to replace those lost in processing, as in milling of cereals. See also fortification.

reticulocyte Immature precursor of the red blood cell (normocyte or erythrocyte) in which the remains of the nucleus are visible as a reticulum. Very few are seen in normal blood as they are retained in the marrow until mature, but on remission of anaemia, when there is a high rate of production, reticulocytes appear in the bloodstream (reticulocytosis).

reticulum See ruminant.

retinal (retinaldehyde), retinene, retinoic acid See vitamin A.

retinoid receptors Intracellular proteins that bind the vitamers of *vitamin A (retinol, retinoic acid, and other *retinoids), resulting in the modulation of gene expression, and hence the basis of the actions of the vitamin other than in vision.

retinoids Compounds chemically related to, or derived from, *vitamin A, which display some of the biological activities of the vitamin, but have lower toxicity; they are used for treatment of serious skin disorders and some cancers.

retinol See vitamin A.

retort In food technology, an *autoclave.

retrogradation *See* staling.

retsina Greek dry white wine, with a strong resinous flavour due to the addition of pine resin as a preservative.

Reuben sandwich American; salt beef (corned beef) with cheese and sauerkraut, on rye bread, served hot. Originated in 1956 as the winner of a competition for novel sandwiches; the origin of the name is unclear.

reverse osmosis *See* osmosis, reverse.

RF heating *See* microwave heating.

rhamnose A methylated pentose (five-carbon) sugar; it has 33% of the sweetness of sucrose, and is widely distributed in plant foods.

rheology Study of deformation and flow of materials; in food technology it involves plasticity of fats, doughs, milk curd, etc. It provides a scientific basis for subjective measurements such as mouth feel, spreadability, pourability.

rhizome Botanical term for swollen stem that produces roots and leafy shoots.

rhizopterin Obsolete name for *folic acid.

rhodopsin The pigment in the cone cells of the retina of the eye, also known as visual purple, consisting of the protein opsin and retinaldehyde, which is responsible for the visual process. In rod cells of the retina the equivalent protein is iodopsin. *See* vitamin A; dark adaptation; vision.

rhubarb Leaf-stalks of the perennial plant, *Rheum rhaponticum*. Has a high content of *oxalate (the leaves contain even more, and hence are toxic). A 200-g portion (stewed without sugar) is a *source of vitamin C; contains 2.5 g of dietary fibre; supplies 15 kcal (65 kJ).

Ribena Trade name for a preparation of *blackcurrant juice; extremely rich source of vitamin C, 200 mg per 100 g, so a 300 mL glassful, diluted 1 : 6 would be a very rich *source of the vitamin.

riboflavin *See* vitamin B_2.

ribonucleic acid (RNA) *See* nucleic acids.

ribose A pentose (five-carbon) sugar which occurs as an intermediate in the metabolism of glucose; especially important in the *nucleic acids and various *coenzymes: occurs widely in foods.

Ribotide Trade name (Japan) for a mixture of the *purine derivatives, disodium inosinate and disodium guanylate, used as a *flavour enhancer for savoury dishes.

rice Grain of *Oryza sativa*; major food in many countries. Rice when threshed is known as paddy, and is covered with a fibrous husk comprising nearly 40% of the grain. When the husk has been removed, brown rice is left. When the outer bran layers up to the endosperm and germ are removed, the ordinary white rice of commerce or polished rice is obtained (usually polished with glucose and talc).

A 200-g portion of boiled brown rice is a good *source of niacin and copper; a source of protein, vitamin B₁, and selenium; provides 1.6 g of dietary fibre; supplies 280 kcal (1180 kJ). A 200-g portion of boiled white rice is a source of niacin and protein; supplies 280 kcal (1180 kJ).

rice, American *See* bulgur.

rice, glutinous For most dishes, separate rice grains that do not stick together in a glutinous mass are preferred. Glutinous rice is rich in soluble starch, dextrin, and maltose and on boiling the grains adhere in a sticky mass; this rice is used for sweetmeats and cakes.

rice grass *See* Indian rice grass.

rice, hungry A variety of *millet, *Digitaria exilis*, important in West Africa.

Rice Krispies Trade name for a breakfast cereal prepared by 'explosion puffing' of rice. A 30-g portion is a rich *source of vitamins B_6, B_{12}, and niacin; a good source of vitamins B_1 and B_2; a source of vitamin D and iron; provides 400 mg of sodium, 0.3 g of dietary fibre; supplies 125 kcal (530 kJ).

rice, maize or mealie *See* maize rice.

rice paper Smooth edible white 'paper' made from the pith of the Taiwanese shrub *Tetrapanax papyriferus* and the Indo-Pacific shrub *Scaevola sericea*. Macaroons and similar biscuits are baked on it and the paper can be eaten with the biscuits.

rice, parboiled *See* parboil.

rice, red West African species, *Oryza glaberrima*, with red bran layer.

rice, synthetic *See* tapioca-macaroni.

rice, unpolished American term; rice that has been under-milled in that the husk, germ, and bran layers have been partially removed.

rice vinegar Japanese; *vinegar prepared from *saké.

rice, wild Also known as zizanie, Tuscarora rice, Indian rice, and American wild rice (American rice is *bulgur); *Zizania aquatica*, native to eastern North America, grows 12 feet high; it has a long, thin, greenish grain; little is grown and it is difficult to harvest, so it is strictly a gourmet food. Higher in protein content than ordinary rice at 14%.

rice wine *See* saké.

Richelieu, à la Dish made with Richelieu sauce (a rich brown Madeira sauce) or garnished with mushrooms, artichoke bottoms, or stuffed tomatoes, etc.

ricin A *lectin in the *castor oil bean.

ricing Culinary term: cutting into small pieces about the size of rice grains.

ricinoleic acid A hydroxylated mono-unsaturated *fatty acid in *castor oil.

rickets Malformation of the bones in growing children due to deficiency of *vitamin D, leading to poor absorption of calcium. In adults the equivalent is osteomalacia.

rickets, refractory *Rickets that does not respond to normal amounts of vitamin D but requires massive doses. Usually a result of a congenital defect in the metabolism of vitamin D, it can also be due to poisoning with strontium.

rickets, vitamin D resistant *See* rickets, refractory.

rickey Long drink made from liqueur or spirit with ginger ale and fresh fruit.

ricotta Italian; *cheese made originally from the *whey left by cheese making, but now often with milk added.

riesling One of the 9 'classic' *grape varieties used for *wine making; the wines have a flowery aroma when young.

riffle flumes Washing equipment consisting of stepped channels along which the product being washed is carried in a flow of water; stones and grit are retained on the steps.

rigor mortis Stiffening of muscle that occurs after death. As the flow of blood ceases, anaerobic metabolism leads to the formation of lactic acid and the soft, pliable muscle becomes stiff and rigid. If meat is hung in a cool place for a few days ('conditioned'), the meat softens again. Fish similarly undergo rigor mortis but it is usually of shorter duration than in mammals. *See also* DFD meat; meat conditioning.

rijstaffel Dutch, Indonesian; meal consisting of a variety of different dishes (twenty or more) served at the same time.

rillauds French; potted pork, goose, or rabbit made from very small pieces, flavoured, seasoned, and cooked very slowly in stock. Rillettes and rillons are modifications of the procedure.

rillettes, rillons *See* rillauds.

rioja Wines from the Rioja region of Spain; white or red. Traditionally matured in oak casks, so have a strong 'oaky' flavour.

risotto Italian; rice dishes cooked with meat, poultry, vegetables, etc.

rissole Small round cake of cooked minced meat, bound with mashed potato, coated in egg and breadcrumb, and fried. Originally enclosed in an envelope of thin pastry before frying.

rissolé Baked or fried and well-browned.

RNA Ribonucleic acid, *see* nucleic acids.

RNI Reference Nutrient Intake, *see* reference intakes; Appendices II–VI.

roast Originally meant to cook meat over an open fire on a spit; now refers to cooking in an enclosed oven, and so is 'dry heating'. With meat the juices are squeezed out and evaporate on the surface, producing the *Maillard complex characteristic of roasted meat.

robert sauce Piquant sauce containing onion, white wine, vinegar, mustard, and espagnole or demi-glace sauce; served with meat.

rocambole Mild variety of *garlic, *Allium scordoprasum*, also called sand leek.

rock cake Plain buns containing fruit and spice, baked in small heaps on a tin or baking sheet.

rock eel, salmon Alternative name for *dogfish.

rocket (French: *roquette*; Italian, *ruchette*.) Cruciferous plant, *Eruca sativa*, with small spear-shaped leaves and peppery taste, eaten raw in salads or cooked. Also called arugula, rucola, Italian cress.

rock lobster *Shellfish, family Palinuridae, *see* lobster.

rock (mint-rock) Traditional English seaside sugar confectionery, made by pulling melted sugar. It is white, with an outer coloured layer (traditionally pink) and an inner ring of coloured sugar that spells out the name of the town.

rocou *See* annatto.

roe Hard roe is the eggs of the female fish. A 100-g portion of (fried) cod roe is a rich *source of protein, vitamins B_1, B_2, and C; a good source of niacin; a source of iron; contains 10 g of fat, of which 10% is saturated and 50% unsaturated; supplies 200 kcal (840 kJ). Soft roe is from the male fish, also known as milt. A 100-g portion of (fried) herring roe is a rich source of protein, vitamin B_2, and niacin; a source of vitamin B_1 and iron; contains 15 g of fat, of which 10% is saturated and 50% polyunsaturated; supplies 240 kcal (1000 kJ). Hard roe of sturgeon and lumpfish are used to make *caviare and mock caviare.

rokelax Scandinavian term for smoked *salmon. *See also* gravadlax; lax; lox.

roller dryer The material to be dried is spread over the surface of internally heated rollers and drying is complete within a few seconds. The rollers rotate against a knife that scrapes off the dried film as soon as it forms. There is little damage to nutrients by this method; for example, roller-dried milk is not scorched, but there is some loss of vitamins B_1 and C, more than in spray drying.

roller mill Pairs of horizontal cylindrical rollers, separated by only a small gap and revolving at different speeds. The material is thus ground and crushed in one operation. Used in flour milling.

rollmop Filleted uncooked *herring pickled in spiced vinegar.

roll-on closure (RO) Aluminium or lacquered tinplate cap for sealing on to narrow-necked bottles with a threaded neck. The unthreaded cap is moulded on to the neck of the bottle and forms an air-tight seal.

roly-poly Sweet suet *pudding filled with jam.

romaine French and American name for cos *lettuce.

romesco sauce Spanish (Catalan); pungent red sauce made from small red peppers, tomatoes, almonds, olive oil, garlic, and cayenne pepper.

rooibos tea Fermented leaves of the South African bush *Aspalathus liniearis*. Contains a unique polyphenol, aspalathin, which becomes red during preparation and produces a reddish herbal tea; free from *caffeine and *theaflavin.

root beer American; non-alcoholic carbonated beverage flavoured with extract of *sassafras root and oil of wintergreen.

ropa vieja *See* old clothes stew.

rope Spore-forming bacteria (*Bacillus mesentericus* and *B. subtilis*) occurring on wheat and hence in flour. The spores can survive baking and then are present in the bread. Under the right conditions of warmth and moisture the spores germinate and the mass of bacteria convert the bread into sticky, yellowish patches which can be pulled out into rope-like threads, hence the term 'ropy' bread. The bacterial growth is inhibited by acid substances. Can also occur in milk, called long milk in Scandinavia.

roquefort Green-blue marbled French *cheese made in Roquefort-sur-Soulzon from cow's milk; ripened in limestone caves where the mould, *Penicillium roquefortii* is present and the cheese thus inoculated. A 30-g portion is a *source of vitamins B_{12}, B_2, and protein, contains 9 g of fat, 200 mg of calcium, 500 mg of sodium; supplies 115 kcal (475 kJ).

rosado Portuguese, Spanish; rosé wines.

rosato Italian; rosé wines (also chiaretto or cerasulo).

rosé Pink-coloured *wines, either made from red grapes, allowing the skin to remain in the fermentation for only 12–36 hours, or by mixing red and white wines. Known as blush wines in the USA.

Rose-Gottlieb test For fat in milk, by extracting the fat with solvent.

rose hips The fruit of the rose (*Rosa* spp.); a rich source of vitamin C. Rose-hip syrup is extract of rose hips with added sugar.

rosella Caribbean plant (*Hibiscus sabdariffa*) grown for its fleshy red sepals, used to make drinks, jams and jelly. Also known as sorrel, flor de Jamaica.

rosemary A bushy shrub, *Rosmarinus officinalis*, cultivated commercially for its essential oil, used in medicine and perfumery. The leaves are used to flavour soups, sauces and meat.

rose water Fragrant water made by distillation or extraction of the *essential oils of rose petals. Used in confectionery (especially *Turkish delight) and baking.

rösti Swiss; potatoes are partly baked or boiled, then sliced and fried in hot fat to form a cake with a golden crust.

rotary louvre dryer A drying process whereby hot air passes through a moving bed of the solid inside a rotating drum.

Roth-Benedict spirometer *See* spirometer.

roti *See* chapatti.

rôtisserie Method of cooking which developed from the traditional rotating spit above an open fire; the food is rotated while roasting, so bastes itself.

rotmos Swedish; mashed boiled potatoes and turnips.

rotten pot *See* Madrid stew.

roughage *See* fibre, dietary.

rouille French (Provençale) sauce made from red chillies, garlic, olive oil, and potatoes or breadcrumbs, served with fish dishes.

roulade French; meat roll or galantine.

roux The foundation of most sauces; prepared by cooking together equal amounts of fat and plain flour, for a short time for white sauces, and longer for blond or brown sauces. The sauce is then prepared by stirring in milk or stock.

Rovimix Trade name for stabilized forms of vitamins, including A, D, and E as beadlets coated with a gelatine-starch mixture, used to enrich foods.

rowan Fruit of the rowan (mountain ash, *Sorbus aucuparia*) can be used to make a bitter-sweet jelly served with *game.

royal icing *See* icing.

royal jelly The food on which bee larvae are fed and which causes them to develop into queen bees. Although it is a rich source of *pantothenic acid and other vitamins, in the amounts consumed it would make a negligible contribution to human intakes. Of its dry weight, 2% is hydroxy-decenoic acid, which is believed to be the active queen substance. Claimed, without foundation, to have rejuvenating properties for human beings.

RPV Relative Protein Value, a measure of *protein quality.

RQ *See* respiratory quotient.

rubané Dish made from food cut into ribbon-like layers.

rubbing-in Method of incorporating fat into flour for pastry, etc.; the fat is cut into small pieces and gently rubbed into the flour by hand.

rubble reel Machine for cleaning materials such as wheat. The material is fed into a long, inclined reel made of perforated metal that rotates inside a frame. The perforations become larger nearer the bottom, so that there is a graded sieving of the material as it passes down the reel.

Rubner factors *See* energy factors.

rum Spirit distilled from fermented sugar cane juice or molasses; may be colourless and light-tasting or dark and with a strong flavour. Traditionally rum is darker and more strongly flavoured the further south in the Caribbean it is made.

There are three main categories: Cuban, Jamaican, and Dutch East Indian; and several types: aguardiente (Spain, Portugal, and S. America), Bacardi (trade name, originally from Cuba), cachaca (Brazil), cane spirit (S. Africa), Demerara rum (Guyana); 35–60% alcohol by volume, 250–420 kcal (1.0–1.8 MJ) per 100 mL.

rumen *See* ruminant.

ruminant Animals such as the cow, sheep, and goat, which possess four stomachs, as distinct from monogastric animals, such as man, pig, dog, and rat. The four are: the rumen, or first stomach, where bacterial fermentation produces volatile fatty acids, and whence the food is returned to the mouth for further mastication (chewing the cud); the reticulum, where further bacterial fermentation produces volatile fatty acids; the omasum; and the abomasum or true stomach. The bacterial fermentation allows ruminants to obtain nourishment from grass and hay which cannot be digested by monogastric animals.

rumpbone Cut of meat: in the USA it is called the aitchbone, in the UK, the loin or haunch.

rush nut *See* tiger nut.

rusk 1 Sweetened biscuit or piece of bread or cake crisped in the oven, especially as food for young children when teething.
2 Cereal added to *sausages and *hamburgers.

russe, à la Containing beetroot and/or sour cream.

Russian dressing *See* salad dressing.

Russian tea Tea without milk, served with lemon. Traditionally it is not sweetened, but is drunk by sucking through a crystal of sugar held between the teeth.

rutabaga American name for *swede.

rutin The disaccharide derivative of *quercitin, containing *glucose and *rhamnose. Found in grains, tomato stalk, and elderberry blossom. Not known to be a dietary essential or to have any function in the body, but once called *vitamin P.

rye Grain of *Secale cereale*, the predominant cereal in some parts of Europe; very hardy and withstands adverse conditions better than wheat. Rye flour is dark and the dough lacks elasticity; rye bread is usually made with *sour dough rather than yeast. *See also* bread, rye; crispbreads; ergot; ergotism; pumpernickel.

rye whisky *See* whisky.

Ryle tube A narrow rubber tube with a blind end containing a lead weight, with holes above this level, for removing samples of the contents of the stomach at intervals after a test meal. *See also* Rehfuss tube.

Ryvita Trade name for a rye *crispbread. A 50-g portion (five biscuits) is a *source of protein, vitamin B_1, iron, and zinc; provides 6 g of dietary fibre; supplies 160 kcal (640 kJ).

S- and R- *See* R- and S-.

sabayon French; *see* zabaglione.

sablé Biscuit paste made with butter and flour; sweet or savoury.

sabra Israeli name for the *prickly pear. Also the name of an Israeli liqueur flavoured with bitter oranges and chocolate.

saccharases Enzymes (including *invertase) that *hydrolyse sugars to liberate their constituent *monosaccharides. *See also* sucrase.

saccharic acid The dicarboxylic acid derived from glucose.

saccharimeter Polarimeter used to determine the purity of sugar; graduated on the International Sugar Scale in degrees sugar (distinct from *saccharometer).

saccharin A synthetic chemical, benzoic sulphimide, 550 times as sweet as sucrose. Soluble saccharin is the sodium salt. It has no food value, but is useful as a sweetening agent for diabetics and slimmers. Discovered in the USA in 1879.

saccharometer Floating device used to determine the specific gravity of sugar solutions (distinct from *saccharimeter).

saccharose *See* sucrose.

sachertorte Austrian; chocolate sponge cake with rich chocolate icing and whipped cream.

sack Old name for a variety of white wines from Spain and the Canaries, e.g. sherry.

sacristan Cake made from trimmings of puff pastry, dusted with sugar, and baked brown in twisted strips.

saddle The whole back of the animal (e.g. *lamb, *venison, *hare), from the end of the loin to the best end of the neck.

safe allowances *See* reference intakes.

safe and adequate intake Where there is inadequate scientific evidence to establish requirements and *reference intakes for a nutrient for which deficiency is rarely, if ever, seen, the observed levels of intake are assumed to be greater than requirements, and thus provide an estimate of intakes that are safe and (more than) adequate to meet needs.

safe level of intake *See* reference intakes.

safflower oil Vegetable oil extracted from the seeds of *Carthamus tinctoria*, 75% polyunsaturated fatty acids. *See also* saffron, Mexican.

saffron Deep orange-red powder from the stigmata of the saffron crocus, *Crocus sativus* (related to the garden crocus); 1 g requires the stigmata of 1500 flowers and yields about 50 mg of extract. Used as natural dyestuff (permitted food colour, with no E-number) and spice. Very soluble in water.

saffron, Indian *See* turmeric.

saffron, Mexican Substitute for *saffron made from the stigmata of *Carthamus tinctoria* (family Compositae), also known as the safflower; the seeds are the source of *safflower oil.

sage Leaf of the Dalmatian sage, *Salvia officinalis*, of the mint family; fragrant and spicy and an important herb used in the kitchen for flavouring meat and fish dishes and in poultry stuffing. Other sages (Greek, Spanish, English) differ in flavour from the Dalmatian variety.

sago Starchy grains prepared from the pith of the swamp sago (*Metroxylon sagu*) and the sugar palm (*Arenga pinnuta*); almost pure starch and sugars (sucrose, glucose, and fructose), free from protein.

St Anthony's Fire *See* ergot.

St Germain, à la Dish made with green peas.

St John's bread *See* carob.

St Raphaël *See* aperitif wines.

saithe Also known as coley and coal fish, *Polachius virens*. Apart from being eaten cooked, it is smoked, salted, and dyed red when it is similar to smoked salmon.

saké Japanese wine made from rice. Cooked whole rice grains are fermented with a yeast-like fungus culture for 10–14 days and stored in wooden barrels. Contains about 17% alcohol, by volume. Normally drunk warm and traditionally served in conical ceramic cups.

salad Originally derived from the Latin *sal* for salt, meaning something dipped into salt. Now normally a dish of uncooked vegetables; either a mixed salad or just one item (commonly lettuce or tomato). In France it can mean a small, hot, savoury dish, e.g. of chicken liver, etc.

salad burnet *See* burnet.

salad, caesar Cos lettuce, fried croûtons, chopped anchovies, Parmesan cheese, and raw egg, tossed in dressing.

salad dressing Emulsions of oil and vinegar, which may or may not contain other flavourings. French dressing (vinaigrette) is a temporary *emulsion of oil and vinegar; heavy French dressing is stabilized with *pectin or vegetable *gum.

Mayonnaise is a stable emulsion of vinegar in oil, made with egg. Salad cream was originally developed as a commercial substitute for mayonnaise (mid-nineteenth century); an emulsion made from vegetable oil, vinegar, salt, spices, emulsified with egg yolk and thickened. Legally, in the UK, it must contain not less than 25% by weight of vegetable oil and not less than 1.35% egg-yolk solids. Mayonnaise usually contains more oil, less carbohydrate and water. By US regulations salad dressing contains 30% vegetable oil and 4% egg yolk; mayonnaise contains 65% oil plus egg yolk.

Red mayonnaise is prepared by adding beetroot juice and the coral (eggs) of lobster to mayonnaise; an accompaniment to lobster and other seafood dishes.

Russian dressing is in fact American; made from mayonnaise with pimento, chilli sauce, green pepper, and celery, or sometimes by mixing mayonnaise with tomato ketchup. Thousand Island dressing is made from equal parts of mayonnaise and Russian dressing, with whipped cream.

salades composées French regional specialities, mixed salads containing meat, fish, eggs, etc., for example, salade Niçoise contains hard-boiled egg, anchovy fillets, tuna and olives as well as lettuce and tomatoes.

salad, Russian Cooked diced vegetables, ham, prawns, etc., in aspic.

salami Type of *sausage speckled with pieces of fat and flavoured with garlic; originally Italian.

salchichón Spanish; *salami.

salep (Greek: *salepi.*) Turkish beverage prepared from orchid tubers; milky white in appearance, with only a slight flavour.

salinometer (salimeter, salometer) Hydrometer to measure concentration of salt solutions by density.

Salisbury steak American; similar to *hamburger, i.e. minced lean beef mixed with bread, eggs, milk, and seasoning, shaped into cakes and fried.

saliva Secretion of the salivary glands in the mouth: 1–1.5 L secreted daily. A dilute solution of the protein mucin (which lubricates food) and the enzyme amylase (which hydrolyses starch), with small quantities of urea, potassium thiocyanate, sodium chloride, and bicarbonate.

salivary glands Three pairs of glands in the mouth, which secrete *saliva: parotid, submandibular, and submaxillary glands.

Sally Lunn A sweet, spongy, yeast cake, named after a girl who sold her tea cakes in Bath in the eighteenth century. In southern states of the USA it refers to a variety of yeast and soda breads.

salmagundi (salamagundi) Old English dish consisting of diced fresh and salt meats mixed with hard-boiled eggs, pickled vegetables, and spices, arranged on a bed of salad.

salmi *Ragoût made from game or poultry.

salmon (French: *saumon*; German: *Lachs.*) Fish of a number of species including Atlantic salmon (*Salmo salar*), and chinook, chum, coho (or silver), pink (or humpback), and sockeye (or red), which are varieties of *Oncorhynchus* and in the UK must be described as red or pink salmon. Although wild salmon are caught on a large scale, much of the salmon available in Europe is farmed in deep inlets of the sea, especially in Scotland and Norway.

A 150-g portion is an exceptionally rich *source of vitamin B_{12}, a rich source of protein, niacin, vitamin B_6, copper, and selenium; a good source of vitamin B_1; a source of vitamin B_2 and folate; contains 160 mg of sodium and 20 g of fat of which 20% is *saturated and 50% is mono-unsaturated; supplies 300 kcal (1260 kJ). Pacific salmon may be a source of vitamin A and a rich source of vitamin D; canned salmon, in which the softened bones are edible, is also a source of calcium.

Salmonella Genus of bacteria of family Enterobacteriaceae. Common cause of *food poisoning. Found in eggs from infected hens, sausages, etc.; can survive in brine and in the refrigerator; destroyed by adequate heating.

salmon, rock Alternative name for *dogfish.

salometer *See* salinometer.

salpicon French; various mixtures of chopped meat, fish, or vegetables in a sauce, used as stuffing or filling.

salsa amarilla Spanish; (literally 'yellow sauce') made from hard-boiled eggs blended with madeira wine, oil, and mustard.

salsa Española Spanish sauce; basically a thick brown roux sauce, diluted with stock made from meat or bones, onion, carrot, garlic, and herbs.

salsa mahonesa Spanish (Balearic) mayonnaise; *see* salad dressing.

salsa romesco *See* romesco sauce.

salsify (oyster plant, vegetable oyster) Long, white, tapering root of the biennial plant *Tragopogon porrifolius*. Black salsify is very similar, the hardy perennial, *Scorzonera hispanica* (sometimes used roasted as coffee substitute).

salt Usually refers to *sodium chloride, common salt or table salt (chemically any product of reaction between an *acid and an *alkali is a salt). The main sources are either mines in areas where there are rich deposits of crystalline salt, or deposits left by the evaporation of sea water in shallow pans (known as sea salt). *See also* sodium; buffers; esters.

'salt-free' diets Diets low in *sodium, for the treatment of *hypertension and other conditions. Most of the sodium of the diet is consumed as sodium chloride or *salt, and hence such diets are referred to as salt-restricted or low-salt diets, or sometimes 'salt-free', to emphasize that no salt is added to foods in preparation or at the table. Since foods naturally contain sodium chloride, a truly salt-free diet is not possible. It is the sodium and not the chloride that is important.

Foods low in salt (0–20 mg/100 g): sugar, flour, fruit, green vegetables, macaroni, nuts. Medium salt (50–100 mg/100 g): chicken, fish, eggs, meat, milk. High salt (500–2000 mg/100 g): corned beef, bread, ham, bacon, kippers, sausages, cheese. *See also* hypertension; sodium.

saltimbocca Italian; thin slices of veal wrapped in ham (literally 'jump in the mouth').

salting Method of preserving meat, fish, and some vegetables using salt and *saltpetre.

saltlicks An adequate intake of *sodium is necessary to all animals. Grass is relatively poor in sodium, and its high potassium content induces excretion of sodium in the urine. This loss causes a craving for sodium which is satisfied by licking on natural outcrops of salt-rich rock or artificial salt crystals.

salt, light (lite) Mixtures of *sodium chloride with potassium chloride and/or other substances to reduce the intake of *sodium.

saltpetre (Bengal saltpetre) Potassium *nitrate.

salts, bile See bile.

salts, Indian Ancient Greek and Roman name for sugar.

sambal South-East Asian; mixture of chillies and spices, or a relish of raw vegetables or fruit in spiced vinegar.

sambol Indian, South-East Asian; *curry of fairly solid consistency.

sambuca Italian; liqueur flavoured with liquorice and *elderberry (*Sambucus nigra*). Traditionally served with coffee beans in the glass, and set alight.

SAMI Socially acceptable monitoring instrument. A small heart-rate counting apparatus used to estimate *energy expenditure of human subjects.

samna Clarified butter fat, see butter.

samosa Indian; deep-fried stuffed pancakes, rolled into a cone or folded into an envelope. The filling is normally spiced; it may be meat or vegetables.

samp Coarsely cut portions of *maize with bran and germ partly removed.

samphire 1 Rock samphire, St Peter's herb, succulent plant of cliffs and salt marshes (*Crithmum maritimum*, member of carrot family); grows on coastal rocks, and has fleshy aromatic leaves which may be eaten raw, boiled, or pickled.
   2 Marsh samphire (glasswort, sea asparagus), *Salicornia* spp., grows in salt marshes, is salty, and is eaten cooked as a vegetable.

samsa See akkra.

Sanatogen Trade name for a preparation of casein and sodium glycerophosphate for consumption as a beverage when added to milk.

sancoche Caribbean (Trinidadian); casseroled salt pork, beef, and vegetables.

sand cake Sponge or madeira cake made with ground rice, cornflour, or potato flour and *matzo meal instead of wheat flour, flavoured with grated lemon rind; a traditional Jewish *Passover delicacy.

sand leek See rocambole.

sandwich Two slices of bread enclosing a filling (meat, cheese, fish, etc.). Invention attributed to the 4th Earl of Sandwich (1718–1792) who spent long periods at the gaming table and carried a portable meal of beef sandwiched with bread.
   Decker sandwiches consist of several layers of bread, each separated by filling; Neapolitan sandwiches are decker sandwiches made with alternating slices of white and brown bread. Open sandwiches (*smørrebrød) consist of a single slice of bread, biscuit, or small roll.

sandwich spread Finely chopped vegetables in salad cream, as a filling for sandwiches.

Sanecta Trade name for *aspartame.

sangaree Caribbean; drink made from spiced and sweetened port and brandy, diluted with crushed ice.

sangiovese A *grape variety widely used for *wine making, although not one of the classic varieties.

sangría Spanish; fruit cup prepared from red wine fortified with brandy, in which fruit has been marinated, diluted with carbonated water and served with ice.

Sanka Trade name for decaffeinated instant coffee. *See* caffeine; coffee, decaffeinated.

sapodilla Fruit of the sapodilla tree (*Achras sapota*); size of a small apple, rough-grained, yellow to greyish pulp. Chicle, the basis of *chewing gum, is made from the latex of the tree.

saponifiable fats *See* saponification.

saponification *Hydrolysis of fat into its constituent *glycerol and *fatty acids by boiling with alkali. The fatty acids will be present as the sodium salts or soaps.

saponins Group of substances that occur in plants and can produce a soapy lather with water. Extracted commercially from soapwort (*Saponaria officinalis*) or soapbark (*Quillaja saponaria*) and used as foam producer in beverages and fire extinguishers, as detergents, and for emulsifying oils. Bitter in flavour. *See also* quillaja.

Saracen corn *See* buckwheat.

saran Generic name for thermoplastic materials made from polymers of vinylidene chloride and vinyl chloride. They are clear, transparent films (cling film) used for wrapping food; resistant to oils and chemicals; can be heat-shrunk on to the product.

sarcolactic acid Obsolete name for (+) lactic acid (which rotates the plane of polarized light to the right), found in muscle, as distinct from the optically inactive *lactic acid (a mixture of (+) and (−) isomers) found in sour milk. Also known as paralactic acid. *See also* DFD meat; meat conditioning; rigor mortis.

sarcolemma *See* muscle.

sarcosine An intermediate in the metabolism of *choline, chemically N-methylglycine. Found in relatively large amounts in starfish and sea urchins, used as an intermediate in the synthesis of antienzyme agents in toothpaste.

sardell *See* anchovy.

sardine Young *pilchard *Sardina* (*Clupea*) *pilchardus*; commonly canned in oil, brine, or tomato paste. Norwegian canned sardines are salted and smoked before canning; French are salted and steamed. A 100-g portion (canned in oil and drained, or canned in brine or tomato sauce) is an exceptionally rich *source of vitamin B_{12}; a rich source of protein, niacin, calcium, selenium, and vitamin D; a good source of vitamins B_2, B_6, iron, zinc, and copper; a source of iodine; contains 13 g of fat of which one-third is *saturated and one third mono-unsaturated; supplies 200 kcal (850 kJ).

Saridele Protein-rich baby food (26–30% protein) developed in Indonesia; extract of soya bean with sugar, calcium carbonate, thiamin, and vitamins B_{12} and C.

sarsaparilla 1 Flavour prepared from oil of *sassafras and oil of wintergreen or oil of sweet birch.

   2 Roots of a South American plant (*Smilax officinalis*); both used to flavour the beverage called sarsparilla.

sassafras American tree (*Sassafras albidum*) with aromatic bark and leaves. The root is used to make *root beer and the young leaves are powdered to make filé powder, an essential flavouring of *gumbo. Sassafras oil from the root-bark is used medicinally and as a flavour in beverages, but banned in some countries because of its toxicity.

saté (sateh, satay) Indonesian, Malaysian; marinated lamb, pork, or chicken, grilled on wooden skewers and served with a peanut sauce.

satiety The sensation of fullness after a meal.

satsuma *See* citrus fruit.

saturated With reference to *fatty acids means that the carbon chain carries its full complement of hydrogen atoms, as compared with mono-unsaturated and polyunsaturated. Where the nutrient content of foods is described in these entries the total amount of fat is listed, together with the proportion of saturates. Where mono-unsaturates are sufficiently important this is also quoted and the polyunsaturates can be calculated by difference from the total. Where the amounts of mono-unsaturates are small the entry lists the proportion of polyunsaturates and the mono-unsaturates can be calculated by difference from the total. *See* e.g. eggs; sunflower oil; Appendix X.

saturates Commonly used short term for saturated *fatty acids.

saturation humidity *See* humidity.

sauce Used to flavour, coat, or accompany a dish, or may be used in the cooking to bind ingredients together; may be sweet or savoury. Thick sauces may be: (1) *roux sauces based on flour heated with fat; (2) thickened with starch (*arrowroot, *cornflour, *custard powder) or *modified starch (gravy granules, thickening granules); (3) thickened with egg (*Hollandaise sauce, *custard); (4) thickened by reduction. *See also* individual sauces.

sauce, table Condiment or relish eaten with food; there are two main types: brown sauce, a (usually secret) blend of herbs, spices, and vegetables in vinegar, and tomato sauce or *ketchup.

sauce, Worcestershire *See* Worcestershire sauce.

sauerbraten German; beef marinated for several days in wine vinegar, then braised and served with sour cream.

sauerkraut German, Dutch, Alsatian; prepared by lactic fermentation of shredded cabbage. In the presence of 2–3% salt, acid-forming bacteria thrive and convert sugars in the cabbage into acetic and lactic acids, which then act as preservatives.

sauerteig Sourdough, *see* bread, sourdough.

sausage (French: *saucisson*; German: *Wurst*.) Chopped meat, mostly beef or pork, seasoned with salt and spices, mixed with cereal (usually wheat rusk prepared from crumbed unleavened biscuits) and packed into casings made from the connective tissue of animal intestines or cellulose.

There are six main types: fresh, smoked, cooked, smoked and cooked, semi-dry, and dry. Frankfurters, Bologna, Polish, and Berliner sausages are made from cured meat and are smoked and cooked. Thuringer, soft salami, mortadella, and soft cervelat are semi-dry sausages. Pepperoni, chorizos, dry salami, dry cervelat are slowly dried to a hard texture.

In the UK pork sausages must be 65% meat and beef sausages 50% meat ('meat' includes flesh and the skin, gristle, rind, and sinew 'naturally associated with the flesh'). A 150-g portion of standard British varieties of pork or beef sausages, grilled, is a rich *source of protein, niacin, and iron; beef sausage contains 25 g of fat of which 40% is saturated and 50% mono-unsaturated; supplies 400 kcal (1700 kJ); pork sausage contains 35 g of fat of which 40% is saturated and 50% mono-unsaturated; supplies 450 kcal (1900 kJ).

sausage casings Natural casings are made from hog intestines for fresh frying sausages, and from sheep intestines for chipolatas and frankfurters. Skinless sausages are prepared in cellulose casing, which is then peeled off.

sausage factor *See* meat factor.

sausage meat Mixture of meats as used to make *sausages, sausage rolls, pies, and stuffing.

sausage toad Sausages baked in batter, also known as toad-in-the-hole.

sauté To toss in hot fat, from the French *sauter*, to jump. Sauté potatoes are usually boiled, cut into slices, and cooked in a little fat until lightly browned.

sauvignon blanc One of the 9 'classic' *grape varieties used for *wine making; the wines are distinctively aromatic and sometimes smokey.

savarin *See* baba.

saveloy Highly seasoned smoked *sausage; the addition of saltpetre gives rise to the bright red colour. Originally a sausage made from pig brains.

savory Herb with strongly flavoured leaves used as seasoning in sauces, soups, and salad dishes. Summer savory is an annual, *Satureja hortensis*; winter savory is a perennial, *Satureja montana*. The plants are cut down at flowering time and dried for later use.

savoury Foods with a savoury or salty flavour; may be small titbits eaten with the fingers (cocktail savouries) or a savoury dish served after the sweet course and before the dessert at a formal banquet. *See also* taste; umami.

savoy Variety of *cabbage (*Brassica oleracea* var. *capitata*) with crimped leaves; said to have a more delicate flavour than ordinary cabbage.

savoy biscuits Small sponge fingers.

Saxin Trade name for *saccharin.

scald 1 To pour boiling water over a food to clean it, loosen hairs (e.g. on a joint of pork), or remove the skin of fruit, tomatoes, etc.
   2 To heat milk almost to boiling point, to retard souring or to make clotted *cream.
   3 Defect occurring in stored apples; the formation of brown patches under the skin, with browning and softening of the tissue underneath. Due to accumulation of gases given off during ripening.

scallion Small onion which has not developed a bulb, widely used in Chinese cooking; also used for shallots and spring onion (especially in the USA). *See also* onion, spring.

scalloped dishes Food (often previously cooked) baked in a scallop shell or similar small container, usually combined with a creamy sauce, topped with breadcrumbs, and surrounded by a border of piped potato.

scalloping A way of decorating the double edge of the pastry covering of a pie by making horizontal cuts with a knife close together round the edge of the pie, then, using the back of the knife, pulling the edge up vertically at regular intervals to form scallops.

scallops (French: *coquille St Jacques*; German: *Pilgermuschel*.) Marine bivalve *molluscs, Pectinidae spp.; Queen scallop is *Chamys opercularis*. A 100-g portion is a rich *source of protein, niacin, and vitamin B$_{12}$; a source of iron; supplies 70 kcal (290 kJ).

scampi *Shellfish, Norway lobster or Dublin Bay prawn, *Nephrops norvegicus*; *see* lobster.

Scenedesmus *See* algae.

Schiedam *See* gin.

Schilling Test A test of *vitamin B$_{12}$ nutritional status and absorption.

schinkenhäger *See* gin.

schmaltz Jewish name for dripping (rendered fat), especially from chicken or goose.

schnapps (snaps) *See* aquavit.

schnitzel Austrian, German; cutlet or escalope of veal or pork. Normally coated in egg and breadcrumbs and fried, then served with various garnishes.
   Bismarck schnitzel is garnished with plovers' eggs, mushrooms, truffles, and tomato sauce; holsteiner schnitzel with fried egg, capers, olives, and anchovies; rahmschnitzel with paprika-flavoured cream sauce; zigeuner schnitzel with tomato sauce, mushrooms, and smoked ox tongue.

schweitzer kraut German; chopped cooked marigold leaves.

scifers Cornish name for Welsh *onion.

scombroid poisoning Apparently caused by bacterial spoilage of fish including many of the Scombridae (*tuna, bonito, *mackerel) but also non-scombroid fish and other foods. Symptoms (including skin rash, nausea, tingling) resemble *histamine poisoning and were previously thought to be due to bacterial formation of histamine, now doubted.

scone A variety of tea cake originally made from white flour or barley meal and sour milk or buttermilk in Scone, Scotland; baked on a griddle and cut in quarters. Drop scone is a small pancake made by dropping spoonfuls of batter on to a griddle.

scorbutic *See* scurvy.

score To make shallow cuts in the surface of food in order to improve its flavour and appearance or to cook more quickly.

scorzonera *See* salsify.

Scotch broth Mutton and vegetable broth with pearl barley.

Scotch bun Spiced plum cake with pastry crust, traditionally eaten in Scotland at Hogmanay (New Year's eve). Also known as black bun.

Scotch egg Hard-boiled eggs cased in seasoned sausage meat and breadcrumbs, fried, and served cold.

Scotch kale Thick broth or soup containing shredded cabbage.

Scotch pancakes Drop-scones cooked by pouring the *batter onto a hotplate or flat pan.

Scotch whisky *See* whisky.

SCP *See* single cell protein.

scrapple American; meat dish prepared from pork carcass trimmings, maize meal, flour, salt, and spices, and cooked to a thick consistency.

scratchings, pork Small pieces of crisply cooked pork skin.

screwdriver A cocktail; half a measure of vodka with four measures of orange juice.

scrod Young *cod.

scrumpy Rough, unsweetened *cider.

scuppernong Name of the most widely cultivated of the muscadine grapes, used chiefly in wine rather than as a dessert grape.

scurvy Deficiency of *vitamin C, fatal if untreated. Nowadays it is extremely rare, but in the past was a major problem in winter, when there were few sources of the vitamin available. It was especially a problem of long sea voyages during the sixteenth and seventeenth centuries; when fresh supplies of fruit and vegetables were not available the majority of the crew often succumbed to scurvy.

scurvy, Alpine *See* pellagra.

scurvy grass A herb, *Cochlearia officinalis*, recommended as far back as the late sixteenth century as a remedy for scurvy.

scutellum Area surrounding the embryo of the cereal grain; scutellum plus embryo is the germ; rich in vitamins.

SDA Specific dynamic action, *see* diet-induced thermogenesis.

SE *See* starch equivalent.

sea crayfish Shellfish, family Palinuridae, *see* lobster.

seafood A general term to include crustaceans and *shellfish, sometimes also *fish.

seafood stick Characteristically pink and white sticks of cooked fish, eaten cold in salads and buffet meals, mainly made from cod or other white fish and containing little or no *shellfish. Also known as crab sticks or fish sticks.

sea kale beet *See* Swiss chard.

sea pie Beef stew with a suet-crust lid.

sear To brown meat quickly in a little fat before grilling or roasting. The term is sometimes used when vegetables are browned in fat before being used in soup or sauce making.

sea slug *See* bêche-de-mer.

seasoning Normally used to mean salt and pepper, but may include any herbs, spices, and condiments added to a savoury dish.

sea truffle *Shellfish, a bivalve *mollusc, *Venus verrucosa*.

seaweed Marine algae of interest as food include *Irish moss, *laver bread and *kelp, which are eaten to some extent in different communities and serve as a mineral supplement in animal feed.

secco Italian; dry wines.

seco Portuguese, Spanish; dry wines.

secretin A peptide *hormone secreted by the intestinal mucosa which stimulates pancreatic secretion.

sedoheptulose (sedoheptose) A seven-carbon sugar which is an intermediate in *glucose metabolism by the pentose phosphate pathway.

seed cake A sponge or madeira cake containing caraway seeds, mace, and nutmeg. Tipperary seed cake contains orange-flower water and caraway seeds, but no mace or nutmeg.

seek kababs Indian; minced meat croquettes shaped over an iron skewer (the seek) and cooked rapidly by grilling.

Seitz filter A filter disc (originally of asbestos) with pores so fine that they will not permit passage of bacteria; thus solutions filtered through a Seitz filter emerge sterile.

sekt German; sparkling *wine, usually dry, made by tank fermentation, not the méthode champenoise.

selenium A dietary essential mineral, which is part of *enzymes glutathione peroxidase and thyroxine deiodinase. Through its role in glutathione peroxidase it acts as an *antioxidant, and to some extent can compensate for *vitamin E deficiency. Similarly, vitamin E can compensate for selenium deficiency to some extent.

Requirements are of the order of 50 µg/day; in parts of New Zealand, Finland, and China soils are especially poor in selenium and deficiency occurs. In China selenium deficiency is associated with Keshan disease.

sesame

Rich *sources include: fish and shellfish, mung (dahl) and red kidney beans, Brazil nuts, bread, kidney, lentils, liver, pork, rabbit, veal.

Selenium is toxic in excess; mild selenium intoxication results in production of foul-smelling hydrogen selenide, which is excreted on the breath and through the skin. Intakes above 450 µg/day are considered hazardous.

self-raising flour See flour, self-raising.

seltzer 1 Effervescent mineral water, originally from Niederselters, Germany. See also soda water.
2 Trade name of effervescent headache cure.

sémillon One of the 9 'classic' *grape varieties used for *wine making, especially the great sauternes, graves, and white bordeaux. Traditionally called riesling in some parts of Australia.

seminose See mannose.

semi-seco Spanish; medium dry wines.

semolina The inner, granular, starchy endosperm of hard or durum wheat (not yet ground into flour); used to make *pasta and semolina milk pudding.

sensory properties See organoleptic.

sequestrants, sequestrol See chelating agents.

sercial See Madeira wines.

serendipity berry Or Nigerian berry, fruit of the West African plant *Dioscoreophyllum cumminsii*. It has an extremely sweet taste; the active principle is a protein, monellin.

serine A non-essential *amino acid.

serotonin See 5-hydroxytryptamine.

serum Clear liquid left after the protein has been clotted; the serum from milk, occasionally referred to as lacto-serum, is whey.

Blood serum is *blood plasma without the fibrinogen. When blood clots, the fibrinogen is converted to fibrin, which is deposited in strands that trap the red cells and form the clot. The clear liquid that is exuded is the serum. See also blood clotting.

serum butter See whey.

serving US food labelling legislation (introduced in 1994) requires that nutrients be shown per standard serving of the food. The Food and Drug Administration has defined serving or portion sizes, based on surveys of amounts customarily eaten, so the definition of portions is not left to the manufacturer.

sesame A tropical and subtropical plant, *Sesamum indicum*. Known as sim-sim in East Africa, benniseed in West Africa, gingelly and til in Asia. Seeds are small and, in most varieties, white; used whole in sweetmeats, in stews, and to decorate cakes and bread, and for extraction of the oil, which is used as a seasoning. The seeds contain 60% oil, of which 15% is saturated and 45% polyunsaturated. It has a strong nutty flavour and is used more as a seasoning than a cooking oil. See also tahini.

Seville orange *See* orange, bitter.

sex hormones *See* hormones, sex.

sfogato Greek; minced meat casserole.

sfumatrice Machine for obtaining the oil from the peel of citrus fruit. Based on the principle that the natural turgor of the oil sacs forces out the oil when the peel is folded.

shaddock *See* pomelo.

shakaria *See* potato, sweet.

shallot Bulb of the plant *Allium escalonium* (*A. cepa aggregatum* group) related to the *onion, with essentially the same flavour but less pungency; each plant has a cluster of small bulbs rather than the single large bulb of the onion.

shandy A mixture of lemonade and *beer, originally shandy-gaff. Ginger beer may be used for ginger beer shandy. Contains 1% *alcohol.

sharon fruit Alternative name for the sweet *persimmon or kaki.

Sharples centrifuge Continuous high-speed centrifuge (15 000–30 000 rpm), consisting of a vertical cylinder. Used to separate liquids of different densities or to clarify by sedimenting solids.

sharps *See* wheatfeed.

shashlik *See* kebab.

shchi Russian; green vegetable soup, sometimes called Russian cabbage soup.

shea butter *See* vegetable butters.

shearling 15–18-month-old sheep. *See* lamb.

sheer (kheer) Indian; creamed-rice dessert.

shellfish, edible A wide range of marine molluscs (*abalone, *clams, *cockles, *mussels, *scallops, *oysters, *whelks, *winkles) and crustacea (members of the zoological order Decapoda: *crayfish, *crabs, *lobsters, *prawns, *shrimps).

shepherd's pie Dish made from minced lamb or mutton with a crust of mashed potato, baked. Cottage pie is made with minced beef.

sherbet 1 Arabic name for water-ice (sugar, water, and flavouring), also known by French name, sorbet, and the Italian name, granita. Used to be served between courses during a meal to refresh the palate.

2 Originally a Middle-Eastern drink made from fruit juice, often chilled with snow. Modern version is made with bicarbonate of soda and tartaric acid (to fizz) with sugar and flavours. Sherbet powder is the same mixture in dry form.

sherry Fortified wines (around 15% *alcohol by volume) from the south-west of Spain, around Jerez and Cadiz. Matured by the solera process rather than by discrete vintages; each year 30% of the wine in the oldest barrel is drawn off for bottling and replaced with wine from the next oldest; this in turn is replaced from the next barrel, and so on.

In order of increasing sweetness, sherries are: fino (very dry); manzanilla; amontillado; oloroso (may be medium-dry or sweetened and more highly fortified); amoroso or cream. Dry sherry contains 1–2% sugar and 100 mL supplies 120 kcal (500 kJ); medium sherry, 3–4% sugar, supplies 125 kcal (530 kJ); sweet sherry, 7% sugar, supplies 140 kcal (590 kJ).

Sherry-type wines are also produced in other countries, including South Africa, Cyprus, and Britain (made from imported grape juice) and may legally be described as sherry as long as the country of origin is clearly shown.

shiitake Or Black Forest mushroom, *Lentinula* (*Lentinus*) *edodes*, see mushrooms.

shir To bake food (usually eggs) in a small shallow container or ramekin dish.

shishkebab See kebab.

shoo-fly pie American; pie with sweet filling made from molasses, brown sugar, and flour.

shortbread Sweet biscuit baked with a high proportion of butter to flour. Sometimes called shortcake in the USA.

shortcake American; rich cake with a filling of fruit and cream. *See also* shortbread.

short crust See pastry.

shortening Soft fats that produce a crisp, flaky effect in baked products. *Lard possesses the correct properties to a greater extent than any other single fat. Shortenings compounded from mixtures of fats or prepared by hydrogenation are still called lard compounds or lard substitutes.

Unlike oils, shortenings are plastic and disperse as a film through the batter and prevent the formation of a hard, tough mass.

showarma Arabic name for *döner kebab.

shoyu See soy sauce.

shred To slice a food such as cheese or raw vegetables into very fine pieces, which often curl as they are cut.

Shredded Wheat Trade name for a breakfast cereal prepared from wheat grains. Two biscuits (44 g) are a *source of protein, niacin, iron, and zinc; provide 4 g of dietary fibre; supply 140 kcal (590 kJ).

shrimp (French: *crevette*; German: *Germale*.) Small shellfish, Paleamonidae and Pandalidae spp. (prawns), *Crangon crangon* (brown shrimp), and *Pandalus montagui* (pink shrimp). A 100-g portion without shell is a rich *source of protein, niacin, vitamin B_{12}, and selenium, a good source of calcium, and a source of iron; contains 400 mg of sodium, 1.3 g of fat of which 8% is saturated; supplies 75 kcal (320 kJ).

shrub A bottled cordial made from various fruits, spirits, and sugar.

sialogogue Substance that stimulates the flow of saliva.

sialorrhoea Excessive flow of saliva.

Sichuan pepper See anise pepper.

sidemeats See offal.

siderophilin *See* iron transport.

siderosis Accumulation of the iron-protein complex, haemosiderin, in liver, spleen, and bone marrow in cases of excessive red cell destruction and on diets exceptionally rich in *iron. It is common among Bantu, apparently owing to intakes of about 100 mg of iron daily from iron cooking pots and *pombé.

sift To shake flour, sugar, etc., through a sieve.

sikor *See* clay.

sild Traditional UK name applied to a mixture of young *herrings and young *sprats when canned, since they are caught together and cannot be separated on a commercial scale. When fresh or frozen the mixture is termed whitebait.

silica gel A drying agent.

silicones Organic compounds of silicon; in the food field they are used as antifoaming agents, as semi-permanent glazes on baking tins and other metal containers, and on non-stick wrapping paper.

sillabub *See* syllabub.

silvaner A *grape variety widely used for *wine making, although not one of the classic varieties.

silver Not of interest in foods apart from its use in covering *non-pareils, the silver beads used to decorate confectionery. Present in traces in all plant and animal tissues but not known to be a dietary essential, and has no known function, nor is enough ever absorbed to cause toxicity. *See also* oligodynamic.

silver beet *See* Swiss chard.

silverside Boned joint of *beef cut from the top part of the hind leg, commonly boiled or salted, although it can be roasted.

simmer A method of cooking in water slightly below boiling point (also known as coddling).

simnel cake Fruit cake with a layer of almond paste on top and sometimes another baked in the middle. Originally baked for Mothering Sunday, now normally eaten at Easter.

Simplesse Trade name for fat substitute made from milk or egg-white. Consists of 0.1–2.0 μm diameter particles which create the feeling of creaminess in the mouth but cannot be used for cooking. Yields 1.3 kcal (5.2 kJ)/g, compared with 9 kcal (37 kJ)/g for fats. *See also* fat replacers.

sim-sim *See* sesame.

singe To pass a plucked bird quickly over a flame to burn off the down.

singing hinnie (singin' hinny) Northern British (Northumberland); large, round, currant scone baked on a girdle or hotplate, usually cut in half, buttered, and eaten hot. The name comes from the hissing noise it makes as it cooks.

single-cell protein Collective term used for biomass of bacteria, algae, and yeast, and also (incorrectly) moulds, of potential use as animal or human food.

sinharanut *See* chestnut.

sippet A small piece of bread, fried or toasted, served as a garnish to a mince or hash.

sirloin Upper part of the hind loin of *beef.

sitapophasis Refusal to eat as expression of mental disorder.

sitology Science of food (from the Greek *sitos*, food).

sitomania Mania for eating, morbid obsession with food; also known as phagomania.

sitophobia Fear of food; also known as phagophobia.

sitosterol The main *sterol found in vegetable oils, similar in structure to cholesterol; may reduce the absorption of cholesterol from the intestinal tract and has been used in treatment of *hyperlipidaemia.

skate Cartilaginous *fish, *Raja undulata*.

skillet Frying pan (especially in the USA).

skim To remove fat from the surface of stock, gravy, stews, etc., or scum from jams, etc., while they are cooking.

skinfold thickness Index of subcutaneous fat and hence body fat content. Measured at four sites: biceps (midpoint of front upper arm), triceps (midpoint of back upper arm), subscapular (directly below point of shoulder blade at angle of 45 degrees), supra-iliac (directly above iliac crest in mid-axillary line). Rapid surveys often involve only biceps. *See also* anthropometry.

skink Irish, Scottish; originally an essence or extract, now a thick soup-stew of meat and vegetables.

skirlie Scottish; cakes of oatmeal and onion fried in pork dripping. Sold commercially in a skin, known as mealie pudding.

skorthalia Greek; sauce with garlic, lemon, and nuts.

skyr *See* milk, fermented.

slapjack *See* flapjack.

Slendid *See* fat replacers.

slimming clubs Groups which provide help and support for *overweight and *obese people trying to lose weight, including nutritional counselling and provision of clear, easy-to-follow, weight-reducing diets. The most successful groups are often those in which the counsellors were once obese people themselves, and understand the problems involved in losing excess weight.

sling Drink made from gin and fruit juice.

slivovitz (sliwowitz) East European (originally Yugoslavian); distilled spirit made from fermented plums; similar to German *quetsch and French *mirabelle. Some of the stones are included with the fruit and produce a characteristic bitter flavour from the hydrocyanic acid (0.008% cyanide is present in the finished brandy).

sloe Wild *plum, fruit of the blackthorn (*Prunus spinosa*) with a sour and astringent flavour; almost the only use for it is for the preparation of *sloe gin.

sloe gin Liqueur made by steeping wild *sloes in gin or neutral spirit. Known in France as prunelle.

sloke See laver.

SMA Trade name (Scientific Milk Adaptation) for a milk preparation for infant feeding modified to resemble the composition of human milk. See milk, humanized.

smallage Wild celery, *Apium graveolens*; its seeds, herb, and root are said to have medicinal properties.

smell See organoleptic.

smetana Thin, sour cream, originally Russian.

smilacin See parillin.

smoked beef See pastrami.

smoke point The temperature at which the decomposition products of frying oils become visible as bluish smoke. The temperature varies with different fats, ranging between 160 and 260 ˚C. See also fire point; flash point.

smoking The process of flavouring and preserving meat or fish by drying slowly in the smoke from a wood fire; the type of wood used affects the flavour of the final smoked product.

smörgåsbord Scandinavian; buffet table laden with delicacies as a traditional gesture of hospitality, a traditional way of serving meals. See also smørrebrød.

smørrebrød Scandinavian; open sandwiches, often on rye bread, with a variety of toppings and garnishes. Literally 'smeared bread'. See also smörgåsbord.

SMS Sucrose monostearate. See sucrose esters.

smut Group of fungi that attack wheat; includes loose or common smut (*Ustilago tritici*) and stinking smut or bunt (*Tilletia tritici*).

snail (French: *escargot*; German: *Weinbergschnecke*.) The small snail eaten in Europe is *Helix pomatia*; giant African snail (which weighs several hundred grams) is *Achatima fulica*. Little information is available about nutrient content other than that a 50-g portion is a *source of protein and iron, and contains about 1 g of fat.

snap pea See mange-tout.

snaps See aquavit.

SNF See solids-not-fat.

snibbing Topping and tailing of *gooseberries.

snow Mixture of sweetened fruit pulp with whisked egg-white, normally served with sponge fingers or biscuits, or on a bed of sponge cake soaked in fruit juice.

snow pea See mange-tout.

SO₂ See sulphur dioxide.

soapbark See quillaja.

soapstock In the refining of crude edible oils the free fatty acids are removed by agitation with alkali. The fatty acids settle to the bottom as alkali soaps and are known as soapstock or 'foots'.

sobresada Spanish (Mallorquin); spiced sausage containing pork, tripe, paprika and cayenne pepper; large in diameter and soft in texture, so it can be spread like a pâté. A firmer variety, which requires cooking, is longaniza.

soda bread Made from flour and whey, or buttermilk, using sodium bicarbonate and acid in place of yeast. Common in Ireland.

soda water Artificially carbonated water, also known as club soda; if sodium bicarbonate is also added, the product is seltzer water.

sodium A dietary essential mineral; requirements are almost invariably satisfied by the normal diet. The body contains about 100 g of sodium and the average diet contains 3–6 g, equivalent to 7.5–15 g of sodium chloride (salt); the requirement is less than 0.5 g sodium/day. The intake varies enormously in different individuals and the excretion varies accordingly. Excessive intake of sodium is associated with high blood pressure, which is hence often treated with low-salt diets.

Sodium controls the retention of fluid in the body, and reduced retention, aided by low-sodium diets, is required in cardiac insufficiency accompanied by *oedema, in certain kidney diseases, toxaemias of pregnancy, and *hypertension. Low-sodium diets are usually about 2.3 g and can be as low as 0.6 g. To improve the palatability of such diets, 'salt' mixtures (*light or lite salt) are available, containing potassium and ammonium chlorides together with citrates, formates, phosphates, glutamates, as well as herbs and spices. Such mixtures may be contra-indicated in conditions where potassium intake also has to be restricted.

See also 'salt-free' diets; salt lick; sodium-potassium ratio; water balance.

sodium bicarbonate Also known as baking soda or bicarbonate of soda (chemically $NaHCO_3$), liberates carbon dioxide when in contact with acid. Used as a raising agent in baking flour confectionery. See also baking powder.

A small pinch of sodium bicarbonate preserves the green colour in cooked vegetables (too much destroys the vitamin C). Also helps to reduce acidity when stewing sour plums or rhubarb.

sodium chloride Common *salt, the commonest form in which *sodium is consumed. See also 'salt-free' diets.

sodium glutamate See glutamate; monosodium glutamate.

sodium-potassium ratio In the body, the ratio of sodium (in the extracellular fluid) to the potassium (in the cell water) is about 2 : 3. The ratio in unprocessed food, no salt added, is much lower, and when salt is added during processing it is much higher. Unproven suggestions have been made for the benefits of controlling the sodium-potassium ratio in the diet.

Fruits and vegetables are relatively low in sodium and rich in potassium. Animal foods are rich in sodium.

sofrito Spanish; sauce prepared from onions, tomatoes, garlic, and other vegetables fried gently in oil.

soft drinks Term applied to non-alcoholic drinks, usually fruit juice or fruit-flavoured, but also a variety of *carbonated beverages. Various concentrations and preparations are termed squash, crush, and cordial, which usually require dilution before drinking; others are ready to drink. In the USA *cider (sometimes soft cider) means unfermented apple juice (a soft drink), while the fermented product is hard cider.

soft swell *See* swells.

sol A colloidal solution, i.e. a suspension of particles intermediate in size between ordinary molecules (as in a solution) and coarse particles (as in a suspension). A jelly-like sol is a gel.

Solanaceae Family of plants including *aubergine (*Solanum melongena*), *Cape gooseberry (*Physalis peruviana*), *potato (*Solanum tuberosum*), *tomato (*Lycopersicon esculentum*).

solanine Heat-stable toxic compound (chemically a *glycoside of the *alkaloid solanidine), found in small amounts in potatoes, and larger and sometimes toxic amounts in sprouted potatoes and in skin when they become green through exposure to light. Causes gastrointestinal disturbances and neurological disorders; 20 mg solanine per 100 g fresh weight of potato tissue is the upper acceptable limit.

sole Flat *fish, *Solea* spp. Dover sole is *Solea solea*.

solera *See* sherry.

solids-not-fat (SNF) Refers to the solids of milk excluding the fat, i.e. protein, lactose, and salts. Used as an index of milk quality, determined by measuring the specific gravity in the *lactometer.

solyanka Russian; fish or meat stew with salted or pickled vegetables.

soondth *See* ginger.

soonf *See* fennel.

sorbet A water-ice containing sugar, water, and flavouring (commonly fruit juice or pulp). Also known as *sherbet (from the Arabic) and granita (Italian).

sorbic acid Chemically hexadienoic acid, $CH_3CH=CH—CH=CH—COOH$. Used together with its sodium, potassium, and calcium salts to inhibit growth of fungi in wine, cheese, soft drinks, low-sugar jams, flour, confectionery, etc. (E-200–203).

Sorbistat Trade name for *sorbic acid and its potassium salt (Sorbistat K).

sorbitol (glycitol, glucitol) A six-carbon *sugar alcohol found in plums, apricots, cherries, and apples and manufactured from glucose. Although it is metabolized in the body, yielding the same amount of energy as other carbohydrates, 4 kcal (16 kJ)/g, it is only slowly absorbed from the intestine and is tolerated by diabetics. It is 50–60% as sweet as sucrose. Used in baked products, jam, and confectionery suitable for diabetics (E-420).

sorcerer's milk *See* witches' milk.

sorghum *Sorghum vulgare, S. bicolor*; cereals that thrive in semi-arid regions and provide important human food in tropical Africa, Central and North India, and China. Sorghum produced in the USA and Australia is used for animal feed. Also known as kaffir corn (in South Africa), guinea corn (in West Africa), jowar (in India), Indian millet, and millo maize. The white-grain variety is eaten as meal; the red-grained has a bitter taste and is used for beer; sugar syrup is obtained from the crushed stems of the sweet sorghum. A 200-g portion is a rich *source of protein, vitamin B_1, niacin, and iron; a good source of zinc; a source of vitamin B_2; provides 14 g of dietary fibre; supplies 660 kcal (2800 kJ). *See also* millet.

sorghum syrup The concentrated juice from a sweet variety of *sorghum.

sorrel A common wild plant (*Rumex acetosa*); the leaves have a strong acid flavour, and are cooked together with spinach or cabbage, used to make soup, and used in salads.

sorrel syrup Caribbean; syrup prepared from *rosella flowers.

soubise Dish flavoured with onion or garnished with onion purée; soubise sauce is a white sauce containing onion.

souchet (souchy) 1 English, nineteenth-century method of poaching fish (especially trout) in the oven with fish stock, onions, and sliced roots of Hamburg parsley.
   2 Fish broth flavoured with onions and thickened with potatoes.

souchong *See* tea.

soufflé Light, fluffy, baked dish of eggs, flour, and butter with various fillings; may be sweet or savoury.

soul food Afro-Caribbean term for food with traditional or cultural links, having emotional significance.

sourballs *See* acid drops.

source In this book foods are listed as sources of nutrients. A rich source of a nutrient means that 30% or more of the recommended daily amount (*see* reference intakes) of the nutrient is supplied in the stated portion; a good source has 20%; and a source, 10%. Although amounts smaller than 10% are not mentioned, the foods may still make a useful contribution to the diet.

sourdough bread *See* bread, sourdough.

soursop *See* custard apple.

sous-vide French-originated term for cooking in special pouches under vacuum, when the food has a shelf-life of weeks; claimed also to retain flavour and nutrients. Derived from the French *cuisine en papillote sous vide*, cooking in sealed container (originally a parchment paper case).

souse To cook or steep food in vinegar; especially oily *fish such as *herring and *mackerel.

Southern Comfort Trade name; liqueur based on American whiskey flavoured with peaches and oranges.

souvlaki, souvlakia Greek; *kebabs, especially shishkebab (from the Greek *souvla*, skewer).

sow thistle A wild plant (*Sonchus oleraceus*); the young leaves can be used in salads, and the roots can be roasted or boiled, and eaten in the same way as *salsify. Also known as milk weed or hare's lettuce.

soya (soy) A *bean (*Glycine max*) important as a source of both oil and protein. The protein is of high *biological value, higher than that of many other vegetable proteins, and is of great value for animal and human food. When raw it contains a *trypsin inhibitor, which is destroyed by heat. Native of China, where it has been cultivated for 5000 years; grows 60–100 cm high with 2–3 beans per pod. Contains indigestible sugars, *stachyose and *raffinose, which can cause *flatulence. A 100-g portion of boiled beans is a good *source of protein and iron; a source of niacin and calcium; provides 6 g of dietary fibre; supplies 140 kcal (590 kJ).

soybean curd *See* tofu.

soybean flour Dehulled, ground *soya bean. The unheated material is a rich source of *amylase and *proteinase and is useful as a baking aid. The heated material has no enzymic activity but is a valuable protein-rich food.

Full-fat soya flour is a rich *source of protein, iron, vitamin B_1, and niacin; a good source of calcium and zinc; a source of vitamin B_2; contains 24 g of fat, of which 15% is saturated and 60% polyunsaturated; provides 10 g of dietary fibre; supplies 450 kcal (1900 kJ). Low-fat flour contains 7 g of fat.

soybean milk Extract of the *soya bean. A 250-mL portion is a rich source of vitamin B_2; a source of vitamin B_1 and protein; supplies 80 kcal (340 kJ).

Soyolk Trade name for full-fat *soya flour.

soy sauce A condiment prepared from fermented soya bean, commonly used in China and Japan. Traditionally the bean, often mixed with wheat, is fermented with *Aspergillus oryzae* over a period of 1–3 years. The modern process is carried out at a high temperature or in an autoclave for a short time.

spaghetti *See* pasta.

spaghetti squash A *gourd, also called cucuzzi, calabash, Suzza melon; often classed as summer squash but not a true *squash. Only after cooking does the flesh resemble spaghetti in appearance.

Spam Trade name for canned pork luncheon meat; a contraction of 'spiced ham'.

Spanish omelette *See* tortilla.

Spanish toxic oil syndrome Widespread disease in Spain during 1981/2, with 450 deaths and many people chronically disabled, due to consumption of an oil containing aniline-denatured industrial rapeseed oil, sold as pure olive oil. The disease appears to be unique and the precise cause is unknown.

Spans Trade name for non-ionic surface agents derived from fatty acids and hexahydric alcohols. They are oil-soluble, in contrast to Tweens which are water-soluble or well-dispersible in water. Used in bread as crumb-softeners (anti-staling) to improve doughs, cakes, and biscuits, and as emulsifiers.

spareribs Pork ribs with most of the surrounding meat removed.

sparkling wine *See* wine, sparkling.

spastic colon *See* irritable bowel syndrome.

spatchcock Small birds split down the back and flattened before grilling. Spitchcock is eel treated similarly.

spätlese *See* wine classification, Germany.

spätzle Austrian, German; very small noodles made by forcing noodle dough through a colander directly into boiling water.

SPE *See* sucrose polyesters.

spearmint *See* mint.

Special K *See* Kellogg's Special K.

specific dynamic action *See* diet-induced thermogenesis.

specificity In relation to enzymes, the ability of an enzyme to catalyse only a limited range of reactions, or, in some cases, a single reaction, and to show considerable specificity for the substances which undergo reaction. Unlike simple chemical catalysts, enzymes readily distinguish between *isomers.

spectrophotometer Instrument that measures the amount of light absorbed at any particular wavelength, which is directly related to the concentration of the material in the solution. Used extensively to measure substances that have specific absorption in the visible, infrared, or ultraviolet range, or can react to form colour derivatives.

spelt Coarse type of wheat, mainly used as cattle feed.

spent wash Liquor remaining in the whisky still after distilling the spirit. A source of unidentified compounds that are growth factors for chicks. When dried it is known as distillers' dried solubles.

sphingomyelins Complex *phospholipids found in cell membranes, and especially in brain and nerve tissue; composed of the base sphingosine plus fatty acids, phosphoric acid, and *choline.

spices Distinguished from *herbs in that part, instead of the whole, of the aromatic plant is used: root, stem, or seeds. Originally used to mask putrefactive flavours. Some have a preservative effect because of their essential oils, e.g. cloves, cinnamon, and mustard.

They are consumed in amounts too small to provide any nutrients except possibly for *curry powder, which may contain 7.5–10 mg of iron in a 10-g portion (possibly arising mainly from the mills in which the spices have been ground).

spina bifida Congenital neural tube defect due to developmental anomaly in early embryonic development. Supplements of *folic acid (400 µg/day), begun before conception, reduce the risk.

spinach Leaves of *Spinacia oleracea*. A 90-g portion is a rich *source of vitamin A (as carotene), folate, and vitamin C; provides 5.4 g of dietary fibre, and supplies 25 kcal (100 kJ). The content of *oxalic acid renders unavailable much of the iron and calcium that are present.

spinach beet *See* Swiss chard.

spinach, Chinese Leaves of *Amaranthus gangeticus*, also known as bhaji and *callaloo.

spinach, Philippine Variety of purslane (*Talinum triangulare*) cultivated in the USA and cooked in the same way as *spinach.

spiny lobster *Shellfish, family Palinuridae, *see* lobster.

spirits Beverages of high *alcohol content made by distillation of fermented liquors, including *brandy, *gin, *rum, *vodka, *whisky; usually 40% alcohol by volume (equivalent to 31.7 g per 100 mL). A standard measure (in the UK) was formerly one-fifth or one-sixth of a gill; now 25 mL.

spirit, silent Highly purified *alcohol, or neutral spirit, distilled from any fermented material.

spirometer Or respirometer, apparatus used to measure the amount of oxygen consumed (and in some instances carbon dioxide produced) from which to calculate the energy expended (indirect calorimetry).

Spirulina Blue-green *alga which can make use of atmospheric nitrogen to form proteins; eaten for centuries round Lake Chad in North Africa, and in Mexico. Many health claims are made, but are negated by the small amounts eaten.

spit Thin metal bar on which meat, poultry, or game is roasted in front of an open fire, and rotated during cooking; now also inside an oven or grill.

spitchcock Eel split down the back and flattened before grilling. *See also* spatchcock.

spleen (French: *rate*; German: *Milz*.) Gland near the stomach with main function of destroying 'worn-out' red blood cells and recycling the iron. As a food it is called melts; A 150-g portion of calf spleen is a rich *source of iron, vitamins B_2, niacin, and C; a good *source of vitamin A; contains 6 g of fat; supplies 150 kcal (630 kJ).

sponge Light-textured *cake made from self-raising flour beaten with butter, eggs, and sugar.

spores In relation to bacteria they are the resting state; they are thick-walled and highly resistant to damage by heat. Under suitable conditions they germinate to produce bacteria. Not all bacteria can form spores; the so-called spore-bearers are a health hazard because they can survive pasteurization and sterilization.

spotted dick (dog) Steamed or boiled suet pudding containing currants and sultanas.

sprat Small oily *fish, *Sprattus* (*Clupea*) *sprattus,* fresh or frozen; young are canned as brisling. *See* herring; whitebait.

spray dryer Equipment in which the material to be dried is sprayed as a fine mist into a hot-air chamber and falls to the bottom as dry powder. The period of heating is very brief and so nutritional and functional damage are avoided. Dried powder consists of hollow particles of low density; widely applied to many foods (e.g. milk) and pharmaceuticals.

springers *See* swells.

spring greens Young leafy *cabbage eaten before the heart has formed, or leaf sprouts formed after cutting off the head. *See also* collard.

spring onion *See* onion, spring.

spring rolls Chinese (and general South-East Asian); pancakes filled with quick-fried vegetables and meat; may be served as soft pancakes prepared at the table, or rolled and deep-fried. Also known as pancake rolls and imperial rolls, as loempia in Indonesian, and nem in Vietnamese cuisine.

sprouts 1 *See* Brussels sprouts.
    2 *See* beansprouts.

spruce beer Western Canadian; branches, bark, and cones of black spruce (*Picea mariana*) boiled for several hours, then put in a cask with molasses, hops, and yeast, and allowed to ferment.

sprue Disease in which the *villi of the small intestine are atrophied and food is incompletely absorbed, followed consequently by undernutrition and weight loss.

sprue, tropical Name given (by Dutch in Java) to a tropical disease characterized by fatty diarrhoea and sore mouth, with signs of undernutrition due to poor absorption of nutrients. Both an unidentified infectious agent and folic acid deficiency have been suggested as causes.

spumante Italian; sparkling wines. *See also* frizzante.

spurtle Scottish; wooden stick traditionally used to stir porridge. Also known as theevil.

squab Young *pigeon; squab pie is a West of England dish made from meat, apples, and onions.

squash Gourds, fruits of *Cucurbita* spp.

squash, fruit *See* soft drinks.

squid (calamar) Marine creature with elongated body and eight arms, *Loligo* and *Illex* spp.

SRD State Registered Dietitian; legal qualification to practice as a dietitian in the UK.

stabilizers Substances that stabilize emulsions of fat and water, e.g. *gums, *agar, egg albumin, *cellulose ethers; used to produce the texture of meringues and marshmallow, *lecithin (E-322) for crumb-softening in bread and confectionery, glyceryl monostearate (E-471) and polyoxyethylene stearate (E-430–436) for crumb-softening. The legally permitted list includes also *superglycerinated fats, propylene glycol alginate and stearate (E-570), methyl-, methylethyl-, and sodium carboxymethyl-celluloses (E-466), stearyl tartrate (E-483), sorbitan esters of fatty acids (E-491–495). Bread may contain only superglycerinated fats and stearyl tartrate.

See also emulsifying agents.

stachyose Tetrasaccharide *sugar composed of two units of *galactose and one each of *fructose and *glucose. Not hydrolysed in the human digestive tract and passes to the large intestine, where it is fermented by bacteria. Present in *soya beans and some other *legumes; gives rise to the flatulence commonly associated with eating beans. Also known as mannotetrose and lupeose.

stachys *See* artichoke, Chinese.

stackburn The deterioration in colour and quality of canned foods which have not been sufficiently cooled after canning, then stored in stacks which cool slowly.

staling Starch has a crystalline structure which is lost during baking. Subsequently the starch recrystallizes, i.e. it retrogrades and, in the instance of bread, the crumb loses its softness and the bread goes stale.

Staling can be delayed by *emulsifiers (crumb softeners) such as polyoxyethylene and monoglyceride derivatives of fatty acids.

Retrogradation of starch also takes place in dehydrated potatoes.

stamp-and-go *See* accra.

stamppot Dutch; vegetable hotpot.

staphylococcal poisoning *See* food poisoning.

staple food The principal food, e.g. wheat, rice, maize, etc.

star anise *See* anise, star.

starch *Polysaccharide, a polymer of *glucose units; the form in which carbohydrate is stored in the plant; it does not occur in animal tissue. (*Glycogen is sometimes referred to as animal starch.) Starch is broken down by acid or enzymic hydrolysis (*amylase), or during digestion, first to maltose and then glucose; it is the principal carbohydrate of the diet and hence the major source of energy for man and animals. Starches from different sources (e.g. potato, maize, cereal, arrowroot, sago, etc.) have different structures, and contain different proportions of two major forms: amylose, which is a linear polymer and amylopectin, which has a branched structure. The mixture of dietary starches consists of about one-quarter amylose and three-quarters amylopectin.

starch, A and B Refers to wheat starch: A, larger granules, 25–35 μm; B, smaller particles, 2–8 μm.

starch, animal *See* glycogen.

starch, arum From the root of the arum lily (*Arum maculatum* and other spp.); similar to *sago and *arrowroot.

starch, derivatized *See* starch, modified.

starch, enzyme-resistant Starch that escapes digestion in the small intestine but can be fermented in the large intestine. According to the

method of analysis used, enzyme-resistant starch may be included with
*dietary fibre. Chemically it is a glucan formed when starch is heated
(apparently formed after gelatinization by spontaneous self-association
of the hydrated amylose component).

starch equivalent A measure of the energy value of animal
feedingstuffs; the number of parts of pure starch that would be
equivalent to 100 parts of the ration as a source of energy.

starches, waxy Those containing a high percentage of *amylopectin;
they form soft pastes rather than rigid gels when *gelatinized. *See also*
maize starches, waxy.

starch, inhibited *See* starch, modified.

starch, modified Starch altered by physical or chemical treatment to
give special properties of value in food processing, e.g. change in gel
strength, flow properties, colour, clarity, stability of the paste. Acid-
modified starch results from acid treatment that reduces the viscosity
of the paste (used in sugar confectionery, e.g. gum drops, jelly beans).

Oxidized starch: peroxide, permanganate, chlorine, etc., alter
viscosity, clarity, and stability of the paste (major use is outside the
food industry).

Derivatized starch: chemical derivatives such as ethers and esters
show properties such as reduced gelatinization in hot water and
greater stability to acids and alkalis ('inhibited' starch); useful where
food has to withstand heat treatment, as in canning or in acid foods.
Further degrees of treatment can result in starch being unaffected by
boiling water and losing its gel-forming properties. *See also* starch,
pregelatinized.

starch, oxidized *See* starch, modified.

starch, pregelatinized Raw starch does not form a paste with cold
water and therefore requires cooking if it is to be used as a food
thickening agent. Pregelatinized starch, mostly maize starch, has been
cooked and dried. Used in instant puddings, pie fillings, soup mixes,
salad dressings, sugar confectionery, and as a binder in meat products.
Nutritional value is the same as that of the original starch. *See also*
starch, modified.

starch, resistant *See* starch, enzyme resistant.

starch syrup *See* syrup.

starter Culture of bacteria used to inoculate or start growth in a
fermentation, e.g. milk for cheese production, or butter to develop the
flavour.

steak Piece of meat cut from the fillet, rump, sirloin, or other lean part
of the animal (normally *beef). Also used for thick sections of fish such
as *salmon and *cod.

steam baking In baking an even temperature is maintained in the
oven by means of closed pipes through which steam circulates. This is
sometimes erroneously taken to mean that the bread is baked in live
steam.

steamed buns Chinese; steamed dough buns containing a savoury meat and vegetable stuffing, also known as pao-tzu. *See also* dim sum.

steaming Method of cooking food in the steam above boiling water; there is less loss of nutrients into the cooking water than with boiling. Steaming is also carried out above 100 °C by means of pressure cookers, *see* autoclave.

stearic acid Saturated *fatty acid with eighteen carbon atoms (chemically octadecenoic acid); is present in most animal and vegetable fats.

steatorrhoea Excretion of faeces containing a large amount of fat, and generally foul-smelling. May be due to lack of *bile, lack of *lipase in the digestive juices, or defective absorption of fat. Treatment is by feeding low-fat diet. *See also* coeliac disease; sprue.

steep The process of leaving a food to stand in water, either to soften it or to extract its flavour and colour. Also the preparation of fruit liqueurs by steeping fruit in *spirit.

steer Bull castrated when very young; if castrated after reaching maturity, it is known as a stag.

steinhäger *See* gin.

stelk Irish; potatoes boiled, then mashed with milk in which spring onions have been simmered. Also called thump.

stercobilin One of the brown pigments of the faeces; formed from the bile pigments, which, in turn, are formed as breakdown products of the *haemoglobin of old red *blood cells.

sterculia gum *See* karaya gum.

stereo-isomerism Occurs when compounds have the same molecular and structural formula, but with the atoms arranged differently in space. There are two subdivisions: optical isomerism (*see* optical activity) and geometrical isomerism (*see* cis-, trans-isomerism).

sterigmatocystin A *mycotoxin.

sterile Free from all micro-organisms, bacteria, moulds, and yeasts. When foods are sterilized, as in canning, they are preserved indefinitely, since they are protected from recontamination in the can, and also from chemical and enzymic deterioration.

sterility, commercial Canned foods that are not *sterile but which will not spoil during storage, because of the high acid content of the food, or the presence of pickling salts, or a high concentration of sugar.

sterilization, cold Applied to preservation with *sulphur dioxide or by *irradiation.

sterilization, radiation *See* irradiation.

steroids Chemically, compounds that contain the cyclopenteno-phenanthrene ring system. All the biologically important steroids are derived metabolically from *cholesterol; they include *vitamin D (chemically a secosteroid rather than a steroid), and hormones including the sex hormones (androgens, oestrogens, and progesterone) and the hormones of the adrenal cortex. *See also* phytosterols; sitosterol.

Toad poisons, cardiac glycosides of the digitalis group, and some of the carcinogenic hydrocarbons are also steroids.

sterols Alcohols derived from the *steroids; including *cholesterol, ergosterol in yeast (the precursor for synthetic *vitamin D_2), sitosterol and stigmasterol in plants, and coprosterol in faeces.

stevia leaves Leaves of the Paraguayan shrub, *Stevia rebaudiana*, the source of *stevioside and *rebaudioside, also known as yerba dulce.

stevioside Naturally occurring *glucoside of steviol, a *steroid derivative, which is 300 times as sweet as sucrose. Isolated from leaves of the Paraguayan shrub, yerba dulce (*Stevia rebaudiana*), the same source as *rebaudioside.

Stevix Trade name (Japan) for mixture of the sweet *glycosides extracted from *stevia leaves.

stew Meat and vegetables cooked together, also known as hotpot. Two main types: brown stew in which meat, vegetables, and flour are fried together before stewing, and white stew in which the ingredients are not fried first. Irish stew is a thin white stew (i.e. not thickened with flour).

stewing Slow cooking in an enclosed pan at a temperature below boiling point, about 90 °C. Such slow cooking is useful for low-quality meat (rich in *connective tissue), since it slowly breaks down the connective tissue to gelatine and so softens the meat. *See also* collagen.

stickwater The aqueous fraction from pressing cooked fish in the manufacture of *fish meal. Contains amino acids, vitamins, and minerals, and is either added to animal feed or mixed back with the fish meal and dried. Also known as fish solubles.

stilboestrol Synthetic substance with potent activity as female sex hormone; the first non-steroid compound developed to have oestrogen activity. Formerly widely used both clinically and for chemical caponization of cockerels and to stimulate the growth of cattle. *See also* capon.

Stilton Semi-hard, creamy white or blue-veined English *cheese made only in a very restricted area of the Vale of Belvoir in Leicestershire, England, but named after the village of Stilton, Huntingdonshire. Matured 3–4 months; for production of blue Stilton the cheese is pricked with stainless steel wires during ripening to encourage growth of the mould *Penicillium roquefortii*. A 30-g portion is a rich *source of vitamin B_{12}, a source of protein and niacin, contains 11 g of fat and supplies 125 kcal (510 kJ).

stiparogenic Foods that tend to cause constipation.

stiparolytic Foods that tend to prevent or relieve constipation.

stirabout Irish name for *porridge.

stir fry Chinese method of cooking; sliced vegetables and meat fried for a short time in a small amount of oil, normally in a *wok, over high heat with constant stirring.

stirrup cup A hot *punch traditionally served to the huntsmen at the start of a hunt.

stobb Strawberry stalk.

stock The juice obtained by boiling meat, fish, or vegetables, used to prepare soups, stews, and gravy. Meat and bone contain *collagen, which is converted into *gelatine by prolonged boiling; hence, the stock may set to a gel on cooling. The main nutritive value of stock is the mineral content.

stock cubes Ready made, dried, preparations of *stock. Most contain relatively large amounts of salt, as well as colouring and flavouring.

stockfish Unsalted fish that has been dried naturally in air and sunshine; mostly prepared in Norway. Contains 12–15% water; 4.5 kg of fresh fish yield 1 kg stockfish.

stollen German; fruit-filled loaves of yeast dough.

storage, gas See gas storage.

stork process The process of ultra-high temperature *sterilization of milk followed by sterilization again inside the bottle.

stout See beer. So-called milk stout merely has added *lactose (milk sugar).

stracciatella Italian; soup into which beaten egg is introduced while boiling, forming curls or strands.

Strasbourg pâté The true gourmet pâté de *fois gras, prepared from the livers of geese which have been force-fed to achieve a very high fat content.

strawberry Fruit of *Fragaria* spp., a perennial herb of American origin, introduced into the UK around 1600. An 80-g portion is a rich *source of vitamin C; provides 1.6 g of dietary fibre and supplies 20 kcal (85 kJ). The alpine strawberry is *Fragaria vesca semperflorens*, a variety of the European wild strawberry.

straw mushroom *Volvariella volvacea*, see mushrooms.

straw potatoes Very thin strips of potato, deep-fried. Also known as pommes *allumettes.

strega Italian; herb-flavoured liqueur.

streptococcal poisoning See food poisoning.

streusel Middle-European; a mixture of flour, sugar, butter, cinnamon, and chopped almonds, sprinkled over cakes and cookies.

stroganoff See beef stroganoff.

stroke Also known as cerebrovascular accident (CVA); damage to brain tissue by hypoxia due to blockage of a blood vessel as a result of thrombosis, atherosclerosis, or haemorrhage. The severity and nature of the effects of the stroke depend on the region of the brain affected and the extent of damage. *Hypertension and *hypercholesterolaemia are major risk factors.

strudel Austrian, German; sweet or savoury pastry made from paper-thin dough.

struvite Small crystals (chemically magnesium ammonium phosphate) that occasionally form in canned fish, and resemble broken glass.

Stubbs and More factor Factor for calculating the amount of fat-free meat in a product from total *nitrogen content. *See also* Kjeldahl determination; nitrogen conversion factor.

stuffing Savoury mixture used to give flavour to a dish; may be placed in a body cavity, as with poultry, laid flat between two portions, or rolled into boneless joint of meat. May be a mixture of breadcrumbs, flour, chestnut, etc., with herbs and spices or may be minced meat. *See also* forcemeat.

stunting Reduction in the linear growth of children, leading to lower height for age than would be expected, and generally resulting in lifelong short stature. A common effect of *protein-energy malnutrition, and associated especially with inadequate protein intake. *See also* anthropometry; Harvard standard; NCHS standards; nutritional status assessment; Tanner standard; Waterlow classification.

sturgeon White *fish of *Acipenser* spp. *See* caviar.

substrate 1 The substance on which an *enzyme acts.
2 The medium on which *micro-organisms grow.

subtilin Antibiotic isolated from a strain of *Bacillus subtilis* grown on a medium containing asparagine. Used as a food preservative (not permitted in the UK), as it reduces the thermal resistance of bacterial *spores and so permits a reduction in the processing time.

Sucaryl Trade name for sodium or calcium salt of cyclohexyl sulphamate (*cyclamate).

succory *See* chicory.

succotash American; sweetcorn (*maize) kernels with green or lima (butter) beans.

succus entericus *See* intestinal juice.

suchar Activated carbon, used to decolorize solutions. *See also* charcoal.

sucking pig Piglet aged 4–5 weeks, usually stuffed and roasted whole.

Sucralose Trade name for synthetic chlorinated sucrose (trichlorogalactosucrose), 2000 times as sweet as sucrose, stable to heat and acid.

sucrase The enzyme that hydrolyses *sucrose to yield *glucose and *fructose (*invert sugar). Also known as invertase or saccharase.

sucrol *See* dulcin.

Sucron Trade name for mixture of *saccharin and *sucrose, four times as sweet as sucrose alone.

sucrose Cane or beet *sugar. A *disaccharide composed of *glucose and *fructose.

sucrose distearate *See* sucrose esters.

sucrose esters Di- and trilaurates and mono- and distearates of sucrose. Used as emulsifiers, wetting agents, and surface active agents, e.g. for washing fruits and vegetables, as anti-spattering agents, anti-foam agents, and anti-staling or crumb-softening agents (E-473).

sucrose intolerance *See* disaccharide intolerance.

sucrose monostearate *See* sucrose esters.

sucrose polyesters (SPE) Mixtures of hexa-, hepta-, and octa-esters of sucrose and common *fatty acids (C-12 to C-20 and above). Can replace fats and oils in foods and food preparation but pass through the gastrointestinal tract without being absorbed, hence known as fat substitutes or *fat replacers.

Sudan gum *See* gum Arabic.

suedoise Moulded fruit purée set with gelatine.

suet Solid white fat around the kidneys of oxen and sheep, used in baking and frying.

suet crust *See* pastry.

sufu Fermented product made by inoculating soybean curd (*tofu) with the mould *Actinomucor elegans*; stored after adding salt and alcohol.

sugar 1 Commonly table sugar or *sucrose, which is extracted from the *sugar beet or *sugar cane, concentrated, and refined. *Molasses is the residue left after the first stage of crystallization and is bitter and black. The residue from the second stage is *treacle, less bitter and viscous than molasses. The first crude crystals are Muscovado or Barbados sugar, brown and sticky. The next stage is light brown, Demerara sugar. Refined white sugar is essentially 100% pure sucrose; technically described as semi-white, white, and extra-white (EU definitions). Yields 3.9 kcal (16 kJ)/g or 24 kcal (100 kJ) per teaspoonful. Soft sugars are fine-grained and moister, white or brown (excluding large-grained Demerara sugar).

2 Chemically a group of compounds of carbon, hydrogen, and oxygen (carbohydrates). The simplest sugars are monosaccharides. They may contain three (triose), four (tetrose), five (pentose), six (hexose), or seven (heptose) carbon atoms, with hydrogen and oxygen in the ratio $C_nH_{2n}O_n$. The nutritionally important monosaccharides are hexoses: glucose (grape sugar), fructose (fruit sugar), and galactose. Two pentoses are also important: ribose and deoxyribose.

Disaccharides consist of two monosaccharide units, linked by condensation (elimination of water). The nutritionally important disaccharides are *sucrose (cane or beet sugar, a disaccharide of glucose + fructose), lactose (milk sugar, a disaccharide of glucose + galactose), and maltose (malt sugar, a disaccharide of glucose).

Trisaccharides consist of three monosaccharide units and tetrasaccharides of four. Larger numbers of monosaccharide units make up oligosaccharides. Most tri-, tetra-, and oligosaccharides are not digested by human enzymes, but are substrates for bacterial fermentation in the large intestine.

sugar alcohols Also called polyols, chemical derivatives of *sugars that differ from the parent compounds in having an alcohol group (CH_2OH) instead of the aldehyde group (CHO); thus *mannitol from *mannose, *xylitol from *xylose, *lacticol from *lactulose (also *sorbitol, *isomalt, and *hydrogenated glucose syrup). Several occur naturally in fruits, vegetables, and cereals. They range in sweetness from equal to sucrose to less than half. They provide bulk in foods such as confectionery (in contrast to intense *sweeteners), and so are called bulk sweeteners. They are slowly and incompletely metabolized so that they are tolerated by diabetics and provide less energy than sucrose: they are less *cariogenic than sucrose, especially hydrogenated glucose syrup, isomalt, sorbitol, and xylitol.

The energy yields differ, but the EU has adopted a value of 2.4 kcal (10 kJ) per gram for all polyols (compared with 4 for carbohydrates). They are considered safe and have no specified *ADI, meaning that they can be used in foods in any required amount; however, a fairly large amount, more than 20–50 g per day (varying with the rest of the diet and the individual) can cause gastro-intestinal discomfort and have a laxative effect. For labelling purposes they are included with carbohydrates, not sugars; they do not ferment and so do not damage teeth. *See also* tooth-friendly sweets.

sugar beet *Beta vulgaris* subsp. *cicla*, a biennial plant related to the garden *beetroot but with white, conical roots; the most important source of *sugar (*sucrose) in temperate countries; contains 15–20% sucrose.

sugar cane The tropical grass, *Saccharum officinarum*; the juice of the stems contains about 15% *sucrose and provides about 70% of the world's sugar production.

sugar, canners' Sugar with a higher standard of microbiological quality control than highly refined table sugar because some bacterial spores can survive the high temperatures of canning and even small numbers can damage canned food. Similarly bottlers' sugar must be virtually free from yeasts, moulds, and certain bacteria.

sugar, caster Ordinary *sugar (sucrose) crystallized in small crystals.

sugar confectionery A range of sugar-based products, including boiled sweets (hard glasses), fatty emulsions (*toffees and caramels), soft crystalline products (fudges), fully crystalline products (fondants), and gels (gums, pastilles, and jellies).

sugar doctor To prevent the crystallization or 'graining' of *sugar in sugar confectionery, a substance called the sugar doctor or candy doctor is added. This may be a weak acid, such as cream of tartar, which 'inverts' (*hydrolyses) part of the cane sugar during the boiling, or invert sugar or starch syrup.

sugar esters *See* sucrose esters.

sugar, icing Powdered *sucrose.

sugaring, of dried fruits A type of deterioration of dried fruit on storage, most frequently on prunes and figs. A sugary substance appears on the surface or under the skin, consisting of glucose and fructose, with traces of citric and malic acids, lysine, asparagine, and aspartic acid. When occurring under the skin of prunes, it is called 'red sugar'.

sugar, London Demerara White sugar coloured with molasses to resemble partly refined sugar.

sugar maple The north American tree *Acer saccharum*; the sap is evaporated down to a syrup, maple syrup, and crystallized to sucrose, maple sugar. Maple-flavoured or pancake syrup is made from flavoured glucose syrup and sugar.

sugar palm *Arenga saccharifera*; grows wild in Malaysia and Indonesia; sugar (sucrose) is obtained from the sap.

sugar pea *See* mange-tout.

Sugar Puffs Trade name for a breakfast cereal made from *puffed wheat. A 40-g portion is a *source of copper; provides 2.4 g of dietary fibre; supplies 145 kcal (610 kJ).

sugar tolerance *See* glucose tolerance.

sugarware Edible seaweed, *Laminaria saccharina*.

sukha bhoona *See* bhoona.

sulphate The mineral *sulphur occurs in foods and in the body in two main forms: as sulphates (salts and esters of sulphuric acid, H_2SO_4); and in the sulphur *amino acids *methionine and *cysteine.

sulphites Salts of sulphurous acid (H_2SO_3) used as sources of *sulphur dioxide (SO_2) (E-221–227).

sulphur An element that is part of the amino acids cystine and methionine and is therefore present in all proteins. It is also part of the molecules of vitamin B_1 and biotin and occurs in foods and in the body as *sulphates. Apart from these amino acids and vitamins, there appears to be no requirement for sulphur in any other form and no deficiency has ever been observed, although it is essential for plants.

   Not only was the old-fashioned remedy of sulphur and molasses (brimstone and treacle) quite unnecessary, but elemental sulphur is not used by the body.

sulphur amino acids *See* methionine.

sulphur dioxide (SO_2) Preservative used in gaseous form or as salts (*sulphites) for fruit drinks, wine, comminuted meat, and as a processing aid to control physical properties of flour; also prevents enzymic and non-enzymic *browning. Protects vitamin C but destroys vitamin B_1. Prepared by ancient Egyptians and Romans by burning sulphur and used to disinfect wine (E-220).

sulphuring Preservation by *sulphur dioxide.

sultanas Made by drying the golden sultana grapes grown in Turkey, Greece, Australia, and South Africa; the bunches are dipped in alkali, washed, sulphured, and dried. Sultanas of the European type produced in the USA are termed seedless raisins. A 20-g portion is a *source of copper; provides 1.4 g of dietary fibre; supplies 50 kcal (210 kJ). *See also* currants, dried; fruit, dried; raisins.

summer pudding Cold sweet of stewed fruit cased in bread or sponge cake; traditionally summer soft fruits such as raspberries, blackberries, strawberries, and currants are used.

sum-sum *See* sesame.

sunchokes *See* artichokes.

sundae Dessert of *ice cream and fruit.

Sunett Trade name for *acesulphame K.

sunflower Annual plant, *Helianthus annuus*. A 50-g portion of seed is a rich *source of vitamin B_1, a good source of protein, iron, and niacin; a source of zinc; contains 25 g of fat of which 10% is saturated and 70% polyunsaturated, provides 3 g of dietary fibre; supplies 290 kcal (1220 kJ).

An important commercial source of edible oil (low in saturates, 12%, approximately 70% polyunsaturated); residual oilseed cake is used as animal feed.

sunlight flavour Name given to unpleasant flavours developing in foods after exposure to sunlight. In milk it is said to be due to the breakdown of *methionine in the presence of vitamin B_2; in beer due to a change in the bitter principles from the hops.

superchill Cool to temperature of −1 to −4 ˚C (chill temperature is usually +2 ˚C).

superglycerinated fats Neutral fats are triacylglycerols, i.e. with three molecules of fatty acid to each molecule of glycerol. Mono- and diacylglycerols (sometimes called mono- and diglycerides) are known as superglycerinated high-ratio fats or fat extenders (E-471).

Glyceryl monostearate (GMS) is solid at room temperature, flexible, and non-greasy; it is used as a protective coating for foods, as a plasticizer for softening the crumb of bread, to reduce spattering in frying fats, as an emulsifier and stabilizer. Glyceryl mono-oleate (GMO) is semi-liquid at room temperature.

supplementation *See* fortification.

suprarenal glands *See* adrenal glands.

suprême French; the best or most delicate part. Also white sauce made with reduced chicken stock, cream, butter, or egg yolk.

suprêmes French; breast and wings of chicken or game birds.

suquet Spanish (Catalan); fish stew.

sur commande French menu term for dishes that take time to prepare and are only cooked when ordered.

surface area *See* body surface area.

surfactants Surface active agents; compounds that have an affinity for fats (hydrophobic) and water (hydrophilic) and so act as emulsifiers, e.g. soaps and detergents. Used as wetting agents to assist the reconstitution of powders, including dried foods, to clean and peel fruits and vegetables, also in baked goods and comminuted meat products.

surimi Water extract of minced flesh of low-oil *fish (mostly myofibrillar protein) with gelling properties, used to prepare a range of foods. It is white, and relatively tasteless and odourless. Introduced from Japan into the United States in 1979, as the basis for *seafood analogues but with broad potentialities.

sur lattes With reference to wines, means storage 'on their side' so that the cork is kept moist and airtight.

surullitos Caribbean (Puerto Rican); small cylindrical biscuits made from corn meal and cheese.

susceptor plates Special metallic films (usually powdered *aluminium) deposited inside the packets of foods intended for microwave cooking; they concentrate the energy on the outside of the food and brown and crisp it.

sushi Japanese; thinly sliced raw fish.

suspensoids *See* colloids, lyophobic.

süss *See* wine, sweetness.

Sussex bread Old English loaf made from wheat and rye flour mixed with grains, given to servants; now revived.

süssreserve Unfermented grape juice added to wines after fermentation to increase sweetness, especially in Germany, England, and New Zealand.

Sustagen Trade name for a food concentrate in powder form, also useable for tube feeding; mixture of whole and skim milk, casein, maltose, dextrins, and glucose.

swainsonine *See* locoweed.

swede Root of *Brassica rutabaga* or Swedish turnip; called rutabaga in the USA. A 150-g portion is a rich *source of vitamin C; a source of vitamin B_1; provides 4.5 g of dietary fibre; supplies 15 kcal (60 kJ).

sweeney *Osteomalacia in livestock due to *phosphate deficiency.

sweetbread Butchers' term for *pancreas (gut sweetbread) or thymus (chest sweetbread).

sweet chervil *See* sweet cicely.

sweet cicely A wild plant (*Myrrhis odorata*) with a smell of aniseed. The aniseed-flavoured leaves are used to flavour fruit cups, fruit salads, and cooked fruit; the main root can be boiled, sliced, and used in salads. Also known as sweet chervil.

sweetcorn *See* maize.

sweeteners Four groups of compounds are used to sweeten foods: (1) The *sugars, of which the commonest is *sucrose. *Fructose has 173% of the sweetness of sucrose; *glucose, 74%; *maltose, 33%; and *lactose, 16%. *Honey is a mixture of glucose and fructose; (2) Bulk sweeteners, including *sugar alcohols; (3) Synthetic non-nutritive sweeteners (intense sweeteners), which are many times sweeter than sucrose, such as *acesulphame K, *aspartame, *cyclamate, *dulcin, *P4000, *saccharin, *sucaryl; (4) Various other chemicals such as *glycerol and *glycine (70% as sweet as sucrose), and certain *peptides.

sweeteners, artificial *See* sweeteners, intense.

sweeteners, bulk Used to replace sucrose and glucose syrups. One example is hydrogenated glucose syrup, in which the free aldehyde groups of glucose have been reduced to sorbitol by catalytic hydrogenation; effectively a mixture of glucose and sorbitol. Used in soft drinks and sugar confectionery, and in some diabetic foods as a partial substitute for sorbitol; is 70–80% as sweet as sucrose. *See also* sugar alcohols.

sweeteners, intense (non-nutritive) Chemical substances that have no calorific value but are intensely sweet and so are useful as a replacement for sucrose in foods intended for diabetics and those on slimming regimes, but unlike bulk sweeteners (*sugar alcohols) do not replace the bulk of sucrose. *See also* acesulphame; aspartame; cyclamate; miracle berry; monellin; neohesperidin; saccharin; stevioside; thaumatin.

sweeteners, non-nutritive *See* sweeteners, intense.

sweetening agents *See* sweeteners.

Sweetex Trade name for *saccharin.

sweet lupin *See* lupins.

sweetness One of the five basic senses of *taste.

sweet pepper *See* pepper.

sweet potato *See* potato, sweet.

sweet sop *See* custard apple.

swells Infected cans of food swollen at the ends by gases produced by fermentation. A 'hard swell' has permanently extended ends. If the ends can be moved under pressure, but not forced back to the original position, they are 'soft swells'. 'Springers' can be forced back, but the opposite end bulges. A 'flipper' is a can of normal appearance in which the end flips out when the can is struck.

Hydrogen swells are harmless, and due to acid fruits attacking the can.

Swiss chard The spinach-like leaves and broad midrib of *Beta vulgaris* var. *cicla*, also known as leaf beet, leaf chard, sea kale beet, silver beet, white leaf beet, spinach beet. A 100-g portion (boiled) is a rich *source of vitamin A (as carotene); a good source of vitamin C; a source of iron; supplies 18 kcal (72 kJ).

The term is also used for blanched summer shoots of globe *artichoke and for inner leaves of *cardoon, *Cynara cardunculus.*

Swiss cheese American term for hard cheese such as Emmental and Gruyère; may be made in the USA or imported from Switzerland.

Swiss roll Thin rectangle of sponge cake, spread with jam or other filling and rolled into a cylinder. Known in the USA as jelly roll.

swordfish Oily *fish, *Xiphias gladius.*

syllabub (sillabub) Elizabethan dish made of cream curdled with wine or cider; the thickened version is used as a dessert and a thinner version as a drink.

synbiotics *See* prebiotics; probiotics.

syneresis Oozing of liquid from gel when cut and allowed to stand (e.g. from jelly or baked custard).

synsepalum *See* miracle berry.

synthetic rice *See* tapioca-macaroni.

synthetic sweeteners *See* sweeteners, intense.

syrah One of the 9 'classic' *grape varieties used for *wine making, important in the red Rhône wines. Also known as shiraz, especially in Australia and California.

syrup A solution of sugar which may be from a variety of sources, such as maple or sorghum, or stages in refining cane and beet sugar such as top syrup, refiners' syrup, sugar syrup, golden syrup, or by hydrolysis of *starch (glucose or corn syrup).

Glucose syrup is the concentrated solution of sugars from the acid or enzymic hydrolysis of starch (usually maize or potato starch); a mixture of varying amounts of glucose, maltose, and glucose complexes. The *Codex Alimentarius definition is: purified, concentrated, aqueous solutions of nutritive saccharides from starch. Usually 70% total solids by weight, containing glucose, maltose, and oligomers of glucose of three, four, or more units. May be in dried form. Used as a sweetening agent in sugar confectionery; also termed corn syrup, corn starch hydrolysate, starch syrup, confectioners' glucose, and uncrystallizable syrup.

Pancake syrup or maple flavour syrup is flavoured glucose syrup.
See also dextrose equivalent value; fructose syrups.

T

T3 Tri-iodothyronine, one of the *thyroid hormones.

T4 Thyroxine (tetra-iodothyronine), one of the *thyroid hormones.

tabasco A thin piquant sauce prepared by fermentation of powdered dried fruits of chilli *pepper, mixed with spirit vinegar and salt. Traditionally used with Mexican and Caribbean foods.

tabbouleh Syrian, Lebanese; salad made with *bulgur, parsley, onion, mint, lemon juice, oil, and spices.

table d'hôte A meal consisting of a set number of courses at a fixed price; there is usually some choice of dishes within each course; a set menu as opposed to à la *carte.

tachycardia Rapid heartbeat, as occurs after exercise; may also occur, without undue exertion, as a result of anxiety, and in *anaemia and *vitamin B_1 deficiency.

tachyphagia Rapid eating.

taco Mexican; *tortilla (maize-meal pancake) filled with meat, beans, and spicy sauce, and fried.

taeniasis Infection with *tapeworms of the genus *Taenia*.

taette *See* milks, fermented.

tafelwein *See* wine classification, Germany.

taffy *See* toffee.

tafia Spirit similar to *rum made from sugar cane.

tagliatelle *Pasta in ribbons 2–3 cm wide.

tahini (tahina) Middle-Eastern; paste made from *sesame seeds, usually eaten as a dip; also used in preparation of *hummus. A 50-g portion is a rich *source of calcium, iron, and vitamin B_1, a good source of niacin; a source of protein and zinc; provides 4 g of dietary fibre; contains 30 g of fat of which 15% is saturated and 45% polyunsaturated; supplies 300 kcal (1250 kJ).

takadiastase Or koji, an enzyme preparation produced by growing the fungus *Aspergillus oryzae* on bran, leaching the culture mass with water, and precipitating with alcohol. Contains a mixture of enzymes, largely diastatic (i.e. *amylases), used for the preparation of starch hydrolysates.

talawa Indian term for deep-fried food.

Talin Trade name for thaumatin, an extract of the berry *Thaumatococcus danielli*, about 3000 times as sweet as sucrose. *See* katemfe.

tallow *See* premier jus.

tallow, rendered Beef or mutton fat prepared from parts other than the kidney, by heating with water in an autoclave. When pressed, separates to a liquid fraction, oleo oil, used in margarine, and a solid fraction, oleostearin, used for soap and candles.

tamal (tamales) Mexican; maize-meal pancake, similar to *tortilla, but made with fat. Traditionally cooked inside the soft husks of maize.

tamarillo *See* tomato, English.

tamarind Leguminous tree, *Tamarindus indica*, with pods containing seeds embedded in brown pulp, eaten fresh, used to prepare beverages and seasonings in oriental cuisine (e.g. the Indian sauce, *imli).

tammy To squeeze a sauce through a fine woollen cloth (a tammy cloth) to strain it.

tandoor Traditional North Indian clay oven.

tandoori (tanduri) Indian term for food cooked in a clay oven (tandoor). The meat is marinated with aromatic herbs and spices before cooking.

tangelo A *citrus fruit, a cross between *tangerine and *pomelo.

tangerine A *citrus fruit, *Citrus reticulata*, also called mandarin; satsuma is a variety of tangerine. One medium-sized tangerine (70 g weighed without the peel) is a rich *source of vitamin C; provides 1.5 g of dietary fibre; supplies 25 kcal (100 kJ).

tangors *See* citrus.

tanier *See* tannia.

tankage Residue from slaughterhouse excluding all the useful tissues; fertilizer or animal feed.

Tanner standard Tables of height and weight for age used as reference values for the assessment of growth and nutritional status in children, based on data collected in England. Now largely replaced by the NCHS (US National Center for Health Statistics) standards. *See also* anthropometry.

tannia (tanier) The corm of *Xanthosoma sagittifolium*; known as new cocoyam or yautia in West Africa; same family as *taro.

tannic acid *See* tannins.

tannins Compounds present in dark-coloured sorghum, carob bean, unripe fruits, tea, etc.; they give an astringent effect in the mouth, precipitate proteins, and are used to clarify beer and wines. Also called tannic acid and gallotannin.

tanrogan Manx name for *scallops.

tansy A herb, *Tanacetum vulgare*. The leaves and young shoots are used for flavouring puddings and omelettes. Tansy cakes made with eggs and young leaves used to be eaten at Easter. Tansy tea made by infusing the herb was formerly used as a tonic and for intestinal worms; may be poisonous in large amounts. The root, preserved in honey or sugar, was used to treat gout.

tapas Spanish; small savoury dishes served with wine in bars.

tapeworm Parasitic intestinal worm; infection is acquired by eating raw or undercooked infected pork (*Taenia solium*), beef (*T. saginata*), or fish

(*Diphyllobothrium latum*). Eggs are shed in the faeces and infect the animal host. Cysticercosis is infection of human beings with the larval stage by ingestion of eggs from faecal contamination of food and water.

tapioca Starch prepared from the root of the *cassava plant (*Manihot utilissima*); there are only traces of nutrients. The starch paste is heated to burst the granules, then dried either in globules resembling *sago or in flakes. The name is also used of starch in general, as in manioc tapioca and potato flour tapioca.

tapioca-macaroni A mixture of either 80–90 parts *tapioca flour, with 10–20 parts of peanut flour; or tapioca, peanut, and semolina, in proportion 60 : 15 : 25; it is baked into shapes resembling rice grains or macaroni; developed in India. Also referred to as synthetic rice.

taramasalata Greek; fish roe (commonly smoked cod roe), whipped with oil, garlic, and lemon juice, then thickened with bread, to make a dip.

taratòr Balkan; cold soup made from yoghurt, cucumber, nuts, and garlic.

tarel *See* apples.

tares Traditional English name for the vetches, which are *pulses.

tarhonya Hungarian; pea-sized balls of egg and flour dough, fried in lard then simmered in water. A staple food of the Hungarian lowland plain.

tarka Indian; foods seared with ghee (clarified butter) and seasoning after cooking. Also known as chamak.

taro Corm of *Colocasia esculenta* and *C. antiquorum*; called eddo or dasheen in the Caribbean, old cocoyam in West Africa.

tarragon Leaves and flowering tops of the bushy perennial plant *Artemisia dracunculus*; the French variety is considered superior to the Russian. Has a mild anise-like flavour and is used to flavour pickles; it is one of the ingredients of *fines herbes. Tarragon vinegar is made by steeping the fresh herb in white wine vinegar and is used in making *sauce tartare and French *mustard.

tart, tartlet Open pastry case filled with fruit, jam, lemon curd, custard, etc.

tartan purry Scottish; finely chopped cooked kale mixed with oatmeal. The name is probably a corruption of *tarte en purée*, suggesting it may originally have been served in a pastry case.

tartar Hard gritty deposit of *plaque and minerals that accumulates on and between teeth. Originally the name given by alchemists to animal and vegetable concretions, such as wine lees, stone, gravel, and deposits on teeth, since they were all attributed to the same cause.

tartar emetic Potassium antimonyl tartrate, produces inflammation of the gastrointestinal *mucosa and used to be used as an emetic.

tartare sauce Mayonnaise flavoured with herbs, chopped capers, gherkins, etc., served with fish. *See also* salad dressing.

tartaric acid A dibasic *acid, chemically dihydroxysuccinic acid. Occurs in fruits, the chief source being grapes; used in preparing lemonade, added to jams when the fruit is not sufficiently acidic (*citric acid also used) and in baking powder (E-334). *Tartar emetic is the potassium antimonyl salt, and Rochelle salt is potassium sodium tartrate (E-337). *See also* cream of tartar.

tarte tatin French; apple pie baked with the pastry uppermost, then inverted before serving.

tartrazine A yellow colour (E-102), called Yellow No. 5 in the USA.

taste The tongue can distinguish five separate tastes: sweet, salt, sour (or acid), bitter, and savoury (sometimes called *umami, from the Japanese word for a savoury flavour), due to stimulation of the *taste buds. The overall taste or flavour of foods is due to these tastes, together with astringency in the mouth, texture, and *aroma.

taste buds Situated mostly on the tongue; about 9000 elongated cells ending in minute hairlike processes, the gustatory hairs.

tatare (steak tatare) Dish prepared from minced beef or other meat, eaten uncooked.

taurocholic acid *See* bile.

tawa Indian; heavy iron griddle.

T-bone steak Cut from the thin fillet end of a sirloin of *beef, containing a T-shaped section of bone.

tea 1 A beverage prepared by infusion of the young leaves, leaf buds, and internodes of varieties of *Camellia sinensis* and *C. assamica*, originating from China. Green tea is dried without further treatment. Black tea is fermented (actually an oxidation) before drying; Oolong tea is lightly fermented. Among the black teas, Flowering Pekoe is made from the top leaf buds, Orange Pekoe from first opened leaf, Pekoe from third leaves, and Souchong from next leaves.
  See also caffeine; herb tea; xanthines.
  2 An afternoon meal; may consist of a light meal (especially in southern Britain) or be a substantial meal (high tea) as in northern Britain.

tea, Brazilian (Paraguayan) *See* maté.

tea, Russian *See* Russian tea.

teacake Flat round cakes made from yeast dough, normally toasted and buttered.

teaseed oil Oil from the seed of *Thea sasangua*, cultivated in China; used as salad oil and for frying; similar in properties to olive oil.

teeth, mottled *See* fluorosis.

TEF Thermic effect of food, *see* diet-induced thermogenesis.

teff A tropical *millet, *Eragrostis abyssinica*, the dietary staple in Ethiopia; little grown elsewhere.

teg A 2-year-old sheep. *See* lamb.

teiglech Jewish; small biscuits made from flour, egg, and ginger, boiled in honey.

tempeh Indonesian; *soya bean fermented by a mould, *Rhizopus* spp.

Templein Trade name for textured vegetable protein.

tempranillo A *grape variety widely used for *wine making, although not one of the classic varieties; the wine of Rioja.

tenderizer Usually refers to the *enzyme *papain (extracted from the *pawpaw), when used to tenderize meat. Similar enzymes occur in *pineapple and *figs. Weak acids such as *vinegar and lemon juice also tenderize meat.

tenderloin Fillet of *beef (especially in the USA) or *pork.

tenderometer Instrument to measure the stage of maturity of peas to determine whether they are ready for cropping. Measures the force required to effect a shearing action.

tenesmus Persistent ineffective spasms of bladder or rectum; intestinal tenesmus commonly occurs in *irritable bowel syndrome.

tenosynovitis Inflammation of a tendon sheath caused by strain, calcium deposits, *hypercholesterolaemia, *gout, rheumatoid arthritis, etc. Claimed to be relieved by high intakes of *vitamin B_6, some 50 times the *reference intake, but there is little evidence. *See also* carpal tunnel syndrome; vitamin B_6 toxicity.

tenuate Anorectic (*appetite suppressing) drug, used in the treatment of *obesity.

tepary bean *Phaseolus acutifolius*, also known as frijole, Mexican haricot bean, or pinto. It is able to grow during drought.

tequila Mexican; *spirit (40–50% alcohol by volume) prepared by double distillation of fermented sap of the cultivated agave or maguey, *Agave tequilana*. Mescal and pulque are similar, made from various species of wild agave, and have a stronger flavour.

teratogen Substance that deforms the foetus in the womb and so induces birth defects.

terpeneless oil *See* terpenes.

terpenes Major components of the *essential oils of citrus fruits; however, they are not responsible for the characteristic flavour, and, since they readily oxidize and polymerize to produce unpleasant flavours, they are removed from citrus oils by distillation or solvent extraction, leaving the so-called terpeneless oils for flavouring foods and drinks.

terrine Oval French earthenware or china dish and also the food cooked in the dish (the latter is technically *pâté en terrine*).

testa The fibrous layer between the pericarp and the inner aleurone layer of a cereal grain.

test meal *See* fractional test meal.

tetany Over-sensitivity of motor nerves to stimuli; particularly affects face, hands, and feet. Caused by reduction in the level of ionized *calcium in the bloodstream and can accompany severe *rickets.

tetracyclines A group of closely related *antibiotics including tetracycline, oxytetracycline (terramycin), and aureomycin. The last two are used in some countries for preserving food and as growth improvers, added to animal feed at the rate of a few mg per tonne.

tetraenoic acid *Fatty acid with four double bonds, e.g. arachidonic acid.

tetramine poisoning Paralysis similar to that caused by curare, caused by a toxin in the salivary glands of the red whelk, *Neptunea antiqua* (distinct from the edible whelk *Buccinum undatum*).

tetrodontin poisoning Caused by a toxin, tetrodotoxin, in fish of the Tetrodontidae family (puffer fish) and amphibia of the Salamandridae family. Occurs in Japan from Japanese puffer fish or fugu (*Fuga rubripes*), eaten for its gustatory and tactile pleasure since traces of the poison cause a tingling sensation in the extremities (larger doses cause respiratory failure).

tetrodotoxin *See* tetrodontin poisoning.

Texatrein Trade name for textured vegetable protein made by extrusion.

Texgran Trade name for textured vegetable protein.

texture Combination of physical properties perceived by senses of kinaesthesis (muscle-nerve endings), touch (including mouth feel), sight, and hearing. Physical properties may include shape, size, number, and conformation of constituent structural elements.

textured vegetable protein Spun or extruded vegetable protein, usually made to simulate meat.

texture profile *Organoleptic analysis of the complex of food in terms of mechanical and geometrical characteristics, fat and moisture content, including the order in which they appear from the first bite to complete mastication.

TGS Trichlorogalactosucrose, *see* sucralose.

thal Indian; platter of brass, copper, or silver on which food is served and eaten; a smaller dish is a thali.

thaumatin The intensely sweet protein of the African fruit, *Thaumatococus danielli*, 1600 times as sweet as sucrose. Called katemfe in Sierra Leone and miracle fruit in the Sudan (not the same as *miracle berry).

theaflavins Reddish-orange pigments formed in *tea during fermentation; responsible for the colour of tea extracts and part of the astringent flavour.

theanine γ-N-Ethylglutamine, the major free amino acid in tea, 1–2% dry weight of leaf.

theevil *See* spurtle.

theine Alternative name for *caffeine.

theobromine An *alkaloid found in cocoa, chemically related to *caffeine, and with similar effects. Theobromine is 3,7-dimethylxanthine; caffeine is trimethylxanthine.

theophylline An *alkaloid found in tea, chemically related to *caffeine, and with similar effects. Theine is 1,3-dimethyl xanthine; caffeine is trimethylxanthine.

therapeutic diets Those formulated to treat disease or metabolic disorders.

thermic effect of food *See* diet-induced thermogenesis.

thermization Heat treatment, less severe than *pasteurization, e.g. heat treatment of milk for cheese-making whereby the number of organisms is diminished.

thermoduric Bacteria that are heat resistant but not *thermophilic, i.e. they survive, but do not develop at, *pasteurization temperatures. Usually not pathogens but indicative of insanitary conditions.

thermogenesis Increased heat production by the body, either to maintain body temperature (by shivering or non-shivering thermogenesis) or in response to food intake, *diet-induced thermogenesis. *See also* brown adipose tissue.

thermogenesis, diet-induced *See* diet-induced thermogenesis.

thermogenic drugs Substances that stimulate body heat output, and thus of interest in 'slimming'.

thermopeeling A method of peeling tough-skinned fruits in which the fruit is rapidly passed through an electric furnace at about 900 °C then sprayed with water.

thermophiles (thermophilic bacteria) Bacteria that prefer temperatures above 55 °C and can tolerate temperatures up to 75–80 °C. Extreme thermophiles can live in boiling water, and have been isolated from hot springs. Thermophilic bacteria are responsible for spontaneous combustion in haystacks.

thiamin *See* vitamin B_1.

thiaminase An *enzyme present in many species of micro-organisms, plants, and fish which splits thiamin (vitamin B_1), forming products that have anti-vitamin activity. Non-enzymic cleavage of thiamin, for example by polyphenols, is also sometimes called thiaminase action. Chastek paralysis in foxes and mink fed diets rich in raw fish, and blind staggers in horses and other animals eating bracken fern, are due to acute vitamin B_1 deficiency caused by dietary thiaminase.

thiobendazole Antifungal agent used for surface treatment of bananas.

thioctic acid *See* lipoic acid.

thirst *See* water balance.

Thousand Island dressing *See* salad dressing.

threonine An essential *amino acid, chemically amino-hydroxybutyric acid. It was the last of the protein amino acids to be discovered, in 1935, in studies of *nitrogen balance on subjects fed mixtures of the then known amino acids in place of proteins.

thrombin Plasma protein involved in the *coagulation of blood.

thrombokinase Or thromboplastin. An enzyme liberated from damaged tissue and blood platelets; it converts prothrombin to *thrombin in the *coagulation of blood.

thromboplastin See thrombokinase.

thrombosis Formation of blood clots in blood vessels.

thump See stelk.

thuricide Name given to a living culture of Bacillus thuringiensis which is harmless to man but kills insect pests. Known as a microbial insecticide. Used to treat certain foods and fodder crops to destroy pests such as corn earworm, flour moth, tomato fruit worm, cabbage looper, etc. The bacillus is mass-produced and stored like a chemical.

thyme The aromatic leaves and flowering tops of Thymus spp. used as flavouring in soup, meat, fish, poultry dressing, and sausages.

thymidine, thymine A pyrimidine; see nucleic acids.

thymonucleic acid Obsolete name for *deoxyribonucleic acid.

thymus (French: riz; German: Bries.) Chest (neck) sweetbread; a ductless gland in the chest, as distinct from gut sweetbread or *pancreas. A 150-g portion is a rich *source of protein, iron, and, unusually for a meat product, of vitamin C; 150 g of calf chest sweetbread contains about 5 g of fat and supplies 170 kcal (700 kJ), beef sweetbread contains about 30 g of fat and supplies 350 kcal (1470 kJ).

thyroglobulin The protein in the thyroid gland which is the precursor for the synthesis of the *thyroid hormones. The thyroid-stimulating hormone of the pituitary gland stimulates hydrolysis of thyroglobulin and secretion of the *hormones into the bloodstream. See also iodine, protein-bound.

thyroid hormones The thyroid is an endocrine gland situated in the neck, which takes up *iodine from the bloodstream and synthesizes two *hormones, tri-iodothyronine (T3) and thyroxine (T4, tetra-iodothyronine). The active hormone is T3; thyroxine is converted to T3 in tissues by the action of a *selenium-dependent enzyme. T3 controls the *basal metabolic rate.

Enlargement of the thyroid gland is *goitre; it may be associated with under- or over-production of the thyroid hormones. Severe iodine deficiency in children leads to *cretinism. See also hypothyroidism; thyrotoxicosis.

thyrotoxicosis Over-activity of the thyroid gland, leading to excessive secretion of *thyroid hormones and resulting in increased *basal metabolic rate. Hyperthyroid subjects are lean and have tense nervous activity. May be due to over-stimulation of the thyroid gland.

Iodine-induced thyrotoxicosis affects mostly elderly people who have lived for a long time in iodine-deficient areas, have had a long-standing goitre, and then have been given extra iodine. Also known as Jodbasedow, Basedow's disease, and Graves' disease.

thyroxine One of the *thyroid hormones.

Tia Maria Trade name; Jamaican rum-based coffee liqueur.

tierce Obsolete measure of wine cask; $^1/_3$ of a *pipe, i.e. about 35 imperial gallons (160 litres).

tiffin Anglo-Indian name for a light midday meal.

tiger nut Tuber of grass-like sedge, *Cyperus esculentus*, also earth or ground almond, chufa nut, rush nut, nut sedge, 5–20 mm long, usually available in partly dried condition. Mainly starch and fat (75% mono-unsaturated); a rich source of dietary fibre (19 g/100 g). *See also* horchata de chufas.

tikka Indian; marinated chicken (or other meat) threaded on skewers and grilled.

til *See* sesame.

timbale Round, fireproof china or tinned copper mould, used for moulding meat or fish mixtures; also the dishes cooked in the mould. For hot timbales the mould is lined with potato, pastry, or pasta; for cold the lining is *aspic.

tin A metal; a dietary essential for experimental animals, but so widely distributed in foods that no deficiency has been reported in man, and its function, if any, is not known. In the absence of oxygen tin is resistant to corrosion; hence widely used in tinned cans for food containers.

tinto Portuguese, Spanish; red wines.

Tipperary seed cake *See* seed cake.

tipsy cake Sponge cake soaked in wine and fruit juice, made into a trifle and reassembled into the original tall shape. The wine and fruit juice may cause the cake to topple sideways in drunken (tipsy) fashion.

tiramisu Italian; dessert made of coffee-flavoured sponge or biscuit filled with sweetened cream cheese (*mascarpone) and cream, doused with syrup.

tisane French term for an infusion made from herbs (camomile, lime blossoms, fennel seeds, etc.), believed to have medicinal properties. *See also* herb tea.

TK$_{ac}$ Transketolase activation coefficient, the result of the *transketolase test for *vitamin B_1 nutritional status, an *enzyme activation assay.

toad-in-the-hole *Sausages cooked in batter, also called sausage toad.

toad skin *See* phrynoderma.

TOBEC Total body electrical conductivity, a method of measuring the proportion of fat in the body by the difference in the electrical conductivity of fat and lean tissue.

tocino Spanish; salted pork fat.

tocol, tocopherol *See* vitamin E.

tocopheronic acid Water-soluble metabolite isolated from the urine of animals fed with tocopherol (*vitamin E); it has vitamin E activity.

tocotrienol *See* vitamin E.

toddy Warming drink made from whisky with hot water and sugar.

toffee A sweet made from butter or other fat, milk, and sugar boiled at a higher temperature than caramels. Called candy or taffy in the USA (originally the UK name). Variants include butterscotch and glessie (Scots). Toffee apples are apples coated with hardened syrup (caramel apples in the USA).

tofu Japanese; soybean curd precipitated from the aqueous extract of the *soya bean. A 200-g portion is a rich *source of protein and calcium; a source of iron and niacin; supplies 8 g of fat (mostly polyunsaturated); supplies 150 kcal (630 kJ). *See also* sufu.

tokay Hungarian sweet white wine made from grapes affected by the '*noble rot'; also a variety of grape used for wine making.

tomatillo Or ground tomato, husk-covered fruit of *Physalis ixocarpa*; resembles a small, green tomato.

tomato The fruit of *Lycopersicon esculentum*. One medium-sized tomato or six cherry tomatoes (85 g) is a good *source of vitamin C; provides 1.3 g of dietary fibre; supplies 13 kcal (54 kJ). A 100-mL portion of tomato juice is a rich source of vitamin C; a source of vitamin A (as carotene); provides 3 g of dietary fibre; supplies 12 kcal (50 kJ).

tomato, English Reddish yellow or purple fruit of *Cyphomandra betacea*, same family as tomato, also called tree tomato and tamarillo; eaten raw or stewed.

tomato, tree *See* tomato, English.

tongue (French: *langue*; German: *Zunge*.) From various animals, e.g. lamb, ox, sheep. A 150-g portion is an exceptionally rich *source of iron, a rich source of protein, niacin, and vitamin B_2; contains about 35 g of fat and supplies 450 kcal (1900 kJ).

tonic water A sweetened, carbonated beverage flavoured with quinine, commonly used as a mixer with *gin or *vodka. Originally invented by the British in India as a pleasant way of taking a daily dose of *quinine to prevent malaria; sometimes known as Indian tonic water.

tonka bean Seed of the S. American tree *Dipteryx odorata* with a sweet, pungent smell, used like *vanilla for flavouring.

tooth-friendly sweets Name given to 'sugar' confectionery made with *sugar alcohols and/or *bulk sweeteners which do not ferment in the mouth and so do not damage teeth; the term originated in Switzerland. Sugar alcohols can have a laxative effect if eaten in large quantities (more than 20–50 g of sweetener per day). *See also* diarrhoea, osmotic.

topepo American; Cross between tomato and sweet pepper.

topfen German; used as a prefix to the names of foods containing curd or cottage cheese.

toppings *See* wheatfeed.

topside Boneless cut of *beef from the top of the hind leg.

torte Open tart or rich cake mixture baked in a pastry case, filled with fruit, nuts, chocolate, cream, etc.

tortilla 1 Mexican; thin maize pancake. Traditionally prepared by soaking the grain in alkali and pressing it to form a dough, which is then baked on a griddle. Tortillas filled with meat, beans, and spicy sauce are *tacos. *See also* tamales.

2 In Spain, an omelette made by frying potatoes and onions with eggs; may be served hot or cold; also used for a variety of filled omelettes.

total parenteral nutrition (TPN) *See* parenteral nutrition.

tournedos Thick steak cut from the 'eye' of the fillet or undercut of beef. *See also* filet mignon.

tourte French; shallow round tart or flan made from pastry, filled with sweet or savoury mixture.

toxic oil syndrome *See* Spanish toxic oil syndrome.

TPN Total parenteral nutrition; *see* parenteral nutrition.

trace elements *See* minerals, trace; minerals, ultra-trace.

tracers *See* isotopes.

traife Foods that do not conform to Jewish dietary laws; the opposite of *kosher.

trans- *See cis-.*

transaminase Any *enzyme that catalyses the reaction of *transamination.

transaminase activation test An *enzyme activation test for *vitamin B_6 nutritional status, based on the fact that *transaminases require the vitamin for activity.

transamination The transfer of the amino group ($=NH_2$) from an amino acid to an acceptor (chemically a keto-acid or oxo-acid). Pyridoxal phosphate, the metabolically active form of *vitamin B_6, acts as the intermediate carrier of the amino group (i.e. it is a *coenzyme). The enzymes catalysing the reaction are known as transaminases or aminotransferases.

transferrin *See* iron, transport.

transketolase test An *enzyme activation test for *vitamin B_1 nutritional status, based on the fact that the *enzyme transketolase in red blood cells requires the vitamin for activity.

Trapistine French; herb-flavoured liqueur made by Trappist monks at the Abbey de la Grace de Dieu.

treacle First product of refining of *molasses from beet or sugar cane extract is black treacle, slightly less bitter; will not crystallize. A 25-g portion is a *source of calcium and iron; supplies 65 kcal (270 kJ).

trebbiano A *grape variety widely used for *wine making, although not one of the classic varieties; makes the relatively thin wines of central Italy if not blended with other varieties.

trehalose Mushroom sugar, also called mycose, a *disaccharide of glucose. Found in some fungi (*Amanita* spp.), *manna, and some insects; hydrolysed to glucose.

trepang *See* bêche-de-mer.

triacylglycerols Sometimes called triglycerides, simple fats or *lipids consisting of glycerol esterified to three *fatty acids (chemically acyl groups). The major component of dietary and tissue fat. Also known as saponifiable fats, since on reaction with sodium hydroxide they yield glycerol and the sodium salts (or soaps) of the fatty acids.

trichinosis (trichinellosis, trichiniasis) Disease that can arise from eating under-cooked pork or pork sausage meat; due to *Trichinella spiralis*, a worm that is a parasite in pork muscle; destroyed by heat and by freezing.

trichlorogalactosucrose *See* sucralose.

trifle Cold sweet made from sponge cake soaked in fruit juice or sweet wine, covered with custard sauce and whipped cream, and decorated.

Trifyba Trade name for processed wheat bran from husk of *Testa triticum tricum*, containing 80 g of dietary fibre/100 g with reduced content of *phytate.

triglycerides Esters of *fatty acids with glycerol, more correctly called *triacylglycerols.

trigonelline A metabolite of *niacin, chemically N-methylnicotinic acid, excreted in the urine in small amounts after consumption of relatively large amounts of nicotinic acid. It also occurs in some foods; it has no vitamin activity, but a considerable amount is converted to active niacin during the roasting of coffee.

tri-iodothyronine One of the *thyroid hormones.

tripa Corsican; pudding made from beetroot, spinach, herbs, and sheep's blood, stuffed into the stomach of a sheep, and boiled.

tripe Lining of the first three stomachs of ruminants, usually calf or ox. Sold 'dressed', i.e. cleaned and treated with lime. According to the part of the stomach there are various kinds, such as blanket, honeycomb, book, monk's hood, and reed tripe. Contains a large amount of *connective tissue which is changed to *gelatine on boiling. A 150-g portion is a good *source of calcium; a source of protein, niacin, iron, zinc, and copper; contains 7 g of fat of which one-fifth is saturated; supplies 150 kcal (630 kJ).

tripeptide *See* polypeptides.

triple sec Sweet orange-flavoured liqueurs such as cointreau and curaçao.

triticale Cross between *wheat (*Triticum* spp.) and *rye (*Secale* spp.) which combines the winter hardiness of the rye with the special baking properties of wheat.

trocken *See* wine, sweetness.

trockenbeerenauslese *See* wine classification, German.

tropical oils Suggested term (USA) for vegetable oils that contain little polyunsaturated fatty acid, such as coconut and palm oils.

tropical sprue *See* sprue.

trout Freshwater oily *fish; brown trout is *Salmo trutta*, rainbow trout is
S. gairdneri. A 150-g portion is a rich *source of protein, vitamin B$_{12}$,
and selenium; a good source of vitamin B$_6$; a source of iron and iodine;
contains 7 g of fat of which 20% is saturated; supplies 200 kcal
(840 kJ).

truffles 1 Edible fungi growing underground, associated with roots of
oak trees; very highly prized for their aroma and flavour. Most highly
prized is the French black or Perigord truffle, *Tuber melanosporum*, added
to pâté de foie gras. Others include: white Piedmontese truffle, *T.
magnatum*; summer truffle *T. aestivum*, and violet truffle *T. brumale*;
see also mushrooms.
   2 Chocolate truffles, a mixture of chocolate, sugar, cream, and
often rum, covered with chocolate strands or cocoa powder.

Trusoy Trade name for full-fat soya flour, heat-treated.

trypsin A *proteolytic enzyme of the pancreatic juice, an
*endopeptidase. Active at alkaline pH (8–11). Secreted as the inactive
precursor, trypsinogen, which is activated by enteropeptidase.

trypsin inhibitors Proteins found in *soya and other beans which
inhibit *trypsin; they are *denatured and hence inactivated by heating.

trypsinogen The inactive precursor of *trypsin, secreted in the
pancreatic juice and activated by *enteropeptidase.

tryptophan An essential *amino acid. In addition to its role in
protein synthesis, it is the precursor of the neurotransmitter
*5-hydroxytryptamine (serotonin) and of *niacin. Average intakes of
tryptophan are more than adequate to meet niacin requirements
without the need for any preformed niacin in the diet.
   It is destroyed by acid, and therefore not measured when proteins
are hydrolysed by acid before analysis; determination of tryptophan
requires alkaline or enzymic hydrolysis of the protein.

TSP Trade name for textured *soya protein, prepared by extrusion
through fine pores to give a fibrous, meat-like texture to the final
product.

tube feeding *See* enteral nutrition.

tuber Botanical term for underground storage organ of some plants, e.g.
*potato, *Jerusalem artichoke, *sweet potato, *yam.

tuberin The major protein of *potato, a globulin.

tumbet Spanish (Balearic); baked vegetables and egg.

tun Obsolete measure; a large cask holding 216 imperial gallons
(972 litres) of ale; 252 gallons (1134 litres) of wine.

tuna *See* prickly pear.

tuna fish (tunny) (French: *thon*; German: *Thunfisch*.) Species of *Thunnus*
and *Neothunnus*, oily *fish. Albacore tuna is specifically *Thunnus alalunga*;
bonita tuna and skipjack tuna are different species. A 100-g portion,
canned, is a rich *source of protein, niacin, and vitamins B$_{12}$ and D;
a source of iodine. When canned in oil and drained it contains about
9 g of fat of which 20% is *saturated and 30% mono-unsaturated;

supplies 200 kcal (840 kJ). When canned in brine the fish contains little fat and the portion supplies 100 kcal (420 kJ).

turkey (French: *dindon*; German: *Truthahn*.) A poultry bird, *Meleagris gallopavo*. A 150-g portion is a rich *source of protein, niacin, and vitamin B_{12}; a good source of vitamin B_6, zinc, and copper; a source of iron, vitamins B_1, B_2, and folate; contains 4 g of fat of which 40% is saturated; supplies 200 kcal (840 kJ).

turkey X disease *See* aflatoxins.

Turkish delight Sweet made from gelatine and concentrated grape juice, flavoured with rose water. Also sometimes made with marshmallow. (Turkish, *rahat lokum*.) *See also* pekmez.

turmeric Dried rhizome of *Curcuma longa* (ginger family), grown in India and South Asia. It is deep yellow and used both as condiment and food colour; used in curry powder and in prepared mustard. Its pigment is used as a dye under the name curcumin or Indian saffron (E-100).

turnip Root of *Brassica campestris* eaten as a cooked vegetable. A 150-g portion is a good *source of vitamin C; provides 3 g of dietary fibre; supplies 20 kcal (85 kJ).

turnip, Swedish *See* swede.

turnip, yellow *See* swede.

turnover Small pie or pasty; the filling is placed on one half of a piece of rolled-out pastry and the other half is folded over to make a semicircular envelope.

turrón Spanish *nougat.

turtle Marine reptile; the main species for food is the green turtle, *Chelonia mydas*, so called because of the greenish tinge of its fat. It is farmed to a small extent, but mainly caught in the wild. *See also* calipash; mock turtle.

Tuscorora rice *See* rice, wild.

tusli *See* basil.

tutti-frutti Mixture of soft fruits bottled in brandy. Also ice cream containing mixed preserved fruit.

tvoroinki Russian; cheese dumplings.

TVP *See* textured vegetable protein.

tweed kettle Scottish; salmon cut into small cubes before poaching. Also called salmon hash.

tyramine The *amine formed by decarboxylation of the amino acid *tyrosine; chemically *p*-hydroxyphenylethylamine.

tyropita Greek; cheese pie prepared with *feta and cottage *cheeses, eggs, and *phyllo pastry.

tyrosinase *Enzyme that oxidizes the *amino acid *tyrosine and other phenolic compounds to form brown and black pigments (melanin). Absent from albinos and the white areas of piebald animals. It is present in some fruits and vegetables, e.g. potato and apple, and is

responsible for the dark colour produced when cut raw food or the
juice is exposed to air.

tyrosine A non-essential *amino acid that can be formed in the body
from the essential amino acid *phenylalanine, hence it has some
sparing action on phenylalanine. In addition to its role in proteins,
tyrosine is the precursor for the synthesis of melanin (the black and
brown pigment of skin and hair), and for *adrenaline and
*noradrenaline.

tzatziki Greek; grated cucumber in yoghurt, flavoured with garlic, olive
oil, and vinegar. A 150-g portion contains 5 g of protein, 7 g of fat,
3 g of carbohydrate, 130 mg of calcium, 550 mg of sodium; supplies
100 kcal (400 kJ).

ubiquinones Coenzymes in the respiratory (electron transport) chain in mitochondria, also known as coenzyme Q or mitoquinones; widely distributed in nature. Chemically derivatives of benzoquinone with isoprene side-chains. There is no evidence that they are dietary essentials; they may have *antioxidant activity.

UFA Unesterified fatty acids; *see* non-esterified fatty acids.

ugli A *citrus fruit, a cross between grapefruit and tangerine, also called tangelo (in the USA); first produced in Jamaica in 1930.

UHT *See* ultra-high-temperature sterilization.

uisge beatha (usquebaugh) *See* whiskey.

uitsmijter Dutch; sandwich of cooked meat or ham and fried egg.

ulcer A crater-like lesion of the skin or a mucous membrane resulting from tissue death associated with inflammatory disease, infection, or cancer. Peptic ulcers affect regions of the *gastro-intestinal tract exposed to gastric juices containing acid and *pepsin: gastric in the stomach and duodenal in the duodenum. Treatment was formerly conservative, with a bland diet, followed if necessary by surgery; specific antagonists of *histamine receptors have improved treatment enormously. May be caused or exacerbated by infection with *Helicobacter pyloris*.

ulcerative colitis *See* colitis.

ullage Liquid left in cask or bottle after some has been removed.

ultra-high-temperature sterilization (UHT) Sterilization at higher temperatures, and for shorter times, than *high-temperature short-time sterilization.

ultrasonic homogenizer High-speed vibrator (above a frequency of 20 000 Hz, hence ultrasonic) giving a cavitation force of 60 tons per square inch (10 000 kg/cm^2) in the liquid. Used to cream soups, disperse dried milk, disperse essential oils in soft drinks, stabilize tomato purée, prepare peanut butter, etc. *See also* homogenization.

ultraviolet (uv) irradiation Light of wavelength below the visible range. Wavelength for maximal germicidal action is 260 nm; it has poor penetrating power and is only of value for surface sterilization or sterilizing air and water. Also used for tenderizing and ageing of meat, curing cheese, and prevention of mould growth on the surface of bakery products.

Ultraviolet from sunlight is responsible for skin tanning, and the formation of *vitamin D from 7-dehydrocholesterol in the skin.

umami Name given to the special taste of *monosodium glutamate, protein, certain amino acids, and the *ribonucleotides (inosinate and guanylate). The Japanese name for a savoury flavour, now considered one of the five basic senses of *taste.

umbles Edible entrails of any animal (more particularly deer) which used to be made into pie, umble pie or humble pie.

uncrystallizable syrup *See* syrup.

Underberg Trade name; German herb-flavoured *bitters, used as an aperitif and digestif.

unesterified fatty acids (UFA) *See* non-esterified fatty acids.

UNICEF The United Nations Children's Fund (UNCF), originally the United Nations International Children's Emergency Fund.

Unicum Trade name; Tyrolean *bitters, slightly sweet, an aperitif and *digestif.

unsaturated fatty acids *See* fatty acids.

uperization A method of sterilizing milk by injecting steam under pressure to raise the temperature to 150 °C. The added water is evaporated off.

upside-down cake A cake or sponge pudding which is baked with a layer of fruit under the sponge mixture, then served upside down, with the fruit uppermost.

urea The end-product of nitrogen metabolism in most mammals, excreted in the urine. Chemically it is $CO(NH_2)_2$. It is synthesized in the liver from ammonia (arising from the deamination of amino acids) and the amino acid *aspartic acid. It is the major nitrogenous compound in urine, and the major component of the non-protein nitrogen in blood plasma.

urethane Ethyl carbamate, used as intermediate in organic syntheses, as a solubilizer, and as the precursor for polyurethane foam. Found in small amounts in liqueurs made from stone fruits, wines, and some distilled spirits where it is formed by reaction between alcohol and nitrogenous compounds; a cause for concern since it is genotoxic.

uric acid The end-product of *purine metabolism in man and other apes; other mammals have the enzyme uricase, which converts the uric acid to allantoin, which is more soluble in water. Gout is the result of excessive formation of uric acid, and/or impaired excretion; it is only slightly soluble in water, and in excess it crystallizes in joints as gouty nodules under the skin, and sometimes in the kidney.

uv *See* ultra-violet.

vacherin 1 Circular cakes of meringue and cream.

2 Range of French mild cheeses made from cows' milk; traditionally moulded in flat circles and wrapped in a border of bark; many are soft enough to eat with a spoon.

vac-ice process Alternative name for *freeze-drying.

vacreation *Deodorization of cream by steam distillation under reduced pressure; developed in New Zealand.

vacuum contact drying Or vacuum contact plate process, a method of drying food in a vacuum oven in which the material is heated by hot plates both above and below. As the material shrinks due to water loss, continuous contact is maintained by closing the plates; supplies heat to the food more effectively than a simple vacuum oven.

valine An essential *amino acid, rarely, if ever, limiting in foods. Chemically, amino-isovaleric acid.

valzin, valzol *See* dulcin.

vanadium A *mineral known to be essential to experimental animals, although sufficiently widespread for human dietary deficiency to be unknown. Its precise function is unknown, although it acts as an activator of a number of enzymes.

vanaspati Indian; purified hydrogenated vegetable oil; similar to *margarine and usually fortified with vitamins A and D. Also used to prepare *ghee (vanaspati ghee).

vanilla Extract of the vanilla bean, fruit of the tropical orchid *Aracus* (or *Vanilla*) *aromaticus* and related species. It was discovered in Mexico in 1571 and could not be grown elsewhere, because pollination could be effected only by a small Mexican bee, until artificial pollination was introduced in 1820. The main growing regions are now Madagascar and Tahiti.

The major flavouring principle is vanillin (chemically methyl protocatechuic aldehyde), but other substances present aid the flavour. Ethyl vanillin is a synthetic substance which does not occur in the vanilla bean; $3^1/_2$ times as strong in flavour, and more stable to storage than vanillin, but does not have the true flavour.

vanilla sugar Sugar flavoured with *vanilla by storing the bean and sugar together.

vanillin *See* vanilla.

vareniki Russian; rounds of noodle dough stuffed with meat, vegetables, curd cheese, etc. Similar to *ravioli.

vareschaga Russian; pork casseroled with beetroot juice and rye breadcrumbs.

variety meat American name for *offal.

vasoconstriction Constriction of the blood vessels; the reverse of *vasodilatation.

vasodilatation (vasodilation) Dilation of the blood vessels; the reverse is *vasoconstriction. Caused by a rise in body temperature; serves to lose heat from the body.

vatana *See* peas.

VCD *See* vacuum contact drying.

VDQS Vins Délimités de Qualité Supérieure. *See* wine classification, France.

Vdt Vini di tavola. *See* wine classification, Italy.

veal (French: *veau*; German: *Kalbfleisch*.) Meat of young calf (*Bos taurus*) $2^{1}/_{2}$–3 months old. A 150-g portion is a rich *source of protein, niacin, iron, vitamin B_{12}, and selenium; a good source of vitamins B_{1}, B_{2}, B_{6}, and zinc; a source of copper; contains about 15 g of fat of which one-third is saturated; supplies 350 kcal (1470 kJ).

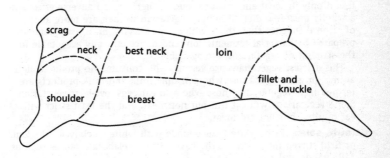

FIGURE 6.

vegans Those who consume no foods of animal origin. (*Vegetarians often consume milk and/or eggs.)

Vegemite Australian; trade name for *yeast extract.

vegetable butters Naturally occurring fats that melt rather sharply because they contain a preponderance of a single *triacylglycerol. Cocoa butter from the *cocoa bean, used in *chocolate; Borneo tallow or green butter from the Malaysian and Indonesian plant, *Shorea stenopiera*, resembles cocoa butter; shea butter from the African plant, *Butyrospermum parkii*, softer than cocoa butter. Mowrah fat or illipé butter from the Indian plant, *Bassia longifolia*, used for soap and candles.

vegetable oyster *See* salsify.

vegetable pepsin *See* papain.

vegetable protein products General term to include textured *soya and other bean products often made to simulate meat. Basic material is termed flour when the protein content is not less than 50%;

concentrate, not less than 65%; isolate, not less than 90% protein. *See also* textured vegetable protein.

vegetables Plants or parts of plants cultivated for food. Some foods that are botanically *fruits, such as tomatoes and cucumbers, and seeds, such as peas and beans, are included with the vegetables; some plants, such as rhubarb, are classed as fruit, although they are not botanically fruits. The distinction in popular usage depends on whether they are eaten as savoury (vegetables) or sweet (fruit) dishes.

As a source of nutrients most of the vegetables are useful sources of *vitamin C and *minerals, the root vegetables supply carbohydrate, but only the seeds are an important source of protein. Green and yellow or orange vegetables and fruits are sources of *vitamin A as *carotene.

vegetable spaghetti *Spaghetti squash, a *gourd (vegetable marrow) with fibrous strands of flesh resembling spaghetti after cooking.

vegetarians Those who do not eat meat, either for ethical/religious reasons or because they believe that a meat-free diet confers health benefits. Apart from a risk of *vitamin B$_{12}$ deficiency (vitamin B$_{12}$ is found only in meat and meat products), there are no adverse effects of a wholly meat-free diet, although vegetarian women are more at risk of *iron deficiency than those who eat meat. Vitamin B$_{12}$ supplements prepared by bacterial fermentation (and hence ethically acceptable to the strictest of vegetarians) are available.

The strictest vegetarians are vegans, who consume no products of animal origin at all. Those who consume milk and milk products are termed lacto-vegetarians; those who also eat eggs, ovo-lacto-vegetarians. Some vegetarians will eat fish but not meat, and the least strict will eat poultry, but not red meat.

velouté sauce Rich, white *sauce made with white stock (veal, chicken, or fish) stirred into a *roux; the basis of more elaborate sauces such as *allemande and *mousseline.

veltol *See* maltol.

vendemmia Italian; the vintage of a wine.

venison (French: *chevreuil, venaison*; German: *Hirsch.*) Meat of deer (*Odocoileus* spp.); traditionally *game, but now mainly farmed. A 150-g portion is a rich *source of protein, niacin, iron, vitamins B$_1$, B$_2$, B$_6$, B$_{12}$, iron, copper, and zinc; contains 10 g of fat of which two-thirds is saturated; supplies 300 kcal (1250 kJ).

verbascose A non-digestible tetrasaccharide, galactose-galactose-glucose-fructose, found in *legumes; it is fermented by intestinal bacteria and causes flatulence.

verdelho *See* Madeira wines.

verjuice Literally 'green juice'; sour juice of crab apples (and sometimes unripe grapes) formerly used in cooking meat, fish, and game dishes. Now normally replaced by lemon juice.

vermicelli *See* pasta.

vermouth Fortified wine (about 16% alcohol by volume) flavoured with herbs and *quinine. French vermouth is dry and colourless; Italian

may be red or white and is sweet. Drunk as an aperitif, either with
soda or with gin or vodka (a *martini). Name originally derived from
German *Wermut* for wormwood, a toxic ingredient that was included in
early vermouths (as in *absinthe). Sweet or Italian vermouth, 15–17%
alcohol (by volume), 12–20% sugar (by weight). Dry or French type,
18–20% alcohol, 3–5% sugar.

véronique Garnish of white grapes.

Versene Trade name for ethylenediamine tetra-acetic acid, *see* EDTA.

vert-pré, au A dish garnished with watercress and straw potatoes, often
served with maître d'hôtel butter; also a dish served with green
mayonnaise.

verveine du Velay French; herb liqueur, strongly flavoured with
verbena; there are two types, yellow and (stronger and sweetened with
honey) green.

very low-density lipoproteins (VLDL) *See* lipids, plasma.

vetch Old term applied generally to *legumes; originally *Vicia* spp., also
called tares.

vichy, à la A dish prepared or garnished with carrots.

vichy carrots Young carrots, lightly scraped, cooked in water and butter
until all the liquid has disappeared and the carrots are glazed with
butter.

vichyssoise Cold leek and potato cream soup.

Vichy water *Mineral water from springs at Vichy in southern France.

vicine One of the toxins in broad beans, responsible for the acute
haemolytic anaemia of *favism.

Vienna bread Loaf with a very crisp, thin, highly glazed crust, with
cuts on the upper surface, coarser than ordinary bread and with gas
holes. It is baked in an oven which retains the steam.

Vienna flour Specially fine flour used to make *strudel pastry, Vienna
bread, and cakes.

Viennese coffee Ground coffee containing dried figs.

villi, intestinal Small, finger-like processes covering the surface of the
small intestine in large numbers (20–40/mm^2), projecting some 0.5–1
mm into the lumen. They provide an enormous surface area (about
300 m^2) for the absorption of digested food from the small intestine.

vinaigrette, à la With a dressing of oil, vinegar, and herbs (French
dressing). *See* salad dressing.

vin classé *See* wine classification, Luxemburg.

vindaloo Indian (especially South India and Sri Lanka); *curry,
marinated and cooked in vinegar; highly spiced with chilli pepper and
hence highly pungent.

vin délimité de qualité supérieure (VDQS) *See* wine classification,
France.

vin de pays, vin de table *See* wine classification, France.

vin de sable French; wines grown on sandy soil; especially the wines of the Languedoc.

vinegar Not less than 4% solution of acetic acid; the product of two fermentations, first with yeast to convert sugars into alcohol, then this liquor, called gyle (6–9% alcohol), is fermented with *Acetobacter* spp. to form acetic acid.

In most countries vinegar is made from grape juice (wine vinegar: may be from red, white, or rosé wine).

Malt vinegar is made from malted barley and may be distilled to a colourless liquid with the same acetic acid content but a more mellow flavour. Cider vinegar (simply known as vinegar in the USA) is made from apple juice; vinegars may be flavoured with a variety of herbs. Non-brewed condiment (once called non-brewed vinegar) is a solution of acetic acid, 4–8%, coloured with caramel. Balsamic vinegar is made from grape juice that has been concentrated over a low flame and fermented slowly in a series of wooden barrels; made only around Modena, Italy.

vinho de mesa *See* wine classification, Portugal.

vinho maduro *See* wine classification, Portugal.

vinho verde Portuguese; literally 'green wine' (white and red) meaning that it is to be drunk when young, i.e. within three years of preparation; light, effervescent wine of relatively low alcohol content (less than 10% by volume).

vini di tavola (con indicazione geografica) *See* wine classification, Italy.

vini tipici *See* wine classification, Italy.

vino gasificado Spanish; sparkling wines produced by adding carbon dioxide.

vin ordinaire *See* wine classification, France.

vinos de la tierra *See* wine classification, Spain.

vintage The year of production of a wine, from the French *vendage*, for grape harvest. Used mainly for superior quality wines, when each year's production is matured separately. Ordinary and table wines (*see* wine classification) are not generally dated, and indeed the production from more than one year may be blended.

viogner A *grape variety widely used for *wine making, although not one of the classic varieties.

violet The sweetly scented flowers of the wild violet (*Viola odorata*) are candied or crystallized and used as decorations in confectionery, or to make a sweet *soufflé. The flowers can be used to flavour syrups, and both flowers and leaves can be used in salads.

viosterol Irradiated ergosterol; *vitamin D_2.

Virginia date *See* persimmon.

Virol Trade name for a vitamin preparation based on malt extract.

viscometer Instrument for measuring the *viscosity of liquids.

viscosity Term used of liquids to define their resistance to flow (i.e. the internal friction).

vision The process of vision is mediated by a pigment derived from *vitamin A bound to a protein (opsin). The pigments are variously known as visual purple (because of the colour), rhodopsin (in the rod cells of the retina) and iodopsin (in the cone cells). The action of light on rhodopsin causes a chemical change, with loss of the purple colour (known as bleaching), which results in the initiation of a nerve impulse from the retina to the brain. *See also* dark adaptation; night blindness.

visual pigments, visual purple *See* vision.

Vita-Wheat Trade name for a *crispbread. A 100-g portion is a good *source of iron; a source of protein; supplies 420 kcal (1760 kJ).

vitamers Chemical compounds structurally related to a *vitamin, and converted to the same overall active metabolites in the body. They thus possess the same kind of biological activity, although sometimes with lower potency.

When there are several vitamers, the group of compounds exhibiting the biological activity of the vitamin is given a *generic descriptor (e.g. *vitamin A is the generic descriptor for retinol and its derivatives as well as several *carotenoids).

vitamin There are thirteen organic substances (thus excluding trace minerals) essential to human life in very small amounts. Eleven of these must be supplied in the diet (vitamins A, B_1, B_2, B_6, B_{12}, C, E, K, folate, biotin, and pantothenate); two (niacin and vitamin D) can be made in the body if there is sufficient of the *amino acid, *tryptophan, and sunlight respectively. *See also* Appendix IX.

The word may be pronounced either 'vaɪtamin' or 'vɪtamin'.

vitamin A Essential in the diet either as the preformed vitamin (retinol) found in animal foods or as a precursor, *carotene, found in plant foods (usually both are present in the diet). Required for control of growth, cell turnover and foetal development, maintenance of fertility, and maintenance of the normal moist condition of epithelial tissues lining the mouth and respiratory and urinary tracts; is essential in *vision.

Deficiency leads to slow adaptation to see in dim light (poor dark adaptation), an early sign of deficiency, and later to night blindness; then drying of the tear ducts (xerophthalmia) and ulceration of the cornea (keratomalacia) resulting in blindness.

Retinol occurs in animal products, especially liver, kidney, fish liver oils, milk, and butter. Carotene is found in green- and orange-coloured vegetables and fruits; especially rich in red *palm oil and *carrots.

The vitamin A content of foods is expressed as retinol equivalents, i.e. retinol plus carotene; 1 μg retinol = 6 μg β-carotene = 12 μg other active carotenoids (in the obsolete nomenclature that is still occasionally used in some countries = 3.33 international units).

vitamin A toxicity Retinol in excess of requirements is stored in the liver, bound to proteins, and is a cumulative poison. When the storage capacity is exceeded, free retinol causes damage to cell membranes. *Carotene is not toxic in excess, since there is only a limited capacity to form retinol from carotene. The recommended upper limits of habitual daily intake of retinol are about 12.5 × *reference intake for adults, but only 2.5 × reference intake for infants. Retinol is also *teratogenic in excess, and for pregnant women the recommended upper limit of daily intake is 3300 μg.

vitamin A₂ Old name for dehydroretinol, the form found in livers of freshwater fish; has 40% of the biological activity of retinol.

vitamin B complex An old-fashioned term for the various B vitamins: *vitamin B₁ (thiamin), *vitamin B₂ (riboflavin), *niacin, *vitamin B₆, *vitamin B₁₂, *folate, *biotin, and *pantothenic acid. These vitamins occur together in cereal germ, liver, and yeast; function as coenzymes; and historically were discovered by separation from what was known originally as vitamin B; hence, they are grouped together as the B complex.

vitamin B₁ Thiamin; essential for the liberation of energy from foods, especially carbohydrates, and for nerve conduction. Deficiency, especially when associated with a carbohydrate-rich diet, results in the disease *beriberi — degeneration of the sensory nerves in the hands and feet fast spreading through the limbs, with fluid retention and heart failure. Relatively acute deficiency, especially associated with alcohol abuse, results in central nervous system damage, the *Wernicke-Korsakoff syndrome.

Good sources are whole grain and enriched bread and cereals, meat (especially liver, kidney, and heart, and pork), yeast, potatoes, and peas; cooking losses can be as much as 50%.

vitamin B₁ dependency syndromes A very small number of children have been reported with a variant form of *maple syrup urine disease in which the defect is in the binding of thiamin diphosphate to the enzyme responsible for the metabolism of the oxo-acids formed from the amino acids leucine, isoleucine, and valine. These children respond well to supplements of large amounts of vitamin B₁, without the need for strict control of their intake of the amino acids.

vitamin B₂ Riboflavin. Involved in a wide range of oxidation reactions, of fats, carbohydrates, and amino acids. Deficiency impairs cell oxidation and results clinically in a set of symptoms known as ariboflavinosis. These include cracking of the skin at the corners of the mouth (angular stomatitis), fissuring of the lips (cheilosis), and tongue changes (glossitis); seborrhoeic accumulations appear round the nose and eyes.

Occurs mainly in yeast, liver, milk, eggs, cheese, and pulses; milk and milk products are probably the most important source in the average diet.

vitamin B₃ Non-existent; term once used for *pantothenic acid and sometimes, quite wrongly, used for *niacin.

vitamin B$_4$ Name given to what was later identified as a mixture of the *amino acids arginine, glycine, and cystine.

vitamin B$_5$ Name given to a substance later presumed to be identical with vitamin B$_6$ or possibly nicotinic acid; also used for *pantothenic acid.

vitamin B$_6$ Generic descriptor for three compounds (chemically derivatives of 2-methylpyridine): (1) the hydroxyl (alcohol) compound, pyridoxine (previously known as adermin and pyridoxol); (2) the aldehyde, pyridoxal; and (3) the amine, pyridoxamine; and their phosphates. All are equally active biologically.

Deficiency causes abnormalities of the metabolism of the amino acids *tryptophan and *methionine; in rats deficiency causes convulsions and skin lesions (acrodynia) and in dairy cows and dogs, anaemia with abnormal red blood cells. Dietary deficiency leading to clinical signs is not known in human beings, apart from a single outbreak in babies fed a severely over-heated preparation of formula milk in the 1950s; they showed abnormalities of amino acid metabolism and convulsions resembling epileptic seizures, which responded to supplements of the vitamin.

Rich sources include nuts, meat, fish, wholegrain cereals, and beans.

vitamin B$_6$ dependency syndromes A very small number of children suffer from *genetic diseases affecting enzymes which require pyridoxal phosphate (*vitamin B$_6$) as coenzyme. The abnormality is corrected by the administration of large supplements of vitamin B$_6$.

vitamin B$_6$ toxicity Very high intakes of supplements of vitamin B$_6$, far in excess of what could be obtained from food, lead to nerve damage.

vitamins B$_7$, B$_8$, and B$_9$ In the early days of nutrition research, when a new factor was discovered which was claimed to be essential for chick growth and feathering, the claimant stated that since nine factors were known the new factors should be called vitamins B$_{10}$ and B$_{11}$. In fact, the B vitamins had been numbered only up to B$_6$, hence B$_7$, B$_8$, and B$_9$ have never existed. B$_9$ is sometimes (incorrectly) used for *folate.

vitamins B$_{10}$ and B$_{11}$ The names given to two factors claimed to be essential for chick growth and feathering; they were later shown to be a mixture of vitamin B$_1$ and folic acid.

vitamin B$_{12}$ A term that covers several chemically related compounds (cobalamins) essential for cell division in tissues where this process is rapid, e.g. in the formation of red blood cells. Deficiency leads to pernicious anaemia when immature red blood cells are released into the bloodstream, and there is degeneration of the spinal cord. This type of anaemia is the same as seen in *folate deficiency. The absorption of vitamin B$_{12}$ requires a particular protein (called the intrinsic factor) which is secreted in the gastric juice and it is a shortage of this protein rather than a dietary deficiency of B$_{12}$ that is the more usual cause of the problem. However, B$_{12}$ is found only in animal foods so *vegans have to rely on special bacterial preparations. The deficiency can be treated with injections of B$_{12}$.

Meat, eggs, and dairy produce are rich sources and dietary deficiency is improbable except among vegans.

vitamin B₁₃ Orotic acid, an intermediate in *pyrimidine synthesis; there is no evidence that it is a dietary essential, and hence not a vitamin.

vitamin B₁₄ Not an established vitamin; name originally given to a substance found in human urine that increases the rate of cell-proliferation in bone-marrow culture.

vitamin B₁₅ *Pangamic acid; no evidence that it has any physiological function in the body, so not a vitamin.

vitamin B₁₆ This term has never been used.

vitamin B₁₇ *Laetrile; there is no evidence that it has any physiological function in the body, so it is not a vitamin.

vitamin B_c Obsolete name for *folic acid.

vitamin B_p Called the antiperosis factor for chicks, but can be replaced by *manganese and *choline (which is not a dietary essential for man).

vitamin B_T *Carnitine; an essential dietary factor for the mealworm, *Tenebrio molitor*, and certain related species, but not a dietary essential for human beings.

vitamin B_w Or factor W; probably identical with *biotin.

vitamin B_x Non-existent; has been used in the past for both *pantothenic acid and *p*-amino benzoic acid.

vitamin C Ascorbic acid. Historically an inadequate intake of vitamin C led to *scurvy, especially common among sailors unable to obtain fruits and vegetables. It has three main areas of function: (1) as a general (non-enzymic) *antioxidant, including the reduction of oxidized *vitamin E in cell membranes; (2) as a coenzyme in the hydroxylation of *lysine and *proline in the synthesis of *collagen, and hence essential for the normal formation of *connective tissue; (3) as a coenzyme in the formation of *noradrenaline.

Deficiency results in scurvy: seepage of blood from capillaries, subcutaneous bleeding, weakness of muscles, soft, spongy gums and loss of dental cement leading to loss of teeth, and, in advanced cases, deep bone pain. A lesser degree of deficiency results in impaired healing of wounds. The requirement to prevent scurvy is less than 10 mg/d; reference intakes are 30 mg/d (FAO); 40 mg/d (UK); 45 mg/d (EU); 60 mg/d (USA and Codex Alimentarius); 85 mg/d (Netherlands). All these differing figures can be justified, depending on the criteria of adequacy adopted and the assumptions made in the interpretation of experimental data. At intakes above 100 mg/d the vitamin is excreted in the urine; there is no evidence of any adverse effects at intakes up to 4000 mg/d.

Losses from foods can be high as they stale; it is easily oxidized, especially in foods kept hot, and it is leached into cooking water. Fruits and vegetables are rich sources. It is also used in curing ham, and as an antioxidant and bread improver. *See also* ascorbic acid; erythorbic acid; iron.

vitamin content of foods According to the UK Code of Practice, no
claims for the presence of a vitamin (or mineral) in a food should be
made unless the amount ordinarily consumed in a day contains one-
sixth of the daily requirements. No claim should be made that the
food is a rich or excellent source unless half of the daily requirement
is present; no reference to the prevention of disease unless the full
day's requirement is present.

EU labelling regulations only permit claims to be made if a food
provides more than 15% of the labelling reference value (*see* Appendix
VI) per 100 g or 100 mL.

vitamin D Vitamin D_3 is calciol or cholecalciferol; formed in the skin by
the action of ultraviolet light on 7-dehydrocholesterol, and hence not
strictly a vitamin. However, in northern latitudes sunlight exposure
may not be adequate to meet requirements, and a dietary source may
become essential. Vitamin D_2 (ercalciol or ergocalciferol) is a synthetic
*vitamer produced by irradiation of ergosterol. The name vitamin D_1
was given originally to an impure mixture and is not used now.

The metabolic function of the vitamin is to control the body's
*calcium metabolism. It stimulates the absorption of dietary calcium
from the intestine and calcium turnover in bone. Deficiency causes
*rickets in young children, *osteomalacia in adults.

It is not widely distributed in foods, but is found in egg yolk, butter,
fatty fish, and enriched margarine. There are no *reference intakes for
adults, since it is assumed that normal sunlight exposure will meet
requirements; for the house-bound elderly the reference intake is
10 µg. The obsolete international unit of vitamin D = 25 ng calciol;
1 mg calciol = 40 iu.

vitamin D resistant rickets *See* rickets, vitamin D resistant.

vitamin D toxicity Excessive intake of vitamin D results in disturbance
of calcium metabolism, resulting in hypercalcaemia, i.e. dangerously
raised blood calcium concentrations leading to raised blood pressure,
the possibility of brain damage, and kidney damage. Excessive exposure
to sunlight does not lead to excessive formation of vitamin D.

vitamin E Generic descriptor for a group of fat-soluble compounds
essential for reproduction in animals. Essential for man (not for
reproduction, so far as is known) but rarely, if ever, deficient in the
diet. Two main groups of compounds have vitamin E activity: the
tocopherols and the tocotrienols; there are 4 isomers of each: α-, β-, γ,
and δ-tocopherols and α-, β-, γ, and δ-tocotrienols, with differing
vitamin potencies.

Vitamin E functions primarily as an *antioxidant in cell membranes,
protecting unsaturated fatty acids from oxidative damage. Deficiency
symptoms vary considerably in different animal species: sterility in
mouse, rat, rabbit, sheep, and turkey; muscular dystrophy in several
species; capillary permeability in chick and turkey; anaemia in
monkey.

The vitamin E content of foods is expressed as mg α-tocopherol
equivalent (based on the different potency of the different vitamers).
The obsolete *international unit of vitamin E activity was equal to

1 mg of synthetic α-tocopherol; on this basis natural-source α-tocopherol is 1.49 iu/mg.

Vegetables, seeds, and most vegetable oils are good sources.

vitamin F Sometimes used for the essential *fatty acids.

vitamin G Obsolete name for *vitamin B_2.

vitamin H *See* biotin.

vitamin K Fat-soluble vitamin essential for the production of prothrombin and several other proteins involved in the *blood clotting system, and the bone protein osteocalcin. Deficiency causes impaired blood coagulation and haemorrhage; sometimes called the antihaemorrhagic vitamin. Two groups of compounds have vitamin K activity: phylloquinones, found in all green plants, and a variety of menaquinones synthesized by intestinal bacteria. Dietary deficiency is unknown, except when associated with general malabsorption diseases. However, some new-born infants are at risk of developing haemorrhagic disease as a result of low vitamin K status, and it is general practice to give a single, relatively large dose of the vitamin by injection.

vitamin L Factors extracted from yeast and thought at the time to be essential for lactation; they have not become established vitamins.

vitamin M Obsolete name for *folic acid.

vitamin P Name given to a group of plant flavonoid substances (sometimes called bioflavonoids) which affect the strength of the walls of the blood capillaries: rutin (in buckwheat), hesperidin, eriodictin, and citrin (a mixture of hesperidin and eriodictin in the pith of citrus fruits). Now considered that the effect is pharmacological and that they are not dietary essentials; indeed, there is little evidence that they can be absorbed through the gut.

It was called vitamin P from the German *permeabilitäts vitamin*, because of the effect on capillary permeability and fragility.

vitamin PP The *pellagra preventing vitamin, an old name for *niacin before it was identified.

vitamin T Factor found in insect cuticle, mould mycelia, and yeast fermentation liquor, claimed to accelerate maturation and promote protein synthesis. Also known as torulitine. Said to be a mixture of folic acid, vitamin B_{12}, and deoxyribosides (DNA); hence not a particular vitamin.

vitaminoids Name given to compounds with 'vitamin-like' activity; considered by some to be vitamins or partially to replace vitamins. Includes bioflavonoids (*vitamin P), *inositol, *carnitine, *choline, *lipoic acid, and the essential *fatty acids. With the exception of the essential fatty acids, there is no evidence that any of them is a dietary essential.

vitamins, fat-soluble Vitamins A, D, E, and K, which are all soluble in lipids, but not in water.

vitamins, water-soluble Vitamin C and the B vitamins (including pantothenic acid, biotin, and folate), which are all soluble in water, but not in lipids.

VLDL Very low-density lipoproteins. *See* lipids, plasma.

vodka Made from neutral spirit, i.e. alcohol distillate mainly from potatoes, with little or no acid, so that there is no ester formation and hence no flavour. Polish vodka is flavoured with a variety of herbs and fruits.

vodkatini A *martini cocktail prepared with *vodka rather than *gin.

vol-au-vent Case of light, rich, puff pastry filled with poultry, fish, vegetables, etc., in a richly flavoured sauce; may be served hot or cold.

vongole Italian; small clams or venus mussels.

votator Machine used for the continuous manufacture of margarine; the fat and water are emulsified, and the subsequent conditioning process carried out in the same machine.

W

wacholder *See* gin.

wafer Very thin, crisp, sweet biscuit, served with ice cream etc. Wafer sandwich biscuits consist of several layers of wafer with a sweet or savoury cream filling.

waffle (French: *gauffe*.) Crisp, golden-brown pancake with deep indentations made by baking batter in a waffle iron which cooks both sides simultaneously.

Waldorf salad Apple, walnuts, and celery with mayonnaise (originated at the Waldorf-Astoria Hotel, New York).

walewska, à la Fish with a lobster sauce and garnish.

walnuts The rough-shelled English walnut (so called because for centuries English ships carried it world-wide), black walnut, hickory nut, and butternut are all botanically walnuts. Common English walnut is *Juglans regia*. A 60-g portion (nine nuts), is a rich *source of vitamin E, copper, and selenium; a good source of protein, niacin, iron, and vitamin B₁; a source of calcium and zinc; contains 40 g of fat of which 10% is *saturated and 75% mono-unsaturated; provides 3 g of dietary fibre; supplies 400 kcal (1670 kJ).

Warfarin A chemical which antagonizes the action of *vitamin K; used to reduce blood clotting in people at risk of *thrombosis and, at much higher doses, as a rat and mouse poison.

wasabe Japanese; condiment prepared from dried *horseradish and *mustard; extremely pungent.

wash, spent *See* spent wash.

wassail 1 Spiced ale, drunk especially on festive occasions.
2 Salutation or toast drunk to a person's health.

water activity (a_w) Ratio between vapour pressure of water in the food and that of pure water at the same temperature. Most bacteria cannot grow at a_w below 0.9, yeasts below 0.85, and moulds below 0.7. So-called dehydrated foods have a_w lower than 0.6.

water balance The balance between intake and excretion of fluids. Average daily intakes are: as drinks, 1–1.5 L; as aqueous part of food, 0.5 L; and formed in the body by oxidation of foodstuffs (*metabolic water), 300–500 mL; total 2–3 L. Losses from the lungs, 400–500 mL; through the skin 400–500 mL; in faeces 80–100 mL; in urine 1–1.8 L.
   Total body water is 40–44 L, as: blood plasma, 2–3 L; extracellular fluid (between cells), 10 L; and intracellular fluid (within cells), 27–30 L. The kidneys control the volume of extracellular water by excreting water. Ingestion of sodium chloride (*salt) raises the *osmotic pressure of the extracellular water, causing thirst.

water biscuit *See* crackers.

water chestnut Seeds of *Trapa natans* and *T. bicornis*; *see* chestnut.

watercress (French: *cresson de fontaine*; German: *Brunnenkresse*.) Leaves of *Nasturtium officinale* (green watercress, remains green in autumn and is susceptible to frost) and *N. microphyllum x officinale* (brown or winter watercress); eaten raw in salads. A 60-g portion is a rich *source of vitamin C; a good source of vitamin A (1300 µg carotene); a source of calcium and iron; provides 1.6 g of dietary fibre; supplies 10 kcal (40 kJ).

water, demineralized Water that has been purified by passage through a bed of *ion-exchange resin which removes mineral salts. Demineralized or de-ionized water is at least as pure as distilled water, and may be purer.

water, extracellular, intracellular *See* water balance.

water hardness Soap-precipitating power of water due to the formation of insoluble calcium and magnesium salts of the soap. Temporary hardness is removed by boiling, permanent hardness is not. May be measured in degrees Clarke; one degree = 1 part of calcium carbonate per 100 000 parts of water.

water-glass Sodium silicate; used at one time to preserve eggs, by forming a layer of insoluble calcium silicate around the shell, and so sealing the pores.

water-ice *See* sorbet.

water lemon *See* passion fruit.

waterless cooking Cooking in a heavy pan with tightly fitting lid, with a steam vent; only a minimal amount of cooking liquid is needed, but the food is not cooked under pressure.

Waterlow classification A system for classifying *protein-energy malnutrition in children based on wasting (the percentage of expected weight for height) and the degree of stunting (the percentage of expected height for age).

watermelon Fruit of *Citrullus vulgaris*, *see* melon.

water, metabolic *See* metabolic water; water balance.

water, mineral *See* mineral water.

water, natural *See* mineral water.

water-soluble vitamins *See* vitamins, water-soluble.

waterzooi (waterzoie, waterzootje) Belgian; chicken or fish simmered in white wine with vegetables.

waxes *Esters of *fatty acids with long-chain monohydric alcohols (fats are esters of fatty acids with the trihydric alcohol glycerol), e.g. beeswax, an ester of palmitic acid with myricyl alcohol; spermaceti, palmitic acid with cetyl alcohol. Animal waxes are often esters of the steroid alcohol *cholesterol.

waxing Coating fruits and vegetables with a thin layer of edible wax. In the case of apples and oranges this replaces the natural wax that is removed when the crop is washed; in the case of vegetables it is an addition; in both instances the waxing prevents loss of moisture, prolongs storage life, and improves the appearance.

weaning foods Foods specially formulated for infants aged between 3 and 9 months for the transition between breast- or bottle-feeding and normal intake of solid foods.

Weende analysis *See* proximate analysis.

weenie American name for small sausages, abbreviation of wienerwurst.

Weetabix Trade name for a breakfast cereal prepared from wheat flakes. Two biscuits (40 g) is a rich *source of vitamin B_2; a good source of vitamin B_1, niacin, iron, and copper; a source of folate; provides 4.8 g of dietary fibre; contains 1.4 g of fat of which 11% is saturated; supplies 140 kcal (590 kJ).

weight, desirable (ideal) Standardized tables of desirable (or idea!) weight for height for adults are based on life expectancy; both undernutrition and obesity are associated with increased risk of premature death. For women desirable weight corresponds to a *body mass index (the ratio of weight in kg/height^2 in m) between 18.7 and 23.5, for men the range is 20.5–25.0. Tables of desirable weight are given in Appendix VII.

weight-for-age An index of the adequacy of the child's nutrition to support growth. Standard weight-for-age is the 50th centile of the weight-for-age curves of well-fed children. *See also* anthropometry.

weight-for-height For children, can be used as an alternative to *weight-for-age as an index of nutritional adequacy; for adults it is the only acceptable way of expressing weight relative to ideal or desirable weight. *See also* weight, desirable; anthropometry.

weight, ideal *See* weight, desirable.

weighting oils *See* brominated oils.

Wellcome classification A system for classifying *protein-energy malnutrition in children based on percentage of expected weight for age and the presence or absence of *oedema. Between 60 and 80% of expected weight is underweight in the absence of oedema, and kwashiorkor if oedema is present; under 60% of expected weight is marasmus in the absence of oedema, and marasmic kwashiorkor if oedema is present.

welschriesling A *grape variety widely used for *wine making, although not one of the classic varieties. Also known as Italian riesling; the wines cannot legally be labelled simply *riesling.

Welsh onion *See* onion, Welsh.

Welsh rarebit (Originally Welsh rabbit), melted cheese, mixed with mustard powder, pepper, and brown ale, served on toast. Buck rarebit is Welsh rarebit topped with a poached egg.

Wernicke-Korsakoff syndrome The result of damage to the brain as a result of *vitamin B_1 deficiency, commonly associated with alcohol abuse. Affected subjects show clear signs of neurological damage (Wernicke's encephalopathy) with psychiatric changes (Korsakoff's psychosis) characterized by loss of recent memory and confabulation (the invention of fabulous stories). *See also* beriberi.

Wetzel Grid Children are grouped by physique into five groups, ranging from tall and thin to short and thick-set. A healthy child will grow, as measured by height and weight, along one of these channels at a standard rate; if he/she deviates from the channel, malnutrition is suspected. *See also* anthropometry.

wey The measure of 48 bushels of oats or 40 bushels of salt or 'corn'.

whale (French: *baleine*; German: *Walfleisch*.) Meat of *Baleanoptera* spp. A 150-g portion is a rich *source of protein, iron, and niacin; a source of vitamin B_2; contains 5 g of fat, of which 25% is saturated, 35% mono-unsaturated; supplies 200 kcal (840 kJ).

wheat The most important of the cereals and one of the most widely grown crops. Many thousand varieties are known but there are three main types: *Triticum vulgare*, used mainly for *bread; *Triticum durum* (durum wheat), largely used for *pasta; and *Triticum compactum* (club wheat), too soft for ordinary bread. The berry is composed of the outer, branny husk, 13% of the grain; the germ or embryo (rich in nutrients), 2%; and the central endosperm (mainly starch), 85%. *See also* flour, extraction rate.

wheatfeed Also called millers' offal and wheat offals; by-product from milling of *wheat, other than the *germ; bran of various particle sizes and varying amounts of attached endosperm.

wheat germ *See* germ, wheat; flour, extraction rate.

wheatmeal, national Name given to the 85% extraction flour (*see* flour, extraction rate) when introduced in the UK in February 1941; later called national flour. The term is now obsolete and replaced by 'brown'.

whelks *Shellfish; several types of spiral-shelled marine *molluscs, *Buccinum undatum, Fusus antiquus*. A 100-g portion of flesh (670 g in the shell) is a rich *source of protein, niacin, vitamin B_{12}, and iron; supplies 100 kcal (420 kJ).

whey The residue from milk after removal of the casein and most of the fat (as in cheese making); also known as lacto-serum. Contains about 1% protein (lactalbumin and lactoglobulin) together with all the lactose and water-soluble vitamins and minerals, and therefore has some food value, although it is 92% water.

Whey cheese can be made by heat coagulation of the protein and whey butter from the small amount of fat (0.25%). Dried whey is added to processed cheese; most whey is fed in liquid form to pigs.

whim-wham Scottish; similar to *syllabub.

whiskey, whisky A grain *spirit distilled from *barley, *rye, *maize, or other cereal which has first been *malted and then fermented. Most brands of whisky are a blend of pure malt whisky with spirit distilled from grain. The distilled spirit is diluted to about 62% alcohol and matured in wooden casks; Irish and Scotch whisky, made from malted barley, are matured for at least three years. Bourbon, made from malted maize, for at least one year. Sour mash bourbon is made from mash that has yeast left in it from a previous fermentation. Other American and Canadian whiskies are made from rye. Diluted after maturation and generally around 40% *alcohol by volume, 220 kcal (920 kJ) per 100 mL.

Both spellings permitted but generally whisky is the Scotch variety and whiskey the Irish and American varieties. Name derived from the Gaelic *uisge beatha*, water of life.

white blood cells *See* leucocytes.

whitebait Traditionally a mixture of young *herrings and young *sprats (fresh or frozen); they are caught together and impossible to separate on a commercial scale.

white cell count *See* leucocytes.

whitecurrants *See* redcurrants.

white foots Fine, white precipitate of calcium and other salts deposited in jars of meat cured with rock salt.

white leaf beet *See* Swiss chard.

white pudding Sausage made from white meat (chicken, rabbit, pork) cereal, and spices. The French version, *boudin blanc*, includes eggs and onions. Irish white pudding is made from flake or leaf lard and oatmeal, spiced; served sliced and fried.

white rice *See* rice.

white spirits Distilled *spirits from fermented fruit; *eau de vie* or *alcool blanc* in French, *schnapps* in German.

whiting White *fish, *Merlangius merlangus*.

WHO World Health Organization; headquarters in Geneva.

wholefoods Foods that have been minimally refined or processed, and are eaten in their natural state. In general nothing is removed from, or added to, the foodstuffs in preparation. Wholegrain cereal products are made by milling the complete grain.

wholesome Description applied to food that is fit for human consumption as far as hygiene is concerned.

whole-wheat meal Flour or meal prepared by milling the whole wheat grain, i.e. 100% extraction rate. *See* flour, extraction rate.

whortleberry *See* bilberry.

williams A variety of pear; *see* poire williams.

windberry *See* bilberry.

wine Fermented juice from grapes (varieties of *Vitis vinifera*), also made with other fruits and even vegetables with the addition of sugar. Red wines are made by fermenting the juice together with the skins at 21–29 °C; white wines normally from white grapes by fermenting the juice alone at 15–17°C; rosé by removing the skins after 12–36 hours, or by mixing red and white wines.

Beverages made by fermenting other fruit juices and sugar in the presence of vegetables, leaves, or roots are also called wines (elderberry, elder flower, parsnip, peapod, rhubarb, etc.), although the legal definition may be restricted to the fermented grape. *See also* alcoholic beverages.

White wines are graded as dry (0.6% sugars), to sweet (6% sugars), on a scale of 1 to 9. Red wines are graded from A (light and dry) to E (full-bodied and heavy). Wines generally contain 9–14% alcohol, dry wines 70 kcal (290 kJ), sweet wines 120 kcal (500 kJ), and about 1 mg of iron per 100 mL; there are only traces of vitamins.

wine, aperitif Slightly bitter-tasting fortified wines drunk before meals; types of *vermouth, including (trade names) Amer Picon, Bonal, Byrrh, Campari, Dubonnet, Fernet-Branca, Martini, Saint Raphaël. Made from red or white wine fortified with spirit and flavoured with herbs and quinine. They contain 15–25% alcohol by volume, 5–10% sugars, 75–130 kcal (320–550 kJ) per 100 mL.

wineberry Orange-coloured fruit of the Japanese and Chinese wild raspberry, *Rubus phoenicolasius*, and now also hybrids with European cultivated raspberries.

wine, British Made in Great Britain from imported grape juice or concentrated grape juice, as distinct from English wine, which is made from grapes grown in England.

wine classification Many of the major wine-producing countries have legally enforced systems of classification of wines based on grape varieties used and regions of production. Other countries have a system of denomination of origin for wines grown in defined regions which may or may not reflect quality. The national classifications are as follows (in increasing order of quality for each country):

wine classification, Austria As for Germany, with an additional classification of QmP wines, ausbruch, intermediate in sweetness between beerenauslese and trockenbeerenauslese.

wine classification, Bulgaria Three grades: wines of declared variety of brand; wine of declared geographical origin (DGO); controliran, specific varieties grown in specific areas. The best of DGO and controliran wines can be offered as reserve, and in exceptional years as special reserve.

wine classification, France Vin de table (or vin ordinaire); vin de pays (subdivided into vin de pays de zone for wines from a single area; départementaux for wines from one département; régionaux for wines from more than one département); vin délimité de qualité supérieure (VDQS); appellation contrôlée (AC) or appellation d'origine contrôlée (AOC) for wines from a specified area, from specified grape varieties grown under controlled conditions.

wine classification, Germany (and Austria) Tafelwein (Deutscher tafelwein is of German origin; wine labelled simply as tafelwein may be of mixed origin); Landwein (dry or half-dry wines from one of fifteen designated areas); Qualitätswein bestimmer Anbaugebeite, QbA (from eleven designated areas and approved grape varieties, sugar may be added to increase sweetness, each bottle carries a batch number (*Amtliche Prüfungsnummer, AP*), as proof that it complies with QbA status);

Qualitätswein mit Prädikat, QmP, with six quality gradings based on the level of natural sugar at harvest (extra sugar may not be added): kabinett, light, fruity, and delicate, usually dry; spätlese, late-picked grapes, dry to sweet; auslese, selected late-picked grapes, rich and sweet; beerenauslese, late-picked grapes affected by *noble rot, always sweet; trockenbeerenauslese, late-picked grapes that have dried to raisins on the vine, strong and sweet; eiswein, rare, made from grapes that have frozen on the vine, very sweet.

wine classification, Italy Vini de tavola (Vdt); vini di tavola con indicazione geografica (from a particular area); vini tipici (equivalent to French vin de pays); denominazione di origine controllata (DOC, from specified areas and grape varieties); denominazione di origine controllata e garantita (DOCG, as DOC but with more stringent regulations and control).

wine classification, Luxemburg Appellation Controlée wines must carry a vintage; bottles carry a neck label awarded by the state-controlled Marque Nationale after tasting, according to the strength of the wine; in order of increasing alcohol content the grades are: non admis, marque nationale, vin classé, premier cru, grand premier cru.

wine classification, Portugal Indicação de proveniencia regulamentada (IPR); região demarcada (RD, the same as AC). Table wines are vinho de mesa, wines aged more than 1 year are vinho maduro.

wine classification, South Africa Classification by variety of grape and area of production; coloured seals used: blue band indicates that origin is certified; red band guarantees vintage year; green band certifies grape varieties; 'estate' certifies that it is from one estate; 'superior' on gold seal indicates superior quality. Wines also carry identification numbers to testify that controls have been adhered to during production.

wine classification, Spain Vinos de la tierra (two-thirds of the grapes must come from the region named on the label); denominacion de origen (DO).

wine classification, USA Each state has its own appellation of origin; in addition 'American wine' or 'vin de table' is blended wine from one area or more; multi-state appellation is wine from two or three neighbouring states (the percentage from each must be shown on the label); for State and County appellation at least 75% must come from the designated area. 'Approved viticultural areas' must have defined boundaries, specific characteristics, and a proven reputation for quality; 85% of the grapes used must come from the defined area; when an individual vineyard is named, 95% of the grapes must have been grown there.

For tax purposes a table wine must be between 10 and 14% alcohol, stronger wines are classified as dessert wines, even if dry; dessert wines between 17 and 21% alcohol are classified by alcoholic strength, not sweetness.

US wines may be sold by a generic classification (e.g. Chablis or Loire); such names are prohibited from export to the EU.

wine, fortified Made by adding *brandy or *spirits to increase the
*alcohol content of the wine to 15–18% and so prevent further
fermentation (to acids) in warm climates, e.g. *Madeira, *marsala,
*port, *sherry.

wine, sparkling Wine containing bubbles of carbon dioxide, bottled
under pressure. There are three methods of production: (1) the
méthode champenoise in which the wine undergoes a second
fermentation in the bottle; wine produced outside the Champagne
region of France may not be called champagne, even if made by this
method; (2) the tank or bulk method, in which the wine is bottled
while still fermenting slightly; (3) the addition of carbon dioxide gas
while bottling.

    Lightly sparkling wines are known as pétillante or frizzante; they are
often young wines, bottled while still fermenting (e.g. *lambrusco,
*vinho verde).

wine, sweetness The UK Wine Promotion Board classifies white and
rosé wines from 1 for very dry wines (0.6% sugars) to 9 (very sweet, 6%
sugars). For red wines the classification is from A (light and dry) to E
(full-bodied heavy wines).

    German and Austrian labelling is: trocken (dry), halbtrocken (half
dry), halbsüss or lieben (medium sweet), and süss (very sweet).

winkle (periwinkle) *Shellfish; small, snail-like, marine *molluscs,
Littorina littorea. A 100-g portion (500 g in the shell) is an exceptionally
rich *source of vitamin B_{12}; a rich source of iron; a good source of
protein and niacin; contains 1000 mg of sodium; supplies 70 kcal
(290 kJ).

winter berry Fruit of the American evergreen shrub *Gaultheria
procumbens*, red, with a spicy flavour; used mainly for pies and sauces.

winterization Applied to edible oils, meaning the removal of the more
saturated glycerides so that the oil remains bright and clear at low
temperatures. The oil is chilled and the solidified palmitates and
stearates filtered off.

wishbone Small, forked bone between the neck and breast of poultry,
also known as merrythought.

witches' milk Secretion of the mammary gland of the newborn of both
sexes; due to the presence of the hormone prolactin that travels from
the blood of the mother into the foetus. Also known as sorcerers' milk.

witchetty grubs Edible grubs, species of longicorn beetle (*Xylentes* spp.);
associated with Australian aborigines.

witloof *See* chicory.

wok Chinese vessel for *stir frying; a shallow, bowl-shaped pan in which
food can be fried rapidly in a small amount of oil over a high heat.

wood alcohol *See* methyl alcohol.

wood blewitt *See* blewitt.

wood-ears Or Chinese black fungus, an edible wild fungus, *Auriculia
polytricha*; *see* mushrooms.

wood grouse *See* capercaillie.

woodruff A wild plant of woodlands on chalk or limestone (*Galium odoratum*); the leaves have the smell and flavour of new mown hay, and are used to flavour alcoholic or fruit drinks, or to make a *herb tea.

wood sugar *See* xylose.

wool green S A green *colour, Green S (E-142).

Worcestershire sauce Characterized by spicy flavour, sediment, and thin supernatant liquid. Recipes are usually secret but basically soya, tamarinds, anchovies, garlic and spices, plus sugar, salt, and vinegar, matured 6 months in oak casks.

work *See* energy.

World Food Programme Part of the Food and Agriculture Organization of the United Nations; intended to give international aid in the form of food from countries with a surplus.

wort *See* beer.

wraplings *See* wuntun.

wuntun (wonton) Chinese; small dough parcels containing meat, boiled or deep-fried, eaten as an accompaniment to a meal or in a soup. Also known as chiao-tzu or wraplings. Sweet wuntun is deep-fried, served with sugar or syrup, and is stuffed with sweetened bean paste.

wurst German; sausage; würstchen are small sausages. Also used generally for salami.

X

xanthan gum Complex polymer made by bacterial fermentation; stable to wide range of pH and temperatures; used as thickening agent to form gels and increase viscosity in foods.

xanthia Cocktail made with equal amounts of yellow Chartreuse, cherry brandy, and gin.

xanthine A *purine, intermediate in the metabolism of adenine and guanine to *uric acid. *Caffeine (in coffee and tea) is 1,3,7-trimethylxanthine; *theophylline (in tea) is 1,3-dimethylxanthine; *theobromine (in cocoa) is 3,7-dimethylxanthine.

xanthophylls Yellow-orange hydroxylated *carotene derivatives; occur in all green leaves together with the chlorophyll and carotene, also present in egg yolk, *Cape gooseberry, *rose hips, etc. Most have no *vitamin A activity. Include flavoxanthin (E-161(a)), lutein (161(b)), cryptoxanthin (E-161(c), which is converted into vitamin A), rubixanthin (161(e)), rhodoxanthin (161(f)), canthaxanthin (161(g)).

xenobiotic Substances foreign to the body, including drugs and some food additives.

xerophilic *See* osmophiles.

xerophthalmia Advanced *vitamin A deficiency in which the epithelium of the cornea and conjunctiva of the eye deteriorates because of impairment of the tear glands, resulting in dryness then ulceration, leading to blindness.

xylitol A five-carbon *sugar alcohol found in raspberries, endive, lettuce, and formed in the body as an intermediate in *glucose metabolism; 80–100% of the sweetness of sucrose; used in sugar-free hard sweets and gelatine gums. Apart from being of low cariogenicity, xylitol is said to have an effect in suppressing the growth of some of the bacteria associated with dental *caries. *See* sugar alcohols; tooth-friendly sweets.

xyloascorbic acid Term used to distinguish *vitamin C (*ascorbic acid) from isoascorbic acid (*erythorbic acid), which is araboascorbic acid and has only slight vitamin C activity.

xylose Pentose (five-carbon) sugar found in plant tissues as complex polysaccharide; 40% as sweet as sucrose. Also known as wood sugar.

Y

yakhni Indian *bouillon or *stock made from meat and bones, sometimes with the addition of vegetables. Garhi yakhni is concentrated and sets to a jelly.

yam Tubers of perennial climbing plants of a number of species of *Dioscorea*: *D. rotundala* white yam, and *D. cayenensis*, yellow or Guinea yam, water, trifoliate, or Chinese yam. A major food in parts of Africa and also the Far East. A 150-g portion is a *source of vitamins B_1 and C; provides 5 g of dietary fibre; supplies 200 kcal (840 kJ). In the United States sweet potatoes are sometimes called yams.

yang *See* macrobiotic diet.

yard-long bean Caribbean name for asparagus bean, *Vigna sesquipedalis*.

Yarmouth bloater *See* red herrings.

yarrow *See* milfoil.

yautia *See* tannia.

yeast Unicellular organisms, grouped with the fungi; they have more complex subcellular organization than *bacteria. Some types are of major importance in the food industry. *Saccharomyces cerevisiae* and *S. carlsbergensis* are used in brewing, wine making, and baking. Varieties such as *Candida utilis* (formerly *Torula utilis*) are grown on carbohydrate or hydrocarbon media as animal feed and potential human food, since they contain about 50% protein (dry weight) and are very rich in B vitamins.

Some yeasts are pathogenic (especially *Candida* spp., which cause thrush); many are used in biotechnology for production of *human hormones and other proteins.

yeast extract A preparation of the water-soluble fraction of autolysed brewers' *yeast, valuable both as a source of the B vitamins and for its strong savoury flavour. Commercial preparations include Marmite, Yeastrel, Yeatex, and Vegemite, used as a drink or a bread spread. A 9-g portion (1 teaspoonful, or the amount spread on two slices of bread) is a rich *source of vitamin B_2, niacin, and folate; a good source of vitamin B_1; supplies 15 kcal (60 kJ).

yeast fermentation, bottom Or deep fermentation; fermentation during the manufacture of *beer with a yeast that sinks to the bottom of the tank. Most beers are produced this way; ale, porter, and stout being the principal beers produced by top fermentation.

Yeastrel Trade name for *yeast extract.

Yeatex Trade name for *yeast extract.

yellow colours *See* colours.

yellow fats *See* fat spread.

yerba dulce The leaves of the Paraguayan shrub, *Stevia rebaudiana*, the source of *stevioside and *rebaudioside.

yerba maté *See* maté.

Yestamin Trade name for a variety of preparations of dried *Saccharomyces* *yeast (debittered brewers' yeast) used to enrich foods.

yin *See* macrobiotic diet.

yiu tiao Chinese; fried dough sticks, generally eaten for breakfast.

yoghurt Milk (from a variety of animals but usually cows) coagulated and fermented with two types of bacteria, *Streptococcus thermophilus* and *Lactobacillus bulgaricus*; may be stirred or set. May be pasteurized, when most of the bacteria are destroyed, otherwise termed live yoghurt. Bioyoghurts also contain *Lactobacillus acidophilus* (*see* acidophilus milk) and *Bifidobacterium bifidum*, which are claimed to enhance the growth of beneficial bacteria in the intestine. A 150-g portion of low-fat, unsweetened (natural) yoghurt is a rich *source of calcium and iodine, a good source of vitamin B_2, a source of protein and vitamin B_{12}; supplies 80 kcal (340 kJ). When sweetened (and usually flavoured), supplies 130 kcal (550 kJ). If made with full-fat milk and sweetened, a portion contains up to 4.5 g of fat, of which half is saturated and supplies 150 kcal (670 kJ). *See also* milk, fermented.

yolk index Index of freshness of an egg; ratio between height and diameter of yolk under defined conditions. As the egg deteriorates, the yolk index decreases.

Yorkshire pudding *Batter cake, traditionally eaten with roast beef.

youngberry A cross between *blackberry and *dewberry.

yuan hsiaos Chinese festival sweet; a small piece of crystallized fruit or ground walnut mixed with sugar, rolled in ground glutinous rice, then boiled and served in the cooking water (which forms a bland soup).

Yuksov disease *See* Haff disease.

Yusho disease Caused by leakage of polychlorinated biphenyls which contaminated edible oil on the Japanese island of Kyushu in 1968.

Z

zabaglione (zabaione) Italian; frothy dessert made from egg yolks, sugar, and wine (usually marsala) whisked over gentle heat until thick. French sabayon is similar.

zakuska Russian appetizer; *caviare, *blinis, smoked sausages, cold meats, pickled fish, and tvoroinki (cheese dumplings).

zarzuela Spanish (Catalan); spiced fish stew served with sauces on a bed of rice.

zearalenone *See* mycotoxins.

zeaxanthin One of the carotenoid pigments in maize, egg yolk, and *Physalis* (*Cape gooseberry); has no vitamin A activity; used as a colouring.

zébrine Variety of *aubergine with purple and white stripes.

zedoary root Root of the Indian plant *Curcuma zedoaria*, a member of the ginger family. Used in the manufacture of flavours and *bitters.

zeera *See* cumin.

zein The major protein of *maize (*Zea mays*), very poor in lysine and tryptophan.

Z-enzyme *Enzyme found associated with *amylases, that attacks the few β-1,3-links present in *amylose. Pure, crystalline β-amylase will convert only 70% of amylose to maltose; it requires the presence of the Z-enzyme for complete conversion.

Zeocarb An *ion exchange resin.

zest Outer skin of citrus fruits. *See* flavedo.

zinc An essential mineral which forms the *prosthetic group of a large number of enzymes, and also the receptor proteins for *steroid and *thyroid hormones and *vitamin A and *vitamin D. Deficiency results in hypogonadism and delayed puberty, small stature, and mild anaemia; it occurs mainly in subtropical regions where a great deal of zinc is lost in sweat, and the diet is largely based on unleavened wholemeal bread, in which much of the zinc is unavailable because of the high content of *phytate.

Meat, fish (especially shellfish), legumes, and (leavened) wholegrain cereals are rich sources.

zinfandel Red grape variety especially grown in California for *wine making. Zinfandel wines may be blush (rosé) or red. White zinfandel wines are really rosé. The wines have a characteristically fruity flavour.

zitoni *See* pasta.

zizanie *See* rice, wild.

zooplankton Wide variety of very small marine crustaceans and other invertebrates, mixed with the young of larger fish, which live upon the *phytoplankton (although some are carnivorous) and serve, in turn, as a food supply of small fish and other marine life.

zubrowka Polish; vodka flavoured with a single sprig of bison grass in each bottle.

zucchini Italian variety of *marrow developed to be harvested when small. American and Australian name for *courgette.

Zucker rat A genetically obese strain of rat used in research.

zuppa inglese Italian; rich cake or *trifle.

z-value *See* decimal reduction time.

zwetschgenwasser (zwetschenwasser) *See* quetsch.

zwieback German name for twice-baked bread or rusk. Ordinary dough plus eggs and butter, baked, sliced, baked again to a rusk, and sometimes sugar-coated. A 100-g portion is a *source of protein and iron; supplies 375 kcal (1580 kJ).

zymase The mixture of *enzymes in *yeast which is responsible for *fermentation.

zymogens The inactive form in which some enzymes, especially the *protein digestive enzymes, are secreted, being activated after secretion. Also called pro-enzymes, or enzyme precursors.

zymotachygraph An instrument that measures the gas produced in a fermenting dough and the amount escaping from the dough, as an index of bread-making properties.

Appendix I. Units of measurement

TABLE 1.1. **Units**

quantity	unit	symbol
length	metre	m
weight (mass)	gram	g
volume	litre	L
energy	calorie	cal
energy	joule	J

TABLE 1.2. **Multiples and submultiples of units**

		name	symbol
a million times	$\times 10^6$	mega	M
a thousand times	$\times 10^3$	kilo	k
a hundred times	$\times 10^2$	centa	ca
ten times	$\times 10$	deca	da
one-tenth	$\times 10^{-1}$	deci	d
one-hundredth	$\times 10^{-2}$	centi	c
one-thousandth	$\times 10^{-3}$	milli	m
one-millionth	$\times 10^{-6}$	micro	μ (or mc)
one-thousand millionth	$\times 10^{-9}$	nano	n
one-million millionth	$\times 10^{-12}$	pico	p

TABLE 1.3. Equivalence of imperial and metric units

imperial	metric	metric	imperial
1 oz	28.35 g (approx 30 g)	100 g	3½ oz
1 lb	454 g (approx 450 g)	1 kg	2.18 lb (35 oz)
1 fl oz	28.35 mL (approx 30 mL)	1 mL	0.035 fl oz
1 pint (20 fl oz)	568 mL (approx 570 mL)	1 L	35 fl oz = 1.75 pints
1 gal	4.5 L		
1 in	2.54 cm	1 cm	0.39 in
1 ft	30.48 cm	1 m	39 in

Appendix II. Estimated average requirements for energy

age	males		females	
	kcal	MJ	kcal	MJ
0–3 m	545	2.28	515	2.16
4–6 m	690	2.89	645	2.69
7–9 m	825	3.44	765	3.20
10–12 m	920	3.85	865	3.61
1–3 y	1230	5.15	1165	4.86
4–6 y	1715	7.16	1545	6.46
7–10 y	1970	8.24	1740	7.28
11–14 y	2220	9.27	1845	7.92
15–18 y	2755	11.51	2110	8.83
19–50 y	2550	10.60	1940	8.10
51–59 y	2550	10.60	1900	8.00
60–64 y	2380	9.93	1900	7.99
65–74 y	2330	9.71	1900	7.96
75+ y	2100	8.77	1810	7.61
pregnant			+200	+0.8
lactating 1 m			+450	+1.9
lactating 2 m			+530	+2.2
lactating 3 m			+570	+2.4

Notes: These figures assume an average level of physical activity; people with a high level of activity have higher requirements, and those with a very sedentary lifestyle have lower requirements.

1 kcal = 4.184 kJ, rounded off to 4.2
1000 kcal = 4200 kJ = 4.2 MJ

Appendix III. EU Population Reference Intakes (PRI) of nutrients, 1993

age	protein g	vit A µg	vit B₁ mg	vit B₂ mg	niacin mg	vit B₆ mg	folate µg	vit B₁₂ µg	vit C mg	calcium mg	phosphorus mg	iron mg	zinc mg	copper mg	selenium µg	iodine µg
6–12 m	15	350	0.3	0.4	5	0.4	50	0.5	20	400	300	6	4	0.3	8	50
1–3 y	15	400	0.5	0.8	9	0.7	100	0.7	25	400	300	4	4	0.4	10	70
4–6 y	20	400	0.7	1.0	11	0.9	130	0.9	25	450	350	4	6	0.6	15	90
7–10 y	29	500	0.8	1.2	13	1.1	150	1.0	30	550	450	6	7	0.7	25	100
males																
11–14 y	44	600	1.0	1.4	15	1.3	180	1.3	35	1000	775	10	9	0.8	35	120
15–17 y	55	700	1.2	1.6	18	1.5	200	1.4	40	1000	775	13	9	1.0	45	130
18+ y	56	700	1.1	1.6	18	1.5	200	1.4	45	700	550	9	9.5	1.1	55	130
females																
11–14 y	42	600	0.9	1.2	14	1.1	180	1.3	35	800	625	18	9	0.8	35	120
15–17 y	46	600	0.9	1.3	14	1.1	200	1.4	40	800	625	17	7	1.0	45	130
18+ y	47	600	0.9	1.3	14	1.1	200	1.4	45	700	550	16*	7	1.1	55	130
pregnant	57	700	1.0	1.6	14	1.3	400	1.6	55	700	550	16*	7	1.1	55	130
lactating	63	950	1.1	1.7	16	1.4	350	1.9	70	1200	950	16	12	1.4	70	160

* 8 mg iron post-menopausally; supplements required in latter half of pregnancy

Appendix IV. UK Reference Nutrient Intakes (RNI), 1991

age	vit B$_1$ mg	vit B$_2$ mg	niacin mg	vit B$_6$ mg	vit B$_{12}$ µg	folate µg	vit C mg	vit A µg	vit D µg	calcium mg	phos mg	magn mg	sodium mg	iron mg	zinc mg	copper mg	selenium µg	iodine µg
0–3 m	0.2	0.4	3	0.2	0.3	50	25	350	8.5	525	400	55	210	1.7	4.0	0.2	10	50
4–6 m	0.2	0.4	3	0.2	0.3	50	25	350	8.5	525	400	60	280	4.3	4.0	0.3	13	60
7–9 m	0.2	0.4	4	0.3	0.4	50	25	350	7	525	400	75	320	7.8	5.0	0.3	10	60
10–12 m	0.3	0.4	5	0.4	0.4	50	25	350	7	525	400	80	350	7.8	5.0	0.3	10	60
1–3 y	0.5	0.6	8	0.7	0.5	70	30	400	7	350	270	85	500	6.9	5.0	0.4	15	70
4–6 y	0.7	0.8	11	0.9	0.8	100	30	500		450	350	120	700	6.1	6.5	0.6	20	100
7–10 y	0.7	1.0	12	1.0	1.0	150	30	500		550	450	200	1200	8.7	7.0	0.7	30	110
males																		
11–14 y	0.9	1.2	15	1.2	1.2	200	35	600		1000	775	280	1600	11.3	9.0	0.8	45	130
15–18 y	1.1	1.3	18	1.5	1.5	200	40	700		1000	775	300	1600	11.3	9.5	1.0	70	140
19–50 y	1.0	1.3	17	1.4	1.5	200	40	700		700	550	300	1600	8.7	9.5	1.2	75	140
50+ y	0.9	1.3	16	1.4	1.5	200	40	700	10	700	550	300	1600	8.7	9.5	1.2	75	140
females																		
11–14 y	0.7	1.1	12	1.0	1.2	200	35	600		800	625	280	1600	14.8	9.0	0.8	45	130
15–18 y	0.8	1.1	14	1.2	1.5	200	40	600		800	625	300	1600	14.8	7.0	1.0	60	140
19–50 y	0.8	1.1	13	1.2	1.5	200	40	600		700	550	270	1600	14.8	7.0	1.2	60	140
50+ y	0.8	1.1	12	1.2	1.5	200	40	600	10	700	550	270	1600	8.7	7.0	1.2	60	140
pregnant	+0.1	+0.3				+100	+10	+100	10									
lactating	+0.1	+0.5	+2		+0.5	+60	+30	+350	10	+550	+440	+50		+6.0	+0.3		+15	

Appendix V. US Recommended Daily Amounts (RDA) of nutrients, 1990

age	protein	vit A	vit D	vit E	vit K	vit C	vit B₁	vit B₂	niacin	vit B₆	folate	vit B₁₂	calcium	phosp	magn	iron	zinc	iodine	selenium
	g	µg	µg	mg	mg	mg	mg	mg	mg	mg	µg	µg	mg	mg	mg	mg	mg	µg	µg
0–6 m	13	375	7.5	3	5	30	0.3	0.4	5	0.3	25	0.3	400	300	40	6	5	40	10
6–12 m	14	375	10	4	10	35	0.4	0.5	6	0.6	35	0.5	600	500	60	10	5	50	15
1–3 y	16	400	10	6	15	40	0.7	0.8	9	1.0	50	0.7	800	800	80	10	10	70	20
4–6 y	24	500	10	7	20	45	0.9	1.1	12	1.1	75	1.0	800	800	120	10	10	90	20
7–10 y	28	700	10	7	30	45	1.0	1.2	13	1.4	100	1.4	800	800	170	10	10	120	30
males																			
11–14 y	45	1000	10	10	45	50	1.3	1.5	17	1.7	150	2.0	1200	1200	270	12	15	150	40
15–18 y	59	1000	10	10	65	60	1.5	1.8	20	2.0	200	2.0	1200	1200	400	12	15	150	50
19–24 y	58	1000	10	10	70	60	1.5	1.7	19	2.0	200	2.0	1200	1200	350	10	15	150	70
25–50 y	63	1000	5	10	80	60	1.5	1.7	19	2.0	200	2.0	800	800	350	10	15	150	70
51+ y	63	1000	5	10	80	60	1.2	1.4	15	2.0	200	2.0	800	800	350	10	15	150	70
females																			
11–14 y	46	800	10	8	45	50	1.1	1.3	15	1.4	150	2.0	1200	1200	280	15	12	150	45
15–18 y	44	800	10	8	55	60	1.1	1.3	15	1.5	180	2.0	1200	1200	300	15	12	150	50
19–24 y	46	800	10	8	60	60	1.1	1.3	15	1.6	180	2.0	1200	1200	280	15	12	150	55
25–50 y	50	800	5	8	65	60	1.1	1.3	15	1.6	180	2.0	800	800	280	15	12	150	55
51+ y	50	800	5	8	65	60	1.0	1.2	13	1.6	180	2.0	800	800	280	10	12	150	55
pregnant	60	800	10	10	65	70	1.5	1.6	17	2.2	400	2.2	1200	1200	320	30	15	175	65
lactating	65	1300	10	10	65	95	1.6	1.8	20	2.1	280	2.6	1200	1200	355	15	19	200	75

Appendix VI. Labelling reference values for vitamins and minerals, EU 1990

The following nutrients may be declared on food labels, with these Reference Intakes; these are the values that have been used in this book to identify foods as rich sources (30%), good sources (20%), or sources (10%) of nutrients in a serving

Nutrient	Reference Intake
Vitamin A	800 µg
Vitamin D	5 µg
Vitamin E	10 mg
Vitamin C	60 mg
Vitamin B_1	1.4 mg
Vitamin B_2	1.6 mg
Niacin	18 mg
Vitamin B_6	2 mg
Folate	200 µg
Vitamin B_{12}	1 µg
Biotin	150 µg
Pantothenic acid	6 mg
Calcium	800 mg
Phosphorus	800 mg
Iron	14 mg
Magnesium	300 mg
Zinc	15 mg
Iodine	150 µg

Appendix VII. Desirable ranges of weight for height for adults

Calculated on the basis of body mass index = 20–25 (which is the desirable range for both men and women)

TABLE 7.1. **Metric units**

height (cm)	desirable range of weight (kg)		
150	45.0	to	56.3
152	46.2	to	57.8
154	47.4	to	59.3
156	48.7	to	60.8
158	49.9	to	62.4
160	51.2	to	64.0
162	52.5	to	65.6
164	53.8	to	67.2
166	55.1	to	68.9
168	56.4	to	70.6
170	57.8	to	72.3
172	59.2	to	74.0
174	60.6	to	75.7
176	62.0	to	77.4
178	63.4	to	79.2
180	64.8	to	81.0
182	66.2	to	82.8
184	67.7	to	84.6
186	69.2	to	86.5
188	70.7	to	88.4
190	72.2	to	90.3
192	73.7	to	92.2
194	75.3	to	94.1
196	76.8	to	96.0
198	78.4	to	98.0

TABLE 7.2. Imperial units

height (ft, in)	desirable range of weight (st, lb)			
4 11	7 0	to	8 10
5 0	7 3	to	9 1
5 1	7 7	to	9 5
5 2	7 10	to	9 9
5 3	8 0	to	10 0
5 4	8 3	to	10 4
5 5	8 7	to	10 9
5 6	8 11	to	10 13
5 7	9 0	to	11 4
5 8	9 4	to	11 9
5 9	9 8	to	11 13
5 10	9 12	to	12 4
5 11	10 2	to	12 9
6 0	10 6	to	13 0
6 1	10 10	to	13 5
6 2	11 0	to	13 11
6 3	11 4	to	14 2
6 4	11 8	to	14 7
6 5	11 13	to	14 12
6 6	12 3	to	15 4

Appendix VIII. Food additives permitted within the European Union

Listed by the numbers by which they may be declared on food labels within the European Union

Colouring materials

Yellow and orange colours

E-100	Curcumin
E-101	Riboflavin, riboflavin phosphate (vitamin B₂)
E-102	Tartrazine (= FD&C Yellow no 6)
E-104	Quinoline yellow
E-110	Sunset yellow FCF or orange yellow S (= FD&C Yellow no 6)

Red colours

E-120	Cochineal or carminic acid
E-122	Carmoisine or azorubine
E-123	Amaranth
E-124	Ponceau 4R or cochineal red A
E-127	Erythrosine BS (= FD&C Red no 3)
E-128	Red 2G
E-129	Allura red (= FD&C Red no 40)

Blue colours

E-131	Patent blue V
E-132	Indigo carmine or indigotine (= FD&C Blue no 2)
E-133	Brilliant blue FCF (= FD&C Blue no 1)

Green colours

E-140	(i) Chlorophylls, (ii) chlorophyllins
E-141	Copper complexes of (i) chlorophylls, (ii) chlorophyllins
E-142	Green S or acid brilliant green BS

Brown and black colours

E-150a	Plain caramel
E-150b	Caustic sulphite caramel
E-150c	Ammonia caramel
E-150d	Sulphite ammonia caramel
E-151	Black PN or brilliant black BN
E-153	Carbon black or vegetable carbon (charcoal)
E-154	Brown FK
E-155	Brown HT (Chocolate brown HT)

Derivatives of carotene

E-160(a)	(i) Mixed carotenes, (ii) β-carotene
E-160(b)	Annatto, bixin, norbixin
E-160(c)	Paprika extract, capsanthin or capsorubin
E-160(d)	Lycopene
E-160(e)	β-apo-8'-carotenal (vitamin A active)
E-160(f)	Ethyl ester of β-apo-8'-carotenoic acid

Other plant colours

E-161(b)	Lutein
E-161(g)	Canthaxanthin
E-162	Beetroot red or betanin
E-163	Anthocyanins

Inorganic compounds used as colours

E-170	(i) Calcium carbonate (chalk), (ii) calcium hydrogen carbonate
E-171	Titanium dioxide
E-172	Iron oxides & hydroxides
E-173	Aluminium
E-174	Silver
E-175	Gold
E-180	Pigment rubine or lithol rubine BK

Preservatives

Sorbic acid and its salts

E-200	Sorbic acid
E-202	Potassium sorbate

E-203   Calcium sorbate

Benzoic acid and its salts

E-210   Benzoic acid

E-211   Sodium benzoate

E-212   Potassium benzoate

E-213   Calcium benzoate

E-214   Ethyl p-hydroxybenzoate

E-215   Ethyl p-hydroxybenzoate sodium salt

E-216   Propyl p-hydroxybenzoate

E-217   Propyl p-hydroxybenzoate sodium salt

E-218   Methyl p-hydroxybenzoate

E-219   Methyl p-hydroxybenzoate sodium salt

Sulphur dioxide and its salts

E-220   Sulphur dioxide

E-221   Sodium sulphite

E-222   Sodium hydrogen sulphite

E-223   Sodium metabisulphite

E-224   Potassium metabisulphite

E-226   Calcium sulphite

E-227   Calcium hydrogen sulphite

E-228   Potassium hydrogen sulphite

Biphenyl and its derivatives

E-230   Biphenyl or diphenyl (for surface treatment of citrus fruits)

E-231   Orthophenylphenol (2-hydroxybiphenyl) (for surface treatment of citrus fruits)

E-232   Sodium orthophenylphenol (sodium biphenyl-2-yl oxide)

Other preservatives

E-233   2-(Thiazol-4-yl) benzimidazole (thiobendazole) (for surface treatment of citrus fruits and bananas)

E-234   Nisin

E-235   Natamycin (NATA) (for surface treatment of cheeses and dried cured sausages)

E-239   Hexamethylene tetramine (hexamine)

E-242   Dimethyl dicarbonate

E-912   Montan acid esters (for surface treatment of citrus fruits)

E-914   Oxidized polyethylene wax (for surface treatment of citrus fruits)

Pickling salts

E-249   Potassium nitrite

E-250   Sodium nitrite

E-251   Sodium nitrate

E-252   Potassium nitrate (saltpetre)

Acids and their salts

E-260   Acetic acid

E-261   Potassium acetate

E-262   (i) Sodium acetate, (ii) sodium hydrogen acetate (sodium diacetate)

E-263   Calcium acetate

E-270   Lactic acid

E-280   Propionic acid

E-281   Sodium propionate

E-282   Calcium propionate

E-283   Potassium propionate

E-284   Boric acid (as preservative in caviare)

E-285   Sodium tetraborate (borax) (as preservative in caviare)

E-290   Carbon dioxide

E-296   Malic acid

E-297   Fumaric acid

Antioxidants

Vitamin C and derivatives

E-300   L-Ascorbic acid (vitamin C)

E-301   Sodium-L-ascorbate

E-302   Calcium-L-ascorbate

E-304   (i) Ascorbyl palmitate, (ii) ascorbyl stearate

E-315   Erythorbic acid (iso-ascorbic acid)

E-316   Sodium erythorbate (sodium iso-ascorbate)

Vitamin E

E-306	Natural extracts rich in tocopherols
E-307	Synthetic α-tocopherol
E-308	Synthetic β-tocopherol
E-309	Synthetic δ-tocopherol

Other antioxidants

E-310	Propyl gallate
E-311	Octyl gallate
E-312	Dodecyl gallate
E-320	Butylated hydroxyanisole (BHA)
E-321	Butylated hydroxytoluene (BHT)
E-322	Lecithins

More acids and their salts

Salts of lactic acid (E-270)

E-325	Sodium lactate
E-326	Potassium lactate
E-327	Calcium lactate
E-585	Ferrous lactate

Citric acid, its salts and esters

E-330	Citric acid
E-331	(i) Monosodium citrate, (ii) disodium citrate, (iii) trisodium citrate
E-332	(i) Monopotassium citrate, (ii) dipotassium citrate, (iii) tripotassium citrate
E-333	(i) Monocalcium citrate, (ii) dicalcium citrate, (iii) tricalcium citrate
E-1505	Triethyl citrate

Tartaric acid and its salts

E-334	L(+)Tartaric acid
E-335	(i) Monosodium tartrate, (ii) disodium tartrate
E-336	(i) Monopotassium tartrate (cream of tartar), (ii) dipotassium tartrate
E-337	Sodium potassium tartrate

Phosphoric acid and its salts

E-338	Phosphoric acid
E-339	(i) Monosodium phosphate, (ii) disodium phosphate, (iii) trisodium phosphate
E-340	(i) Monopotassium phosphate, (ii) dipotassium phosphate, (iii) tripotassium phosphate
E-341	(i) Monocalcium phosphate, (ii) dicalcium phosphate, (iii) tricalcium phosphate
E-450	Diphosphates: (i) disodium diphosphate, (ii) trisodium diphosphate, (iii) tetrasodium diphosphate, (iv) dipotassium diphosphate, (v) tetrapotassium diphosphate, (vi) dicalcium diphosphate, (vii) calcium dihydrogen diphosphate
E-451	Triphosphates: (i) pentasodium triphosphate, (ii) pentapotassium triphosphate
E-452	Polyphosphates: (i) sodium polyphosphate, (ii) potassium polyphosphate, (iii) sodium calcium polyphosphate, (iv) calcium polyphosphate
E-540	Dicalcium diphosphate
E-541	Sodium aluminium phosphate, acidic
E-542	Edible bone phosphates (bone meal, used as anti-caking agent)
E-544	Calcium polyphosphates (used as anti-caking agent)
E-545	Ammonium polyphosphates (used as anti-caking agent)

Salts of malic acid (E-296)

E-350	Sodium malate
E-351	Potassium malate
E-352	Calcium malate

Other acids and their salts

E-353	Metatartaric acid
E-354	Calcium tartrate
E-355	Adipic acid
E-356	Sodium adipate

E-357	Potassium adipate
E-363	Succinic acid
E-370	1,4-Heptonolactone
E-375	Nicotinic acid
E-380	Triammonium citrate
E-381	Ammonium ferric citrate
E-385	Calcium disodium EDTA

Emulsifiers and stabilisers

Alginates

E-400	Alginic acid
E-401	Sodium alginate
E-402	Potassium alginate
E-403	Ammonium alginate
E-404	Calcium alginate
E-405	Propane-1,2-diol alginate

Other plant gums

E-406	Agar
E-407	Carrageenan
E-410	Locust bean gum (carob gum)
E-412	Guar gum
E-413	Tragacanth
E-414	Gum acacia (gum Arabic)
E-415	Xanthan gum
E-416	Karaya gum
E-417	Tara gums
E-418	Gellan gums

Fatty acid derivatives

E-431	Polyoxyethylene (40) stearate
E-432	Polyoxyethylene (20) sorbitan monolaurate (Polysorbate 20)
E-433	Polyoxyethylene (20) sorbitan mono-oleate (Polysorbate 80)
E-434	Polyoxyethylene (20) sorbitan monopalmitate (Polysorbate 40)
E-435	Polyoxyethylene (20) sorbitan monostearate (Polysorbate 60)
E-436	Polyoxyethylene (20) sorbitan tristearate (Polysorbate 65)

Pectin and derivatives

E-440	(i) Pectin, (ii) amidated pectin

Other compounds

E-442	Ammonium phosphatides

E-444	Sucrose acetate isobutyrate
E-445	Glycerol esters of wood rosins

Cellulose and derivatives

E-460	(i) Microcrystalline cellulose, (ii) powdered cellulose
E-461	Methyl cellulose
E-463	Hydroxypropy cellulose
E-464	Hydroxypropylmethyl cellulose
E-465	Ethylmethyl cellulose
E-466	Carboxymethylcellulose, sodium carboxymethylcellulose

Salts or esters of fatty acids.

E-470a	Sodium, potassium and calcium salts of fatty acids
E-470b	Magnesium salts of fatty acids
E-471	Mono- and diglycerides of fatty acids
E-472a	Acetic acid esters of mono- and diglycerides of fatty acids
E-472b	Lactic acid esters of mono- and diglycerides of fatty acids
E-472c	Citric acid esters of mono- and diglycerides of fatty acids
E-472d	Tartaric acid esters of mono- and diglycerides of fatty acids
E-472e	Mono- and diacetyl tartaric esters of mono- and diglycerides of fatty acids
E-472f	Mixed acetic and tartaric acid esters of mono- and diglycerides of fatty acids
E-473	Sucrose esters of fatty acids
E-474	Sucroglycerides
E-475	Polyglycerol esters of fatty acids
E-476	Polyglycerol esters of poly-condensed esters of castor oil (polyglycerol polyricinoleate)
E-477	Propane-1,2-diol esters of fatty acids
E-479b	Thermally oxidized soya bean oil interacted with mono- and diglycerides of fatty acids
E-481	Sodium stearoyl-2-lactylate
E-482	Calcium stearoyl-2-lactylate

E-483   Stearyl tartrate
E-491   Sorbitan monostearate
E-492   Sorbitan tristearate
E-493   Sorbitan monolaurate
E-494   Sorbitan mono-oleate
E-495   Sorbitan monopalmitate
E-1518   Glyceryl triacetate (triacetin)

Acids and salts used for special purposes

Carbonates

E-500   (i) Sodium carbonate,
          (ii) sodium bicarbonate
          (sodium hydrogen carbonate),
          (iii) sodium sesquicarbonate

E-501   (i) Potassium carbonate,
          (ii) potassium bicarbonate
          (potassium hydrogen
          carbonate)

E-503   (i) Ammonium carbonate,
          (ii) ammonium hydrogen
          carbonate

E-504   (i) Magnesium carbonate,
          (ii) magnesium hydrogen
          carbonate (magnesium
          hydroxide carbonate)

Hydrochloric acid and its salts

E-507   Hydrochloric acid
E-508   Potassium chloride
E-509   Calcium chloride
E-510   Ammonium chloride
E-511   Magnesium chloride
E-512   Stannous chloride

Sulphuric acid and its salts

E-513   Sulphuric acid
E-514   (i) Sodium sulphate,
          (ii) sodium hydrogen sulphate
E-515   (i) Potassium sulphate,
          (ii) potassium hydrogen
          sulphate
E-516   Calcium sulphate
E-517   Ammonium sulphate
E-518   Magnesium sulphate
E-520   Aluminium sulphate
E-521   Aluminium sodium sulphate

E-522   Aluminium potassium sulphate
E-523   Aluminium ammonium
          sulphate

Alkalis

E-524   Sodium hydroxide
E-525   Potassium hydroxide
E-526   Calcium hydroxide
E-527   Ammonium hydroxide
E-528   Magnesium hydroxide
E-529   Calcium oxide
E-530   Magnesium oxide

Other salts

E-535   Sodium ferrocyanide
E-536   Potassium ferrocyanide
E-538   Calcium ferrocyanide
E-540   Dicalcium diphosphate
E-541   Sodium aluminium phosphate,
          acidic

Compounds used as anti-caking agents, and other uses

E-542   Edible bone phosphate (bone
          meal)
E-544   Calcium polyphosphates
E-545   Ammonium polyphosphates

Silicon salts

E-551   Silicon dioxide (silica)
E-552   Calcium silicate
E-553a   (i) Magnesium silicate,
          (ii) magnesium trisilicate
E-533b   talc
E-554   Sodium aluminium silicate
E-555   Potassium aluminium silicate
E-556   Calcium aluminium silicate

Other compounds

E-558   Bentonite
E-559   Kaolin (aluminium silicate)
E-570   Fatty acids
E-574   Gluconic acid
E-575   Glucono-δ-lactone
E-576   Sodium gluconate
E-577   Potassium gluconate
E-578   Calcium gluconate

E-579	Ferrous gluconate
E-585	Ferrous lactate

Compounds used as flavour enhancers

E-620	L-Glutamic acid
E-621	Monosodium glutamate (MSG)
E-622	Monopotassium glutamate
E-623	Calcium diglutamate
E-624	Monoammonium glutamate
E-625	Magnesium diglutamate
E-626	Guanylic acid
E-627	Disodium guanylate
E-628	Dipotassium guanylate
E-629	Calcium guanylate
E-630	Inosinic acid
E-631	Disodium inosinate
E-632	Dipotassium inosinate
E-633	Calcium inosinate
E-634	Calcium 5'-ribonucleotides
E-635	Disodium 5'-ribonucleotides
E-636	Maltol
E-637	Ethyl maltol
E-640	Glycine and its sodium salt
E-900	Dimethylpolysiloxane

Compounds used as glazing agents

E-901	Beeswax
E-902	Candelilla wax
E-903	Carnauba wax
E-904	Shellac
E-912	Montan acid esters
E-914	Oxidized polyethylene wax

Compounds used to treat flour

E-920	L-Cysteine hydrochloride
925	Chlorine
926	Chlorine dioxide

Propellant gases

E-938	Argon
E-939	Helium
E-941	Nitrogen
E-942	Nitrous oxide

E-948	Oxygen

Sweeteners and sugar alcohols

E-420	(i) Sorbitol, (ii) sorbitol syrup
E-421	Mannitol
E-422	Glycerol
E-927a	Azodicarbonamide
E-927b	Carbamide
E-950	Acesulfame K
E-951	Aspartame
E-952	Cyclamic acid and its sodium and calcium salts
E-953	Isomalt
E-954	Saccharine and its sodium, potassium and calcium salts
E-957	Thaumatin
E-959	Neohesperidine dichalcone
E-965	(i) Maltitol, (ii) maltitol syrup
E-966	Lactitol
E-967	Xylitol

Miscellaneous compounds

E-999	Quillaia extract
E-1105	Lysozyme (EC 3.2.1.17)
E-1200	Polydextrose
E-1201	Polyvinyl pyrrolidone
E-1202	Polyvinyl polypyrrolidone
E-1505	Triethyl citrate
E-1518	Glyceryl triacetate (triacetin)

Modified starches

E-1404	Oxidized starch
E-1410	Monostarch phosphate
E-1412	Distarch phosphate
E-1413	Phosphated distarch phosphate
E-1414	Acetylated distarch phosphate
E-1420	Acetylated starch
E-1422	Acetylated starch adipate
E-1440	Hydroxypropyl starch
E-1442	Hydroxypropyl distarch phosphate
E-1450	Starch sodium octanoyl succinate

Appendix IX. The vitamins

vitamin		functions	deficiency disease
A	retinol β-carotene	visual pigments in the retina; cell differentiation; β-carotene is an antioxidant	night blindness, xerophthalmia; keratinization of skin
D	calciferol	maintenance of calcium balance; enhances intestinal absorption of Ca^{2+} and mobilizes bone mineral	rickets = poor mineralization of bone; osteomalacia = bone demineralization
E	tocopherols tocotrienols	antioxidant, especially in cell membranes	extremely rare, a serious neurological dysfunction
K	phylloquinone menaquinones	coenzyme in formation of carboxyglutamate in enzymes of blood clotting and bone matrix	impaired blood clotting, haemorrhagic disease
B_1	thiamin	coenzyme in pyruvate and 2-oxo-glutarate dehydrogenases, and transketolase; poorly defined function in nerve conduction	peripheral nerve damage (beriberi) or central nervous system lesions (Wernicke- Korsakoff syndrome)
B_2	riboflavin	coenzyme in oxidation and reduction reactions; prosthetic group of flavoproteins	lesions of corner of mouth, lips and tongue, seborrhoeic dermatitis
niacin	nicotinic acid nicotinamide	coenzyme in oxidation and reduction reactions, functional part of NAD and NADP	pellagra: photosensitive dermatitis, depressive psychosis
B_6	pyridoxine pyridoxal pyridoxamine	coenzyme in transamination and decarboxylation of amino acids and glycogen phosphorylase; role in steroid hormone action	disorders of amino acid metabolism, convulsions
	folic acid	coenzyme in transfer of one- carbon fragments	megaloblastic anaemia
B_{12}	cobalamin	coenzyme in transfer of one- carbon fragments and metabolism of folic acid	pernicious anaemia = megaloblastic anaemia with degeneration of the spinal cord
	pantothenic acid	functional part of CoA and acyl carrier protein	peripheral nerve damage (burning foot syndrome)
H	biotin	coenzyme in carboxylation reactions in gluconeogenesis and fatty acid synthesis	impaired fat and carbohydrate metabolism, dermatitis
C	ascorbic acid	coenzyme in hydroxylation of proline and lysine in collagen synthesis; anti-oxidant; enhances absorption of iron	scurvy: impaired wound healing, loss of dental cement, subcutaneous haemorrhage

Appendix X. Fatty acids commonly found in foods

	no. of carbon atoms	no. of double bonds	first double bond	shorthand code
saturated fatty acids				
butyric	4	0	—	C4 : 0
caproic	6	0	—	C6 : 0
caprylic	8	0	—	C8 : 0
capric	10	0	—	C10 : 0
lauric	12	0	—	C12 : 0
myristic	14	0	—	C14 : 0
palmitic	16	0	—	C16 : 0
stearic	18	0	—	C18 : 0
arachidic	20	0	—	C20 : 0
behenic	22	0	—	C22 : 0
lignoceric	24	0	—	C24 : 0
mono-unsaturated fatty acids				
palmitoleic	16	1	6	C16 : 1 ω6
oleic	18	1	9	C18 : 1 ω9
cetoleic	22	1	11	C22 : 1 ω11
nervonic	24	1	9	C24 : 1 ω9
polyunsaturated fatty acids				
linoleic	18	2	6	C18 : 2 ω6
α-linolenic	18	3	3	C18 : 3 ω3
γ-linolenic	18	3	6	C18 : 3 ω6
arachidonic	20	4	6	C20 : 4 ω6
eicosapentaenoic	20	5	3	C20 : 5 ω3
docosatetraenoic	22	4	6	C22 : 4 ω6
docosapentaenoic	22	5	3	C22 : 5 ω3
docosapentaenoic	22	5	6	C22 : 5 ω6
docosahexaenoic	22	6	3	C22 : 6 ω3

OXFORD

MORE OXFORD PAPERBACKS

This book is just one of nearly 1000 Oxford Paperbacks currently in print. If you would like details of other Oxford Paperbacks, including titles in the World's Classics, Oxford Reference, Oxford Books, OPUS, Past Masters, Oxford Authors, and Oxford Shakespeare series, please write to:

UK and Europe: Oxford Paperbacks Publicity Manager, Arts and Reference Publicity Department, Oxford University Press, Walton Street, Oxford OX2 6DP.

Customers in UK and Europe will find Oxford Paperbacks available in all good bookshops. But in case of difficulty please send orders to the Cash-with-Order Department, Oxford University Press Distribution Services, Saxon Way West, Corby, Northants NN18 9ES. Tel: 01536 741519; Fax: 01536 746337. Please send a cheque for the total cost of the books, plus £1.75 postage and packing for orders under £20; £2.75 for orders over £20. Customers outside the UK should add 10% of the cost of the books for postage and packing.

USA: Oxford Paperbacks Marketing Manager, Oxford University Press, Inc., 200 Madison Avenue, New York, N.Y. 10016.

Canada: Trade Department, Oxford University Press, 70 Wynford Drive, Don Mills, Ontario M3C 1J9.

Australia: Trade Marketing Manager, Oxford University Press, G.P.O. Box 2784Y, Melbourne 3001, Victoria.

South Africa: Oxford University Press, P.O. Box 1141, Cape Town 8000.

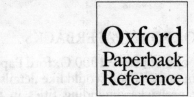

Oxford
Paperback
Reference

OXFORD PAPERBACK REFERENCE

From *Art and Artists* to *Zoology*, the Oxford Paperback Reference series offers the very best subject reference books at the most affordable prices.

Authoritative, accessible, and up to date, the series features dictionaries in key student areas, as well as a range of fascinating books for a general readership. Included are such well-established titles as Fowler's *Modern English Usage*, Margaret Drabble's *Concise Companion to English Literature*, and the bestselling science and medical dictionaries.

The series has now been relaunched in handsome new covers. Highlights include new editions of some of the most popular titles, as well as brand new paperback reference books on *Politics*, *Philosophy*, and *Twentieth-Century Poetry*.

With new titles being constantly added, and existing titles regularly updated, Oxford Paperback Reference is unrivalled in its breadth of coverage and expansive publishing programme. New dictionaries of *Film*, *Economics*, *Linguistics*, *Architecture*, *Archaeology*, *Astronomy*, and *The Bible* are just a few of those coming in the future.

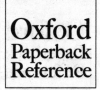

Oxford
Paperback
Reference

THE OXFORD DICTIONARY OF PHILOSOPHY

Edited by Simon Blackburn

* **2,500 entries covering the entire span of the subject including the most recent terms and concepts**

* **Biographical entries for nearly 500 philosophers**

* **Chronology of philosophical events**

From Aristotle to Zen, this is the most comprehensive, authoritative, and up to date dictionary of philosophy available. Ideal for students or a general readership, it provides lively and accessible coverage of not only the Western philosophical tradition but also important themes from Chinese, Indian, Islamic, and Jewish philosophy. The paperback includes a new Chronology.

'an excellent source book and can be strongly recommended . . . there are generous and informative entries on the great philosophers . . . Overall the entries are written in an informed and judicious manner.'
Times Higher Education Supplement

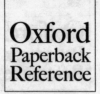

Oxford
Paperback
Reference

THE CONCISE OXFORD DICTIONARY
OF POLITICS

Edited by Iain McLean

Written by an expert team of political scientists from Warwick University, this is the most authoritative and up-to-date dictionary of politics available.

* Over 1,500 entries provide truly international coverage of major political institutions, thinkers and concepts

* From Western to Chinese and Muslim political thought

* Covers new and thriving branches of the subject, including international political economy, voting theory, and feminism

* Appendix of political leaders

* Clear, no-nonsense definitions of terms such as veto and subsidiarity

Oxford Paperback Reference

CONCISE SCIENCE DICTIONARY

New edition

Authoritative and up to date, this bestselling dictionary is ideal reference for both students and non-scientists. Fully revised for this third edition, with over 1,000 new entries, it provides coverage of biology (including human biology), chemistry, physics, the earth sciences, astronomy, maths and computing.

* 8,500 clear and concise entries

* Up-to-date coverage of areas such as molecular biology, genetics, particle physics, cosmology, and fullerene chemistry

* Appendices include the periodic table, tables of SI units, and classifications of the plant and animal kingdoms

'handy and readable . . . for scientists aged nine to ninety'
Nature

'The book will appeal not just to scientists and science students but also to the interested layperson. And it passes the most difficult test of any dictionary—it is well worth browsing through.'
New Scientist

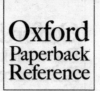

Oxford
Paperback
Reference

THE CONCISE OXFORD DICTIONARY
OF MATHEMATICS

New Edition

Edited by Christopher Clapham

Authoritative and reliable, this is the ideal reference guide for students of mathematics at school or in the first year at university. Nearly 1,000 entries have been added for this new edition and the dictionary provides clear definitions, with helpful examples, of a wide range of mathematical terms and concepts.

* **Covers both pure and applied mathematics as well as statistics.**

* **Entries on the great mathematicians**

* **Coverage of mathematics of more general interest, including fractals, game theory, and chaos**

'the depth of information provided is admirable'
New Scientist

'the style encourages browsing and a desire to find out more about the topics discussed'
Mathematica

Oxford
Paperback
Reference

THE CONCISE OXFORD DICTIONARY
OF OPERA

New Edition

Edited by Ewan West and John Warrack

Derived from the full *Oxford Dictionary of Opera*,
this is the most authoritative and up-to-date dictionary of opera available in paperback. Fully revised
for this new edition, it is designed to be accessible to
all those who enjoy opera, whether at the opera-
house or at home.

* **Over 3,500 entries on operas, composers, and
  performers**

* **Plot summaries and separate entries for well-
  known roles, arias, and choruses**

* **Leading conductors, producers and designers**

From the reviews of its parent volume:

'the most authoritative single-volume work of its
kind'
Independent on Sunday

'an invaluable reference work'
Gramophone

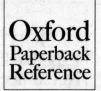

Oxford
Paperback
Reference

THE CONCISE OXFORD DICTIONARY
OF MUSIC

New Edition

Edited by Michael Kennedy

Derived from the full *Oxford Dictionary of Music*
this is the most authoritative and up-to-date dictionary of music available in paperback. Fully revised
and updated for this new edition, it is a rich mine of
information for lovers of music of all periods and
styles.

* **14,000 entries on musical terms, works, composers, librettists, musicians, singers and or-
chestras.**

* **Comprehensive work-lists for major composers**

* **Generous coverage of living composers and performers**

'clearly the best around . . . the dictionary that
everyone should have'
Literary Review

'indispensable'
Yorkshire Post

OXFORD

RETHINKING LIFE AND DEATH
THE COLLAPSE OF OUR TRADITIONAL ETHICS

Peter Singer

A victim of the Hillsborough Disaster in 1989, Anthony Bland lay in hospital in a coma being fed liquid food by a pump, via a tube passing through his nose and into his stomach. On 4 February 1993 Britain's highest court ruled that doctors attending him could lawfully act to end his life.

Our traditional ways of thinking about life and death are collapsing. In a world of respirators and embryos stored for years in liquid nitrogen, we can no longer take the sanctity of human life as the cornerstone of our ethical outlook.

In this controversial book Peter Singer argues that we cannot deal with the crucial issues of death, abortion, euthanasia and the rights of nonhuman animals unless we sweep away the old ethic and build something new in its place.

Singer outlines a new set of commandments, based on compassion and commonsense, for the decisions everyone must make about life and death.

PAST MASTERS

PAST MASTERS

A wide range of unique, short, clear introductions to the lives and work of the world's most influential thinkers. Written by experts, they cover the history of ideas from Aristotle to Wittgenstein. Readers need no previous knowledge of the subject, so they are ideal for students and general readers alike.

Each book takes as its main focus the thought and work of its subject. There is a short section on the life and a final chapter on the legacy and influence of the thinker. A section of further reading helps in further research.

The series continues to grow, and future Past Masters will include **Owen Gingerich** on *Copernicus*, **R G Frey** on *Joseph Butler*, **Bhiku Parekh** on *Gandhi*, **Christopher Taylor** on *Socrates*, **Michael Inwood** on *Heidegger*, and **Peter Ghosh** on *Weber*.